Head and Neck Cancer

Guest Editor

LILLIAN L. SIU, MD, FRCPC

HEMATOLOGY/ONCOLOGY CLINICS OF NORTH AMERICA

www.hemonc.theclinics.com

December 2008 • Volume 22 • Number 6

SAUNDERS an imprint of ELSEVIER, Inc.

W.B. SAUNDERS COMPANY
A Division of Elsevier Inc.

1600 John F. Kennedy Blvd. ● Suite 1800 ● Philadelphia, PA 19103-2899

http://www.theclinics.com

HEMATOLOGY/ONCOLOGY CLINICS OF NORTH AMERICA Volume 22, Number 6
December 2008 ISSN 0889-8588, ISBN 13: 978-1-4160-6308-7, ISBN 10: 1-4160-6308-0

Editor: Kerry Holland

Hematology/Oncology Clinics (ISSN 0889-8588) is published bimonthly by Elsevier Inc., 360 Park Avenue South, New York, NY 10010-1710. Months of issue are February, April, June, August, October, and December. Business and Editorial Offices: 1600 John F. Kennedy Blvd., Suite 1800, Philadelphia, PA 19103-2899. Customer Service Office: 11830 Westline Industrial Drive, St. Louis, MO 63146. Periodicals postage paid at New York, NY and additional mailing offices. Subscription prices are $283.00 per year (domestic individuals), $439.00 per year (domestic institutions), $141.00 per year (domestic students/residents), $321.00 per year (Canadian individuals), $537.00 per year (Canadian institutions) $382.00 per year (international individuals), $537.00 per year (international institutions), and $191.00 per year (international and Canadian students/residents). International air speed delivery is included in all *Clinics* subscription prices. All prices are subject to change without notice. **POSTMASTER:** Send address changes to *Hematology/ Oncology Clinics of North America*, 11830 Westline Industrial Drive, St. Louis, MO 63146. Customer Service (orders, claims, online, change of address): Elsevier Periodicals Customer Service, 11830 Westline Industrial Drive, St. Louis, MO 63146. Tel: 1-800-654-2452 (U.S. and Canada). Fax: 314-523-5170. E-mail: journalscustomerservice-usa@ elsevier.com (for print support); journalsonlinesupport-usa@elsevier.com (for online support).

Reprints. For copies of 100 or more, of articles in this publication, please contact the Commercial Reprints Department, Elsevier Inc., 360 Park Avenue South, New York, New York 10010-1710; Tel.: 212-633-3813, Fax: 212-462-1935, E-mail: reprints@elsevier.com.

Hematology/Oncology Clinics of North America is covered in *MEDLINE/PubMed (Index Medicus), EMBASE/ Excerpta Medica, and BIOSIS.*

Printed in the United States of America.

Contributors

GUEST EDITOR

LILLIAN L. SIU, MD, FRCPC
Associate Professor, Princess Margaret Hospital, University of Toronto, Toronto, Ontario, Canada

AUTHORS

FRANCO BERRINO, MD
Director, Department of Preventive and Predictive Medicine, Fondazione IRCCS, Istituto Nazionale dei Tumori, Milan, Italy

JACQUES BERNIER, MD, PD
Department of Radio-Oncology, Genolier Swiss Medical Network, Genolier, Switzerland

BRYAN H. BURMEISTER, MB ChB, FF Rad(T) SA, FRANZCR, MD
Division of Cancer Services, Princess Alexandra Hospital, Woolloongabba; Associate Professor, University of Queensland, School of Medicine, Brisbane, Queensland, Australia

ANTHONY T. CHAN, MD, FRCP
Department of Clinical Oncology, Prince of Wales Hospital, Shatin, New Territories, Hong Kong SAR; Professor and Chair, Department of Clinical Oncology, Sir Y K Pao Center for Cancer, Hong Kong Cancer Institute, Li Ka Shing Institute for Health Sciences, State Key Laboratory in Oncology in South China, Chinese University of Hong Kong, Hong Kong

ERIC X. CHEN, MD, PhD
Drug Development Program, Department of Medical Oncology and Hematology, Princess Margaret Hospital, University of Toronto, Toronto, Ontario, Canada

ROGER B. COHEN, MD
Senior Member, Department of Medical Oncology, Fox Chase Cancer, Philadelphia, Pennsylvania

ANDREW COLEMAN, MBBS, MSc, FRANZCR
Division of Radiation Oncology, Peter MacCallum Cancer Centre, Melbourne, Australia

MARION E. COUCH, MD, PhD, FACS
Associate Professor, Department of Otolaryngology–Head & Neck Surgery, University of North Carolina at Chapel Hill; Lineberger Comprehensive Cancer Center, Chapel Hill, North Carolina

EUROCARE WORKING GROUP
Austria, M Hackl (Austrian National Cancer Registry); Germany, H Ziegler (Saarland Cancer Registry); Italy, M Federico (Modena Cancer Registry); V De Lisi (Parma Cancer Registry); R Tumino (Cancer Registry Azienda Ospedaliera "Civile M.P.Arezzo" Ragusa, Italy); F.Falcini, (Romagna Cancer Registry- I.R.S.T); E Paci, (Tuscan Cancer Registry); Poland, J Rachtan (Cracow Cancer Registry); Slovenia, M Primic-Žakelj (Cancer Registry of Slovenia); Sweden, Å Klint (Cancer Registry of Sweden); Switzerland, M Usel (Geneva Cancer Registry); SM Ess (St. Gall Cancer Registry); The Netherlands, O Visser (Amsterdam Cancer Registry); UK (Scotland), DH Brewster (Scottish Cancer Registry); UK (Wales), JA Steward (Welsh Cancer Intelligence and Surveillance Unit)

GEMMA GATTA, MD
Research Assistant, Department of Preventive and Predictive Medicine, Fondazione IRCCS, Istituto Nazionale dei Tumori, Milan, Italy

MAURA L. GILLISON, MD, PhD
Associate Professor of Oncology and Epidemiology, Johns Hopkins Medical Institutions, Baltimore, Maryland

RALPH W. GILBERT, MD, FRCSC
Professor, Department of Otolaryngology/Head and Neck Surgery, University of Toronto, Princess Margaret Hospital, University Health Network, Wharton Head and Neck Centre, Toronto, Ontario, Canada

ROBERT I. HADDAD, MD
Dana Farber Cancer Institute, Boston, Massachusetts

DAVID NEIL HAYES, MD, MPH
Assistant Professor, Department of Medicine, Division of Hematology/Oncology, University of North Carolina at Chapel Hill; Lineberger Comprehensive Cancer Center, Chapel Hill, North Carolina

RODNEY J. HICKS, MBBS, MD, FRACP
Centre for Molecular Imaging, Peter MacCallum Cancer Centre, St Andrews Place, East Melbourne, Victoria; Professor of Medicine and Radiology, Department of Medicine, University of Melbourne, Parkville, Victoria, Australia

SEBASTIEN J. HOTTE, MD
Assistant Professor, Department of Oncology, McMaster University; Juravinski Cancer Centre at Hamilton Health Sciences, Hamilton, Ontario, Canada

GREGORY J. KUBICEK, MD
Department of Radiation Oncology, Jefferson Medical College; Kimmel Cancer Center; Bodine Center for Cancer Treatment, Thomas Jefferson University, Philadelphia, Pennsylvania

CHRISTOPHE LE TOURNEAU, MD, PhD
Drug Development Program, Department of Medical Oncology and Hematology, Princess Margaret Hospital, University of Toronto, Toronto, Ontario, Canada

LISA LICITRA, MD
Director, Head and Neck Medical Oncology Unit, Fondazione IRCCS, Istituto Nazionale dei Tumori, Milan, Italy

HERBERT H. LOONG, MBBS, MRCP
Medical Officer, Department of Clinical Oncology, Prince of Wales Hospital, Shatin, New Territories, Hong Kong SAR

JOCHEN H. LORCH, MD
Dana Farber Cancer Institute, Boston, Massachusetts

BRIGETTE B. MA, MBBS, FRACP
Department of Clinical Oncology, Prince of Wales Hospital, Shatin, New Territories, Hong Kong SAR; Associate Professor, Department of Clinical Oncology, Sir Y K Pao Center for Cancer, Hong Kong Cancer Institute, Li Ka Shing Institute for Health Sciences, State Key Laboratory in Oncology in South China, Chinese University of Hong Kong, Hong Kong

MITCHELL MACHTAY, MD
Department of Radiation Oncology, Jefferson Medical College, Thomas Jefferson University; Kimmel Cancer Center, Thomas Jefferson University, Philadelphia, Pennsylvania

ROSEMARY MARTINO, MA, MSc, PhD
Assistant Professor, Department of Speech Language Pathology, University of Toronto; Health Care and Outcomes Research, Toronto Western Research Institute, Toronto, Ontario, Canada

RANEE MEHRA, MD
Associate Member, Department of Medical Oncology, Fox Chase Cancer Center, Philadelphia, Pennsylvania

MIHIR R. PATEL, MD
Department of Otolaryngology–Head & Neck Surgery, University of North Carolina at Chapel Hill, Chapel Hill, North Carolina

SANDRO V. PORCEDDU, BSc, MBBS, FRANZCR
Division of Cancer Services, Princess Alexandra Hospital, Woolloongabba; Associate Professor, University of Queensland, School of Medicine, Brisbane, Queensland, Australia

MARSHALL R. POSNER, MD
Dana Farber Cancer Institute, Boston, Massachusetts

JOLIE RINGASH, BSc, MD, MSc
Associate Professor, Department of Radiation Oncology, The Princess Margaret Hospital; The University of Toronto, Toronto, Ontario, Canada

DANNY RISCHIN, MBBS, MD, FRACP
Department of Medical Oncology, Peter MacCallum Cancer Centre, Melbourne; University of Melbourne, Victoria, Australia

MARIA-JOSÉ SÁNCHEZ, MD, PhD
Coordinator of Research Projects, Andalusian School of Public Health-Granada, CIBER Epidemiología y Salud Pública (CIBERESP, Spain), Granada, Spain

MICHAEL E. STADLER, MD
Department of Otolaryngology–Head & Neck Surgery, University of North Carolina at Chapel Hill, Chapel Hill, North Carolina

LAURA VIDAL, MD
Clinical Research Fellow, Department of Medical Oncology, Princess Margaret Hospital, Toronto, Ontario, Canada

LORI J. WIRTH, MD
Dana Farber Cancer Institute, Boston, Massachusetts

JAMES R. WRIGHT, MD
Associate Professor, Department of Oncology, McMaster University; Juravinski Cancer Centre at Hamilton Health Sciences, Hamilton, Ontario, Canada

GIULIA ZIGON, PhD
Statistician, Department of Preventive and Predictive Medicine, Fondazione IRCCS, Istituto Nazionale dei Tumori, Milan, Italy

Contents

> Patients present with a differential baseline risk of cancer based on normal and expected variations in genes associated with cancer. The baseline risk of developing cancer is acted on throughout life as the genome of different cells interacts with the environment in the form of exposures (eg, toxins, infections). As genetic damage is incurred throughout a lifetime (directly to DNA sequences or to the epigenome), events are set in motion to progressively disrupt normal cellular pathways toward tumorigenesis. This article attempts to characterize broad categories of genetic aberrations and pathways in a manner that might be useful for the clinician to understand the risk of developing cancer, the pathways that are disrupted, and the potential for molecular-based diagnostics.

> Strong epidemiologic and molecular data now support the conclusion that human papillomavirus (HPV) infection is responsible for a distinct form of head and neck squamous cell carcinoma (HNSCC), independent from the traditional risk factors of tobacco and alcohol use. Patients with HPV-positive HNSCC have a different clinical presentation and better clinical outcomes than those with HPV-negative HNSCC. A diagnosis of HPV-positive HNSCC is associated not only with therapeutic relevance, but also has important implications for future prevention and screening strategies.

> The aim of this study was to assess incidence and survival of human papillomavirus–related and unrelated head and neck squamous cell carcinoma sites from 15 European population-based cancer registries. This analysis was performed on 29,265 adult (aged approximately 15 years) cancer patients diagnosed in the period from 1988 to 2002. The human papillomavirus–unrelated cancer sites had an age-standardized incidence higher than the human papillomavirus–related cancer cases (3.8 versus 2.5/100,000 year). Incidence rates of head and neck squamous cell carcinomas increased more for human papillomavirus-related than unrelated

cancer sites. Three-year survival rates improved more in human papillomavirus-related than unrelated cancer sites, and women had better rates of survival than men.

Locally advanced squamous cell cancer of the head and neck is a major contributor to morbidity and mortality worldwide. Despite progress through the use of multimodality treatment involving surgery, radiotherapy, and chemotherapy in recent years, the survival remains poor, and treatment-related morbidity—mainly caused by radiation-induced effects such as soft tissue scarring, esophageal stenosis, xerostomia, dental decay, and osteoradionecrosis—is a major problem in long-term survivors. Data from early trials and encouraging results from meta-analyses have revived interest in the use of neoadjuvant or induction chemotherapy before definitive local treatment. Recent randomized trials have demonstrated marked improvements in survival with the addition of the taxane docetaxel (Taxotere) to the traditional induction regimen consisting of cisplatin and 5FU (TPF) compared with cisplatin and 5FU (PF) alone and have established a new standard of care. The newer TPF induction chemotherapy regimens also appear to be tolerated better than PF when accompanied by adequate supportive measures. Studies to enhance the efficacy of TPF induction chemotherapy by adding new targeted agents, such as the EGF-R inhibitors cetuximab and panitumumab, are underway.

Radiotherapy has an integral role in the treatment of head and neck cancer. Although radiotherapy has the potential to cure patients with advanced disease it also carries the potential for significant long-term morbidity. New technologies in the setting of head and neck radiotherapy are emerging, which have the potential to increase the cure rate and decrease toxicity. These new technologies include improved radiotherapy treatment design (intensity modulated radiation therapy) and improved planning and implementation (image-guided radiation therapy). Some of these advances are discussed in this article.

The surgical management of head and neck tumors continues to evolve with a focus on reducing treatment-related morbidity. The major changes in the past two decades have been the introduction of function-preserving, minimally invasive surgical approaches and a dramatic change in the ability to reconstruct ablative defects and restore form and function. The future certainly will include better evidence regarding the efficacy and appropriate application of these new techniques. Reconstructive techniques will continue to evolve with introduction of tissue engineering and cell therapy to further improve the quality of life of patients afflicted with head and neck malignancies.

Molecular markers will become increasingly important in directing treatment approaches in locally advanced squamous cell carcinomas of the head and neck (HNSCC). Several predictive markers have been identified that may be useful for selecting tumors most likely to respond to radiotherapy or chemotherapy. However, few markers have potential as therapeutic targets. The epidermal growth factor receptor (EGFR) is the most extensively investigated of these targets in the clinical setting. EGFR inhibitors have demonstrated activity in several studies and the monoclonal antibody cetuximab is currently the only biologic agent approved for the treatment of locally advanced HNSCC in combination with radiotherapy. Another potentially promising approach is the inhibition of vascular endothelial growth factor, alone or in combination with EGFR inhibition.

Proof of principle that molecularly targeted therapy is a valid therapeutic approach for squamous cell carcinoma of the head and neck (SCCHN) has emerged with epidermal growth factor receptor targeting agents. Other interesting targets, such as Src, insulin-like growth factor 1 receptor, and the proteasome, have been shown in vitro to play key roles in SCCHN, and their inhibition is currently being studied in phase II trials. Identification of predictive biomarkers of resistance or sensitivity to these therapies remains one of the main challenges in the optimal selection of patients most likely to benefit from them. However, clinical trials with these novel agents need to be designed rationally to improve the overall outcome of patients. Given the emerging evidence that human papilloma virus–related SCCHN is a distinct disease, it should be studied in specific trials.

Positron emission tomography (PET) has emerged as an integral diagnostic tool in the management of head and neck squamous cell carcinoma (HNSCC). This article reviews the usefulness and ongoing dilemmas of fluorine-18 fluorodeoxyglucose (18-F FDG) PET and FDG PET/CT in HNSCC. In addition, it examines the potential role of novel markers and biologic characterization of disease, which in the future may assist in targeted therapeutic strategies.

Common concerns of head and neck squamous cell cancer patients include concerns about illness and their future, general physical and emotional well being, speech, body image, and financial issues. Patients receiving radiotherapy report high levels of problems with swallowing, eating, and dry mouth. This article focuses on several of the most common and severe lasting issues for head and neck squamous cell cancer patients: impairments of overall quality of life, xerostomia, speech, and swallowing, focusing primarily on the tools and techniques for measuring such effects.

Clinical trials evaluating therapies in patients who have head and neck cancer are often challenged by low power and competing clinical outcomes, which makes interpretation difficult. Meta-analyses that combine the results of independent trials have the potential to provide high-quality, evidence-based information on what should be considered best practice beyond that of any one trial. In this summary of published meta-analyses, the authors review the evidence supporting the use of concurrent chemotherapy and fractionated radiotherapy for patients who have locally advanced squamous cell carcinoma of the oral cavity, oropharynx, hypopharynx, and larynx.

Despite being potentially curable at an early stage, more than 50% of patients who have nasopharyngeal carcinoma present with advanced locoregional disease, which results in a poor prognosis. This article discusses key advancements in the management of nasopharyngeal cancer, including the incorporation of concurrent chemoradiotherapy, new radiotherapy delivery techniques in the form of conformal and intensity-modulated radiotherapy, and salvage options for locoregional recurrence. New cytotoxic and targeted therapies that have resulted in improved survival in the metastatic setting are also described. The use of Epstein-Barr virus DNA for the prognostication and monitoring of nasopharyngeal cancer and the role of new diagnostic imaging techniques are also discussed.

The treatment of relatively rare malignancies, such as those of the salivary glands and iodine refractory thyroid cancer, has been invigorated by the development of novel molecular targeting agents. Accrual to clinical trials for these disease sites continues to be limited by their relatively low incidence. Nonetheless, multicenter collaborations have contributed greatly to the development of a number of emerging systemic therapies. This article briefly summarizes the epidemiology and pathogenesis of salivary gland and thyroid cancer, and then describes some of the new drugs under evaluation for these malignancies.

The sinonasal malignancies of putative neuroendocrine origin—esthesio-neuroblastoma, sinonasal neuroendocrine carcinoma, sinonasal undifferentiated carcinoma, and sinonasal small cell carcinoma—are uncommon malignancies that frequently present with locally advanced disease. Pathologic distinction between these entities can be difficult, but is important to guide management. These malignancies require complex multimodality treatment and are best managed by multidisciplinary teams in major centers that have expertise in sinonasal malignancies.

FORTHCOMING ISSUES

February 2009
Gastrointestinal Stromal Tumors
Jay Trent, MD and
Shreyaskumar Patel, MD
Guest Editors

April 2009
Bone Marrow Failure Syndromes
Grover Bagby, MD
Guest Editor

June 2009
Melanoma
David Fisher, MD
Guest Editor

RECENT ISSUES

October 2008
Non-Hodgkin's Lymphomas: New Insights
and Therapeutic Strategies
Bruce D. Cheson, MD
Guest Editor

August 2008
Integrative Medicine in Oncology
Moshe Frenkel, MD and
Lorenzo Cohen, PhD, MD
Guest Editors

June 2008
Thymic Epithelial Neoplasms:
A Comprehensive Review of Diagnosis
and Treatment
Cesar A. Moran, MD and Saul Suster, MD
Guest Editors

RELATED INTEREST
Otolaryngology Clinics of North America, February 2005 (Vol. 38, No. 1)
Contemporary Diagnosis and Management of Head and Neck Cancer
Jeffrey Spiegel, MD, FACS and Scharukh Jalisi, MD, *Guest Editors*

THE CLINICS ARE NOW AVAILABLE ONLINE!

Access your subscription at:
www.theclinics.com

Preface

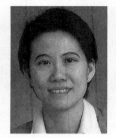

Lillian L. Siu, MD, FRCPC
Guest Editor

This issue of *Hematology/Oncology Clinics of North America*, entitled "Head and Neck Cancer," provides a timely update of the substantial knowledge that has been gained in the diagnostic and therapeutic areas of head and neck malignancies over the past decade. Advances in molecular biology have elucidated cellular proteins and pathways that play critical roles in the pathogenesis and progression of head and neck cancers. The identification of human papilloma virus (HPV) as an etiologic pathogen in an increasing subgroup of head and neck cancer patients has led to a growing body of scientific and epidemiologic literature on this disease entity. Innovations in surgical techniques, radiation delivery, systemic therapy (including chemotherapy sequencing and incorporating of targeted agents), and diagnostic imaging constantly are challenging existent standards of care.

Among the contributors to this issue are field experts from otolaryngology, radiation and medical oncology, diagnostic imaging, speech language pathology, and biostatistics, which highlights the relevance of a multidisciplinary approach in the management of this disease. Furthermore, the representation of authors from Asia, Australia, Europe, and North America underscore that head and neck cancer is a worldwide health issue.

The first three articles focus on the molecular, biological, and epidemiologic advances that have furthered understanding of the pathogenesis and progression of head and neck squamous cell cancer (HNSCC). The article by Drs. Stadler, Patel, Couch, and Hayes (entitled "Molecular Biology of Head & Neck Cancer: Risks and Pathways") offers a comprehensive overview of various cellular molecules and pathways, perturbations of which have putatively culminated in the hallmark processes of cancer. In their article entitled "Human Papilloma Virus in Head and Neck Squamous Cell Cancer – Recognition of a Distinct Disease Type," Drs. Vidal and Gillison succinctly summarize the body of evidence supporting the etiologic role played by HPV in a subset of HNSCC, predominantly in the oropharyngeal area. The article by Drs. Licitra, Zigon, Gatta, Sánchez, Berrino, and the EUROCARE Working Group (entitled "Human Papilloma Virus in Head and Neck Squamous Cell Cancer: A European Epidemiological Perspective") analyzes data from 15 population-based cancer

Hematol Oncol Clin N Am 22 (2008) xiii–xv
doi:10.1016/j.hoc.2008.10.001   hemonc.theclinics.com

registries in Europe to assess the incidence and survival of HNSCC related and unrelated to HPV. Similarities and differences are highlighted in comparison to the trends that have been published based on the US Surveillance Epidemology and End Results database.

The next six articles share the common theme of innovative strategies that have been incorporated into clinical practice or are undergoing definitive evaluations for implementation. The article by Drs. Lorch, Posner, Wirth and Haddad, "Induction Chemotherapy in Locally Advanced Head and Neck Cancer: A New Standard of Care?," discusses the renewed interest in induction chemotherapy, which is administered in combination with concurrent chemoradiation as a sequential therapeutic approach. Comparison of the therapeutic ratios between sequential therapy and concurrent chemoradiotherapy in HNSCC awaits the completion of randomized controlled trials. Drs. Kubicek and Machtay, in their article "New Advances in High-Technology Radiotherapy for Head and Neck Cancer," showcase new radiotherapy technologies, such as intensity modulated radiation therapy and image-guided radiation therapy, which promise to deliver improved tumor locoregional control while reducing toxicity. In his article entitled "Innovation in the Surgical Management of Head and Neck Tumors," Dr. Gilbert describes some of the newer surgical procedures that aim to minimize morbidity and maximize functional preservation. Dr. Bernier, in his article "Incorporation of Molecularly Targeted Agents in the Primary Treatment of Squamous Cell Carcinomas of the Head and Neck," provides a detailed and authoritative review of the current use of molecularly targeted therapy, especially inhibitors of the epidermal growth factor receptor, in the locally advanced disease setting. The article by Drs. Le Tourneau and Chen ("Molecularly Targeted Agents in the Treatment of Recurrent or Metastatic Squamous Cell Carcinomas of the Head and Neck") focuses primarily on the development of novel agents in the palliative setting and uses, as a benchmark, the anti-epidermal growth factor receptor antibody ceutuximab, which has been approved in platinum-refractory recurrent or metastatic HNSCC. The last article of this group, eloquently written by Drs. Porceddu, Burmeister and Hicks, entitled "Role of Functional Imaging in Head and Neck Squamous Cell Carcinoma: FDG PET and Beyond," provides an up-to-date overview of the use of FDG PET scans in the diagnosis and management of head and neck cancer.

The next two articles offer insights into other important aspects of head and neck cancer management. In their article "Evaluation of Quality of Life and Organ Function in Head and Neck Squamous Cell Carcinoma," Drs. Martino and Ringash underscore the relevance of these patient-reported outcomes in the multidisciplinary care of HNSCC and provide guidance on the tools and techniques used to evaluate these endpoints. The article by Drs. Hotte and Wright, "Understanding the Results of Meta-Analyses in the Treatment of Head and Neck Squamous Cell Cancer," give expert interpretations of published results of landmark meta-analyses on the use of concurrent chemotherapy and fractionated radiotherapy.

The final three articles are unique, because they concentrate on other epithelial cancers of the head and neck besides HNSCC. Drs. Loong, Ma, and Chan provide their perspectives on the latest diagnostic and therapeutic strategies in nasopharyngeal cancer, in their article entitled "Update on the Management and Therapeutic Monitoring of Advanced Nasopharyngeal Cancer." In their article, "New Agents in the Treatment for Malignancies of the Salivary and Thyroid Glands," Drs. Mehra and Cohen give a state-of-the-art summary of the current knowledge in the molecular biology and clinical experience of these two tumor types, with particular emphasis on the use of molecularly targeted therapy. Lastly, in their article "Sinonasal Malignancies of Neuroendocrine Origin," Drs. Rischin and Coleman provide a comprehensive overview and clarify the distinguishing features of these related but uncommon tumor types.

These 14 articles, contributed by the various experts, have encapsulated the recent progresses made in the molecular, epidemiologic, and clinical understanding of head and neck cancer. These collaborative efforts have formulated an excellent and knowledge-laden issue of *Hematology/Oncology Clinics of North America*.

Lillian L. Siu, MD, FRCPC
Princess Margaret Hospital
University of Toronto
610 University Avenue, Suite 5-718
Toronto, Ontario M5G 2M9, Canada

E-mail address:
lillian.siu@uhn.on.ca (L.L. Siu)

Molecular Biology of Head and Neck Cancer: Risks and Pathways

Michael E. Stadler, MD[a], Mihir R. Patel, MD[a],
Marion E. Couch, MD, PhD, FACS[a,b], David Neil Hayes, MD, MPH[b,c],*

KEYWORDS

- Head and neck neoplasms • Cancer • Review
- Molecular biology • Pathway

There is a remarkably diverse array of anatomy and tumor morphologies, with at least 10 anatomic subsites of the head and neck, challenging all members of the multidisciplinary team to precisely define the extent of a patient's disease (**Fig. 1**). Although most of the histopathology consists of squamous cell carcinoma (SCC), there are dozens of other pathologic diagnoses. Accordingly, a broad spectrum of treatment modalities is offered, frequently in combination, including chemotherapy, radiation (including intensity-modulated radiation therapy), and surgery with and without reconstruction. Historically, the treating teams have labored to join the anatomic and morphologic considerations of a patient's disease (and patient preference and comorbidities) to select the appropriate range of treatment options. Increasingly, clinicians are also required to consider a new set of issues—the so-called "molecular determinants" of head and neck cancer. In the sections that follow, the authors attempt to highlight the spectrum of these targets that are most likely to impact clinicians and patients in the coming years. The authors touch briefly on inherited and somatic aberrations that predispose to tumorigenesis (genetic and epigenetic) and on a number of specific cancer pathways as targets of tumorigenesis and therapeutics. Finally, the role of new and developing molecular diagnostics in the management of patient care is considered.

[a] Department of Otolaryngology–Head & Neck Surgery, University of North Carolina at Chapel Hill, CB #7070, Chapel Hill, NC 27599, USA
[b] Lineberger Comprehensive Cancer Center, Room 11-130, Chapel Hill, NC 27599, USA
[c] Department of Medicine, Division of Hematology/Oncology, University of North Carolina at Chapel Hill, 450 West Drive, CB #7295, Chapel Hill, NC 27599, USA
* Corresponding author. Department of Medicine, Division of Hematology/Oncology, University of North Carolina at Chapel Hill, 450 West Drive, CB #7295, Chapel Hill, NC 27599.
E-mail address: hayes@med.unc.edu (D.N. Hayes).

Hematol Oncol Clin N Am 22 (2008) 1099–1124
doi:10.1016/j.hoc.2008.08.007
0889-8588/08/$ – see front matter © 2008 Elsevier Inc. All rights reserved.

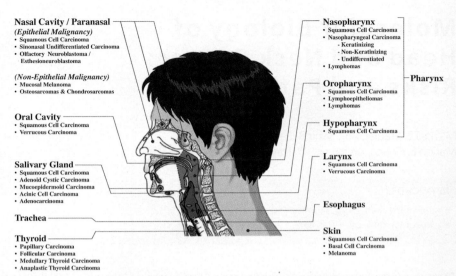

Fig. 1. Diversity of head and neck cancer. Histopathologic diagnoses that present at the various subsites in the head and neck.

MOLECULAR BASIS OF RISK FACTORS FOR DEVELOPMENT OF HEAD AND NECK CANCER

The most well known risk factor for developing head and neck cancer is the deleterious effects of tobacco. Indeed, head and neck SCC (HNSCC) was one of the first carcinomas to be linked with *p53* mutations caused by tobacco usage.[1] Alcohol use is synergistic with tobacco in causing HNSCC. There are other cultural habit-forming risk factors that have an association with HNSCC. Betel nut, a fruit that is the basic ingredient of a stimulant chew, is used by an estimated 200 to 400 million people throughout Southeast Asia.[2] Betel nut is incorporated into Asian medicines to treat a variety of complaints, from headaches to rheumatism.[3] The odds ratio of developing leukoplakia and submucous fibrosis from using betel nut is 5 compared with 1 in nonchewers.[4] The addition of tobacco raises the risk threefold.[4] The duration and frequency of betel nut use increase the risk of developing cancer, suggesting a dose-response relation.[5]

Tobacco smoke is associated with structural changes in DNA, particularly those induced by oxidative damage. Benzo[a]pyrene diol epoxide (BPDE), a known tobacco carcinogen, induces genetic damage by forming covalently bound DNA adducts throughout the genome, including *p53*.[6] Damage induced by BPDE and other such carcinogens can be repaired through the nucleotide excision repair (NER) system. Along with the NER system, the base excision repair (BER) system is another set of multistep enzymatic complexes involved in the repair of nonspecific DNA damage, including gamma and ultraviolet radiation, cross-linking, and chemical intra-/interstrand adduct formation. The BER system handles the largest number of cytotoxic and mutagenic base lesions by specifically removing alterations of a single base pair that has been methylated, oxidized, or reduced and corrects single-strand interruptions in DNA.[7] Therefore, individual variations in NER/BER is one of the factors that may influence tobacco smoking–related cancer risks like HNSCC.

Several studies have demonstrated that sequence variations in NER/BER genes contribute to HNSCC susceptibility.[8-11] The ERCC1 gene product is a key enzyme in the NER system, and one particular polymorphism at the ERCC1 gene (C8092A) may affect its mRNA stability, resulting in impaired DNA repair capacity.[12] Two single-nucleotide polymorphisms (SNPs) in the XPD gene (Asp312Asn and Lys751Gln), also part of the NER cascade, have been associated with suboptimal DNA repair capacity.[13] There are conflicting data regarding SNPs in the BER system and the predilection for developing HNSCC. Li and colleagues,[9] in one of the largest case-control studies of 830 patients who had HNSCC and 854 cancer-free control subjects, evaluated the progression to HNSCC based on polymorphisms in three BER nonsynonymous SNPs. Although the BER system enzyme XRCC1 (Arg399Gln) inconsistently increases the risk of HNSCC in Caucasians,[13-16] Li and colleagues[9] concluded that polymorphisms in the ADPRT enzyme of the BER system are associated with HNSCC and demonstrated that individuals who have the ADPRT 762Ala/Ala and Ala/Ala1Val/Ala genotypes are at lower risk of developing HNSCC compared with individuals who have the Val/Val genotypes. Further studies to elucidate the genetic predisposition of developing HNSCC in the face of total tobacco burden may provide preventative health benefits in the future to those who have susceptible polymorphisms.

Marijuana is the most commonly used illegal drug in the United States and the second most commonly smoked substance after tobacco.[17] Habitual marijuana smoking manifests with similar signs and symptoms associated with chronic tobacco use.[18,19] Furthermore, the carcinogenic properties of marijuana smoke are similar to those of tobacco, and numerous studies parallel the use of cannabinoids to cancer development.[20-22] Marijuana has been shown to induce cytogenic changes consisting of chromosomal breaks, deletions, and translocations in mammalian cells in vivo.[23] Until recently, there was not enough evidence to suggest a causative relation with oropharyngeal HNSCC, especially those cases caused by tobacco use;[24] however, HNSCC caused by human papilloma virus (HPV) may be associated with marijuana (see later discussion).

Clearly, normal variation in patient genotype for genes in DNA repair pathways appears to modify baseline risk for cancer development, especially when impacted by environmental toxins such as smoking. In parallel, there is a range of germline variants that are more rare than SNPs and accordingly called mutations. These rare heritable events can be sporadic or conserved in families and are frequently recognized due to the high penetrance of one of a number of recognized familial cancer syndromes. Fanconi's anemia, known for the risk of developing lymphoreticular malignancies due to germline mutations in the caretaker genes FAA, FAD, and FCC, carries a risk for developing second primary cancers in the tongue, pyriform sinus, and postcricoid region.[25] Patients who have Bloom syndrome are characterized to have mutations in the helicase genes and are predisposed to developing solid tumors in a number of anatomic sites, 6% and 8% of which arise from the tongue and larynx, respectively.[26] Homozygotes who have ataxia telangiectasia who survive into their 20s and 30s are at increased risk of developing chronic T-cell leukemia and solid malignancies of the oral cavity, breast, stomach, pancreas, ovary, and bladder.[27] Xeroderma pigmentosum, an autosomal recessive disorder of one or more of the XP genes in the NER system, manifests second primaries within the oral cavity in addition to the known risks of skin malignancies.[26,28] Other such syndromes and affected genes (indicated in parentheses) with primary manifestations in the head and neck include Cowden disease (PTEN), multiple endocrine neoplasia type I (MEN I), multiple endocrine neoplasia type II (MEN II), neurofibromatosis type II (NF-2), and retinoblastoma (Rb).

Genetic cancer syndromes are generally recognized by the early age of onset of malignancies in impacted individuals and by specific or unusual patterns of tumors. Cancer syndrome tumors are of scientific importance out of proportion to their incidence in that they point clearly at specific pathways and targets that are key to the development of malignancy, in contrast to sporadic tumors in which the causative lesion may be difficult to identify. For example, a relatively rare cancer syndrome, multiple endocrine neoplasia, type IIA, is well known for its association with germline mutation of the RET proto-oncogene. Although MEN IIa is rare, the RET gene has relevance in a wide variety of tumors and is targeted by anti-cancer drugs, such as vandetanib.[29,30]

VIRAL ASSOCIATIONS AND NEW EPIDEMIC OF HEAD AND NECK SQUAMOUS CELL CARCINOMA CAUSED BY HUMAN PAPILLOMAVIRUS

Recently, HPV infection has been identified as an etiologic agent for oropharyngeal carcinoma, a subset of SCCs that comprises the tongue base and tonsil. Patients who have oropharyngeal SCCs and have the HPV genes incorporated in their tumor genome are younger in age (by 3–5 years) and are less likely to have a history of tobacco and alcohol use.[31]

What is most disconcerting is that although the overall incidence of HNSCC (1973–2004) has steadily declined according to the Surveillance Epidemiology and End Results database, the incidence of oropharyngeal cancer is increasing among younger age groups.[32–35] The unsettling implication is that the incidence of HPV-related HNSCC of the oropharynx could overtake HPV-unrelated HNSCC, which is thought to be associated more with traditional risk factors.

There is substantial evidence that infection with high-risk HPV subtypes, in particular HPV-16, is a risk factor for the development of oropharyngeal cancers.[36–47] In fact, Gillison and colleagues[48] claimed that HPV-positive and HPV-negative HNSCC of the oropharynx should be classified as two distinct cancers based on the clinical and molecular risk factors and etiology. According to their case-controlled study, patients at risk for HPV-16–positive oropharyngeal SCC were more likely to be white ($P = .06$), married ($P<.001$), college educated ($P = .03$), and have an annual income over $50,000 ($P<.01$); intensity or duration of tobacco smoking or alcohol consumption did not increase the odds ratio of HPV-16–positive HNSCC.[48] Although case-control studies have not linked marijuana use to HPV-negative HNSCC, Gillison and colleagues[48] demonstrated a strong association of marijuana use and HPV-16–positive HNSCC and further theorized plausible mechanisms of cannabinoid modulation of the immune system.

High-risk HPV strains (HPV-16 and HPV-18) associated with oropharyngeal SCC (and cervical cancer) manipulate cellular pathways within affected cells to activate cell growth and suppress apoptosis. Malignant transformation begins with inactivation of the p53 tumor suppressor gene by E6, whereas a second HPV protein, E7, inactivates the retinoblastoma tumor suppressor protein (Rb). The HPV E6 and E7 proteins, encoded in the HPV-16 genome, functionally disrupt regulatory cell-cycle and DNA-repair pathways that drive genetic or epigenetic changes during molecular progression of HNSCC.[49] E6 targets the cellular ubiquitin-protein ligase E6-AP, which then targets p53 for ubiquitination and degradation, leaving cell growth unregulated. E7 associates with Rb and p21, blocking the interaction of Rb with E2F and initiating uncontrolled cell division.[50]

Not only is the nascent HPV-positive tumor subject to inactivation of tumor suppression genes from the viral genome, but several genes involved in transcription and cell cycle regulation are among the most prominent up-regulated genes in these tumors. One such cell cycle inhibitor is CDKN2A, which encodes the p16^{INK4A} tumor suppressor protein that functions as a cyclin-dependent kinase inhibitor in the Rb tumor suppressor pathway. Increased expression of p16^{INK4A} may potentially reflect loss of a negative feedback loop associated with inactivation of Rb by HPV E7.[51] Overexpression of p16^{INK4A} is strongly correlated with HPV infection in head and neck carcinomas and has been used as a surrogate marker for HPV.[52]

Detecting high-risk HPV using in situ hybridization from ethanol-fixed and Papanicolaou-stained smears after fine-needle aspiration has a 93% correlation to corresponding tissue sections positive for HPV-16 with polymerase chain reaction.[53] Of interest, HPV-positive tumors are associated with nonkeratinizing cytomorphology.[53] A recent meta-analysis showed that 26% of HNSCCs from all subsites contain HPV genomic DNA,[54] and it is now estimated that over 50% of oropharyngeal HNSCCs are related to HPV infection.[55] Although in situ hybridization and polymerase chain reaction techniques are available, there are no standardized clinical tests approved by the Food and Drug Administration for HPV-positive HNSCC tumors.

TUMORIGENESIS/CARCINOGENESIS

In the case of HPV, a virus can usurp normal cellular processes, whereas in the case of most patients, the development of carcinoma is the result of a stepwise accumulation of genetic alterations.[56] Three main steps include initiation, promotion, and progression. For this multiple-step process to succeed, numerous cellular processes and derangements must occur. The creation of an initial, critical, early genetic change helps set into motion the carcinogenic process.[57] Exposure to carcinogenic factors may lead to the abnormal expression of tumor suppressor genes, proto-oncogenes, or both, which in turn activate pathways that lead to the malignant transformation of cells. Oftentimes, this abnormal expression may include a sporadic mutation, deletion, loss of heterozygosity, overexpression, or epigenetic modification such as hypermethylation. For example, telomerase, an enzyme involved in immortalization, has been shown to be reactivated in roughly 90% of HNSCCs, whereas a deletion of 9p21 is found in 70% to 80% of these cases. Various point mutations in TP53 and the loss of heterozygosity of 17p are shown to exist in over 50% of HNSCC lesions.[58] When this occurs, secondary genetic changes create greater genetic instability, shifting the cell toward a more malignant phenotype (**Fig. 2**). Specifically, inactivation of tumor-suppressor genes allows for cellular proliferation to continue with unregulated and autonomous, self-sufficient growth. Proto-oncogenes also play a key role in tumorigenesis by helping the cell attain a malignant phenotype.

Six hallmarks of cancer cells have been described that distinguish them from their normal counterparts: (1) self-sufficiency in growth signals, (2) insensitivity to growth-inhibitory signals, (3) evasion of programmed cell death, (4) immortality or unlimited replicative potential, (5) sustained angiogenesis, and (6) tissue invasion and metastasis.[59] In the following sections, the authors discuss major pathways, receptors, and proteins implicated in the initiation or progression of HNSCC as they relate to aspects of all six of these hallmarks. It is the accumulation of specific abnormalities such as those described, likely along with other genetic events and alterations, that accounts for the process of carcinogenesis in HNSCC.

FIELD CANCERIZATION

Although it is unclear exactly why HPV appears to target certain subsites in the head and neck, the pattern is clear. In contrast, there seems to be a more general phenomenon seen in smokers in whom broad regions of tissue appear to be damaged, giving

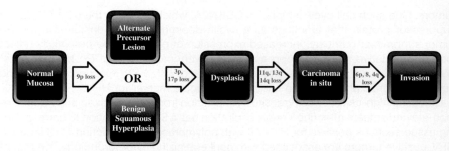

Fig. 2. Genetic progression of HNSCC. Genetic changes associated with the histologic progression of HNSCC based on loss of chromosomal material (allelic loss). Genetic alterations have been placed before the lesion where the frequency of the particular event plateaus. It is the accumulation and not necessarily the order of genetic events that determines the progression. A small fraction of benign squamous hyperplastic lesions contain 9p21 or 3p21 loss, suggesting that an unidentified precursor lesion (or cells) may also give rise to dysplasia. Candidate tumor suppressor genes include p16 (9p21), p53 (17p), and Rb (13q), and a candidate proto-oncogene includes cyclin D1 (11q13). (*Courtesy of* Joseph A. Califano, MD, Baltimore, MD.)

rise to multiple premalignant and frankly invasive tumors. In 1953, Slaughter and colleagues[60] first hypothesized that primary tumors emerge from a layer of precancerous tissue and coined the term "field cancerization" after demonstrating histopathologic changes consistent with genetic aberration from normal mucosa. Forty years after Slaughter and colleagues proposed field cancerization, Califano and colleagues[49] demonstrated the molecular basis for histopathologic changes. Samples of dysplastic mucosa and benign hyperplastic lesions displayed loss of heterozygosity at specific loci (9p21 [20%], 3p21 [16%], 17p13 [11%]). In particular, loss of 9p21 or 3p21 is one of the earliest detectable events leading to the progression to dysplasia. From dysplasia, further genetic alteration in 11q, 13q, and 14q creates carcinoma in situ (see **Fig. 2**).

The high rate of recurrence in the location of the primary tumor is thought to be a result of the fact that 30% of histopathologically benign squamous cell epithelium consists of a clonal population, with genetic alterations seen in HNSCC.[61] Studies using microsatellite analysis and X chromosome inactivation have verified that metachronous and synchronous lesions from distinct anatomic sites in HNSCC often originate from a common clone.[62] This evidence confirms that genetically altered mucosa is difficult to cure in the HNSCC patient because it is on the path to tumorigenesis. Indeed, second primaries are common in patients who have HNSCC.

EPITHELIAL-TO-MESENCHYMAL TRANSITION

There is evidence that suggests that fundamental changes to the programming of cells, including stem cells, may also be involved in tumorigenesis. One program that is particularly dangerous is the epithelial-to-mesenchymal transition (EMT), a phenotypic change in cells that provides them with the ability to escape from the constraints of surrounding tissue architecture. It has been postulated that EMT is the means by which epithelial tumors invade and metastasize to other tissues. As defined by Hugo and colleagues,[63] EMT is a culmination of protein modifications and transcriptional events in response to extracellular stimuli. These changes lead to long-term yet sometimes reversible cellular changes. Abnormalities in cadherins, tight junctions, and desmosomes lead to a decrease in cell–cell adherence and loss of polarity in the cells, increasing the mobility of these cells. More specifically, epithelial cells disassemble their junctional structures, undergo extracellular matrix remodeling, begin to express proteins of mesenchymal origin, and subsequently become migratory.[64] This process has been postulated to be a part of normal embryogenesis, the inflammatory process, and wound healing.[63] When the process of EMT becomes pathologic, it lacks the tight coordination and regulatory checkpoints that are normally present. Specifically, in the carcinogenic process, EMT causes changes in tumor cell properties that contribute to tumor invasion and metastasis, enabling cancer cell dissemination and self-renewal capabilities.[65] In HNSCC, EMT has been found to play a role, especially in high-risk tumor subtypes. Chung and colleagues[66] showed that genes involved in EMT and nuclear factor–kappaB (NF-κB) signaling deregulation were the most prominent molecular characteristics of the high-risk tumors in the subset they examined. Although it is clear that EMT plays a role in tumorigenesis in many cancers, the complete clinical significance of this process is yet to be fully defined.

EPIGENETIC MODIFICATION

Many programs (such as those discussed in **Fig. 2**) are the result of direct damage to the genome; however, there are other mechanisms of heritable somatic changes in gene expression that do not require direct alteration of the DNA sequence itself. The DNA molecule can be modified, such as by the addition or subtraction of methyl groups, without a change in the base composition. Similarly, histones, the structural proteins found in close association with DNA, can be modified by acetylation, methylation, or ubiquitylation. These non-DNA encoded modifications can result in heritable changes in gene expression that are clinically significant, including in the setting of cancer. Different cancers display varying behaviors, likely due to the multiple epigenetic changes and genetic mutations that occur within a tumor environment. Hypermethylation is one such type of epigenetic modification that is increasingly well characterized. Recently identified as a probable component in the development of carcinoma, hypermethylation in certain promoter regions of a gene can lead to repression of transcription.[67] Numerous studies have implicated this process of aberrant methylation in many tumor suppressor genes, causing them to become inactive.[67]

MOLECULAR PATHWAYS INVOLVED IN HEAD AND NECK SQUAMOUS CELL CARCINOMA

Increasingly, model systems and other research techniques have helped to decipher pathways of importance for patients (**Fig. 3**). Knowledge of these pathways has led investigators to interrogate key pathway components for tumor-specific gene mutations, and many have been reported in head and neck tumors (**Table 1**). Initial clarity in the activated pathways and mutated genes of head and neck tumors resulted in clinical trials of a host of targeted therapies, such as those documented in **Table 2**. The most promising pathways and agents from this inventory are discussed in the following paragraphs.

Epidermal Growth Factor Receptor

Epidermal growth factor receptor (EGFR) signaling has been strongly implicated in carcinogenesis, tumor progression, and response to therapy in HNSCC (reviewed by Thariat and colleagues).[68] The ErbB family of proteins, a family of four structurally related receptor tyrosine kinases, comprises four receptors (ErbB 1–4, also known as HER 1–4) and 13 polypeptide extracellular ligands.[69] In the literature, ErbB2 is synonymous with HER2/neu, whereas ErbB1 is commonly referred to as EGFR.

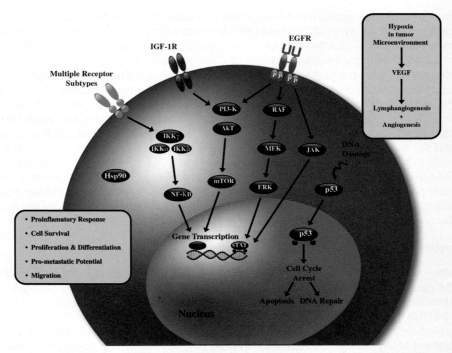

Fig. 3. Molecular pathways contributing to the promotion and progression of tumorigenesis in head and neck cancer. Akt, protein kinase B; EGFR, epidermal growth factor receptor; ERK, extracellular signal–related kinase; Hsp90, heat shock protein 90; IGF-1R, insulin-like growth factor-1 receptor; IKKα, inhibitor κB kinase alpha; IKKβ, inhibitor κB kinase beta; IKKγ, inhibitor κB kinase gamma; JAK, Janus kinase; MEK, mitogen-activated protein kinase; mTOR, mammalian target of rapamycin; PI3-K, phosphatidylinositol-3-kinase; STAT, signal transducers and activators of transcription; VEGF, vascular endothelial growth factor.

When ligands bind to one of the ErbB receptors, a dimer forms and the receptor's intracellular tyrosine residues then undergo ATP-dependent autophosphorylation. Currently, there are 12 different ligands that are known to activate four known ErbB receptors.

When phosphorylated, the receptor has the potential to trigger a number of different intracellular downstream pathways that can eventually arrest apoptosis, promote cellular proliferation, stimulate tumor-induced neovascularization, and activate carcinoma invasion and metastasis.[69] The Ras/mitogen-activated protein kinase/extracellular signal–related kinase (Ras-MAPK-ERK) pathway is known to control gene transcription, cell proliferation, and cell-cycle progression, whereas the phosphatidylinositol-3-kinase/protein kinase B (PI3K/Akt) pathway has been shown to stimulate numerous antiapoptotic signals within the cell. The Janus kinase/signal transducers and activators of transcription (STAT) and phospholipase-Cγ/protein kinase C pathways are also activated in association with EGFR phosphorylation.[70] Thus, EGFR plays a role in carcinoma growth and survival through a multitude of oncogenic downstream signaling pathways.

EGFR mRNA and protein are known to be preferentially expressed in HNSCC compared with surrounding normal tissues, suggesting a significant role in carcinogenesis. Similarly, most epithelial carcinomas overexpress and possess functional activation of the EGFR family of receptors.[71] In HNSCC, EGFR is overexpressed in up to 80% to

Table 1
Limited listing of the most common somatic mutations of various head and neck subsites

Head and Neck Subsite[a]	Gene	Sample Positive/Total (% Positive)
Larynx	CDKN2A	45/262 (17)
	PTEN	10/43 (23)
	EGFR	5/82 (6)
	KRAS	4/166 (2)
	HRAS	2/96 (2)
Oral cavity	CDKN2A	98/508 (19)
	HRAS	67/494 (13)
	FGFR3	44/136 (32)
	PIK3CA	18/145 (12)
	KRAS	14/497 (2)
Oropharynx	MET	33/156 (21)
	CDKN2A	19/173 (10)
	PTEN	7/27 (25)
	KRAS	3/105 (2)
	BRAF	3/52 (5)
Tonsil	EGFR	7/45 (15)
	CDKN2A	0/3 (0)
	HRAS	0/3 (0)
	KRAS	0/3 (0)
	NRAS	0/3 (0)
Sinonasal cavity	KRAS	4/121 (3)
	HRAS	2/11 (18)
	NRAS	2/11 (18)
	STK11	2/7 (28)
	EGFR	1/5 (20)
Esophagus (upper one third)	TP53	4/4 (100)
	KRAS	1/4 (25)
	CDKN2A	1/3 (33)
	PIK3CA	1/3 (33)
	CTNNB1	0/9 (0)
Thyroid	BRAF	2013/4793 (41)
	RET	274/706 (38)
	NRAS	132/1962 (6)
	KRAS	80/1878 (4)
	HRAS	56/1844 (3)
Salivary gland	HRAS	17/90 (18)
	PTEN	5/13 (38)
	DTNNB1	2/44 (4)
	KRAS	1/40 (2)
	CDKN2A	1/8 (12)

Although the capability exists to detect these mutations within tumor samples, their full clinical relevance has yet to be fully realized.

[a] SCC was the only histology tested for in the larynx, oral cavity, oropharynx, tonsil, sinonasal cavity, and esophagus. A wider range of histologic variants was included for the analysis of thyroid and salivary gland subsites.

Table 2
Limited listing of selected targeted agents that are currently undergoing clinical trials for the treatment of head and neck cancer

Drug Name (Trade Name)	Target	Phase of Study in Head and Neck Cancer
Cetuximab (Erbitux)	EGFR	III
Gefitinib (Iressa)	EGFR	I/II/III
Erlotinib (Tarceva)	EGFR	I/II/III
Panitumumab (Vectibix)	EGFR	I/II/III
BIBW 2992 (Tovok)	EGFR, HER-2/neu	II
Zalutumumab (HuMax-EGFr)	EGFR	I/II/III
Trastuzumab (Herceptin)	HER-2/neu	II
Lapatinib (Tykerb)	EGFR, HER-2/neu	I/II/III
Cediranib (Recentin)	VEGF	I/II
Sorafenib (Nexavar)	Raf, VEGF	I/II
Semaxanib	VEGF	I/II
Pazopanib	VEGF	II
Sunitinib (Sutent)	VEGF	I/II
Bevacizumab (Avastin)	VEGF	I/II/III
Romidepsin	Histone deacetylase	I/II
Vorinostat (Zolinza)	Histone deacetylase	I/II
Dasatinib (Sprycel)	Tyrosine kinases	II
Imatinib (Gleevec)	Tyrosine kinases	II
Pazopanib	VEGF, tyrosine kinases	II
Vandetanib (Zactima)	VEGF, EGFR	I/II
XL880	VEGF, tyrosine kinases	II
Perifosine (KRX-0401)	AKT	II
Bortezomib (Velcade)	NF-kB, tyrosine kinases	I/II
Lonafarnib (Serasar)	Farnesyl transferase	I/II
Tanespimycin (KOS-953)	Hsp90	I/II
AZD0530	Src/Abl kinase	II

This partial list was obtained through an extensive and comprehensive search on www.clinicaltrial.gov.

Abbreviations: Akt, protein kinase B; EGFR, epidermal growth factor receptor; Hsp90, heat shock protein 90; VEGF, vascular endothelial growth factor.

100% of tumors, some of the highest rates of any human carcinoma.[72,73] There are regional differences among tissues in the head and neck that express EGFR, with relatively lower levels associated with laryngeal tumors compared with those of the oral cavity and oropharynx.[74]

EGFR demonstrates increased overexpression in the more advanced-stage carcinomas and in those carcinomas found to be poorly differentiated.[70] In addition, EGFR overexpression is associated with decreased patient survival rates and has been demonstrated by some groups to confer resistance to various therapeutic modalities, including targeted therapy.[70,75–79] Although the association with poor patient prognosis has not been as clearly established, specific mutations of the EGFR receptor have also been studied. The most common mutation of EGFR is likely *EGFRvIII*, occurring in up to 40% of HNSCC.[80] This mutant receptor is found only in cancer cells and manifests from an in-frame deletion of exons 2 to 7, which encodes the receptor's extracellular domain, thus resulting in a constitutively active receptor that is completely independent of any activation by way of ligand binding.[80] The fact that *EGFRvIII* is not found in normal tissues makes this a very intriguing, highly specific target for therapy, given that it would not interfere with the normal EGFR signaling in noncancerous tissues (see **Table 1**).

In addition to overexpression, other pathologic manifestations of EGFR can be performed through mutational activation, amplification, and transactivation by other tyrosine kinases.[81] The potential, constitutive activation of several different oncogenic pathways, by way of EGFR-independent mechanisms, likely explains the lack of response that is commonly appreciated in patients being treated with EGFR inhibitor therapy.[70]

With the prominent role that EGFR is known to play in tumorigenesis, this family of proteins was a logical choice in pursuing a new class of targeted cancer therapy. Currently, there are several EGFR antagonists available for clinical use in the treatment of four metastatic epithelial carcinomas, including non–small cell lung cancer, colorectal cancer, pancreatic cancer, and HNSCC. The two classes of therapies that exist to date are monoclonal antibodies to EGFR receptor subunits and small-molecule EGFR tyrosine kinase inhibitors. In simplest terms, the monoclonal antibodies probably act by binding the conserved extracellular domain of EGFR and by blocking the ligand-binding region by competitive inhibition, which in turn blocks ligand-induced autophosphorylation through the inability to stimulate tyrosine kinase. The EGFR tyrosine kinase inhibitors function by way of a separate mechanism. They act by reversibly competing with ATP in its binding site to the intracellular catalytic domain of tyrosine kinase, therefore inhibiting autophosphorylation of EGFR and its subsequent downstream signaling.[71]

Akimoto and colleagues[82] were the first to provide evidence that EGFR expression may have an effect on radiation sensitivity, a result that has been validated clinically.[75,83] EGFR overexpression in head and neck cancer cell lines was found to have greater radioresistance compared with cell lines that had relatively lower levels of EGFR expression. It was also found that following radiation, EGFR becomes upregulated within the tumor, leading to increased activation of its downstream signaling pathways.[84,85] This work culminated in the landmark 2006 publication of the randomized trial by Bonner and colleagues[86] that showed an overall and progression-free survival advantage with the addition of cetuximab to standard radiation therapy.

At least 40 trials involving patients who have HNSCC are currently investigating various "targeted agents" including tyrosine kinase inhibitors and antibody therapy.[87] More than 10 different EGFR-targeting agents are in development for the treatment of various carcinomas. Although a great deal of effort has gone into the development and validation of predictive biomarkers, it remains difficult to determine a priori who will benefit from these therapies. In some studies, EGFR expression is an independent predictor of response, whereas in others, no relationship is appreciated.[75,88–91] The search for molecular predictors of clinical outcome that would potentially optimize patient selection and therapeutic efficacy continues to be an area of intense ongoing investigation.

Insulin-Like Growth Factor-1 Receptor

An emerging potential target for directed, molecular-based cancer therapy is the insulin-like growth factor (IGF) signaling axis. Numerous preclinical and clinical studies have implicated the IGF-1 receptor (IGF-1R) and its ligands, IGF-1 and IGF-2, in the development and progression of a number of human cancers.[92–94] IGF-1R is a transmembrane heterotetramer receptor that consists of two α and two β subunits. Like the insulin receptor, IGF1-R possesses tyrosine kinase activity. With activation of the receptor, downstream signaling events include phosphorylation of insulin receptor substrate-1, activation of MAPKs, and stimulation of the PI3K pathway.[95] This activation of the Ras-MAPK-ERK and PI3K/Akt pathways is similar to the downstream signaling seen with EGFR autophosphorylation and activation. Six IGF binding proteins (IGFBPs) are known to exist in humans. These proteins have been shown to help modulate the effects of IGF-1 by way of multiple unique mechanisms. In humans, IGF-1 is bound to one of the IGFBPs over 95% of the time, with IGFBP-3 accounting for roughly 85% of this binding.[96]

In vitro and in vivo studies have shown that IGF-1R encourages cellular growth and protects cells from apoptosis.[97] This phosphorylation cascade leads to the activation of various transcription factors involved in cellular proliferation and transformation.[98–102] Constitutive activation and overexpression of IGF-1R has been associated with malignant transformation, involving glioblastoma, melanoma, pancreatic, breast, colon, and ovarian carcinoma models.[103–105] The receptor has been closely linked to the metastatic properties of tumor cells, with studies showing that the receptor to signal pathways are linked to tumor invasiveness and angiogenesis.[106,107] IGF-1R signaling has also been shown to influence and promote focal adhesion stability, cell-to-cell contact, and cellular motility.[108] Numerous studies have also shown that enhanced IGF-1R activation is associated with resistance to certain cytotoxic chemotherapy regimens, hormonal agents, biologic anticancer therapies, and radiation therapy.[109–117]

Although Ouban and colleagues[118] showed only 13% immunostaining positivity for IGF-1R in 31 different human HNSCC tissue samples, other studies have shown much higher levels of expression. IGF-1R is ubiquitously expressed at varying levels in cancerous tissues, and plays an intricate role in the regulation of cellular proliferation and differentiation even at very low levels of expression.[95,118]

As mentioned previously, the IGF-1R and the EGFR signaling pathways are intricately associated with one another, regulating overlapping downstream signaling pathways. Increased IGF-1R expression has been reported to mediate resistance to anti-EGFR–based therapies in certain solid tumors, including glioblastoma, pancreatic, and breast carcinoma.[119–122] It has been found that the use of both antibodies in combination was more effective in reducing cancer cell growth than the use of either single agent alone.[123] There may be a potential benefit in the use of combined anti–tyrosine kinase receptor–directed therapies to treat HNSCC. Slomiany and colleagues[124] also demonstrated the potential for the cotargeting of IGF-1R and EGFR signaling pathways in HNSCC.

Design of IGF-1R inhibitors has proved to be somewhat problematic, due to the close homology (60%–70% amino acid homology) with the insulin receptor;[125] however, specific inhibitors have recently been developed. Several approaches to tumor growth inhibition have been undertaken, including IGF-1R dominant mutants, IGF-1R blocking antibodies, and oligonucleotides aimed at down-regulating IGF-1R expression, but little success has been achieved in terms of improved clinical outcomes. The first IGF-1R tyrosine kinase inhibitor demonstrating in vivo therapeutic potential (NVP-AEW541 [Novartis]), however, has been shown to enhance tumor cell chemosensitivity and inhibit tumor growth in human fibrosarcoma, myeloma, and Ewing's sarcoma models.[125,126] Studies with the inhibitor have yet to be undertaken in an HNSCC model.

Phosphatidylinositol-3-Kinase/Protein Kinase B Pathway

The PI3-K/Akt signal transduction pathway has been shown to regulate numerous cellular processes, including apoptosis, proliferation, cell cycle progression, cytoskeletal stability and motility, and energy metabolism.[127,128] Activated Akt induces increased expression of numerous proliferative and antiapoptotic proteins, including Bcl-2, Bcl-x, and NF-kB.[127] The pathway has been shown to be activated in up to 50% to 80% of HNSCCs.[78] The PI3-K/Akt pathway is one of the main downstream signaling pathways activated by the ErbB/tyrosine kinase receptor family of receptors. After ligand binding, the cytoplasmic domain of the EGFR undergoes tyrosine phosphorylation and subsequently activates PI3-K.[129] Activation of the PI3-K/Akt pathway, however, is not entirely dependent on the tyrosine kinase family of receptors. In certain carcinoma models, it has been shown to be activated through direct mutation or amplification of PI3-K, amplification of Akt, activation of the RAS oncogene, or decreased expression of the tumor-suppressor protein phosphatase and tensin homolog (PTEN), a known inhibitor of the PI3-K/Akt pathway.[129] Loss of PTEN expression, along with Akt activation, correlates with worse clinical outcomes in patients who have SCC of the tongue.[130,131] This pathway has also been found to be overexpressed and activated in a number of different carcinomas, including HNSCC. In a study conducted by Massarelli and colleagues,[132] it was shown that disease-free survival was significantly decreased in cases of SCC of the tongue that stained positive for activated Akt (p-Akt). The comparatively poor outcome that was associated with p-Akt expression was also found to be independent of cancer stage and nodal status. Akt activation has also been correlated with the squamous cell progression and transformation—from normal epithelial tissue, to dysplasia, and even to invasive SCC.[133]

The PI3kK/Akt pathway has also been shown to be up-regulated following radiation therapy. Bussink and colleagues[129] described how the pathway is intricately involved with resistance to radiation therapy by way of multiple mechanisms. The *RAS* oncogene is a well-known contributor to the intrinsic radioresistance of tumor cells, mediated at least partially through its downstream signaling through the PI3-K/Akt pathway.[129] In addition, this pathway is involved in DNA repair by way of EGFR signaling, with multiple studies showing that with EGFR blockade, the PI3-K/Akt pathway–mediated DNA repair process is altered. When combined with radiation therapy, this decreased DNA repair leads to greater levels of tumor cell apoptosis and subsequent improved locoregional control compared with radiation therapy alone.[129]

Although this pathway is most often activated through EGFR, EGFR-independent activation is also common and of clinical relevance.[129] Using tissue microarray technology, Molino and colleagues[134] showed that the PI3-K/Akt/mammalian target of rapamycin (mTOR) pathway was frequently activated in HNSCC samples and that this was often independent of any associated EGFR activation. There has also been a strong and independent correlation between expression of activated Akt (pAkt) and treatment outcome in laryngeal and oropharyngeal HNSCC.[132,135] Similarly, enhanced Akt activity has been independently associated with more-advanced tumor stage and progression in a number of different malignancies.[136] Knowing this information, further study of this pathway (independent of EGFR) is needed so that it can be used in regard to treatment and prognostic markers for HNSCC.

A recent phase II trial conducted by Karamouzis and colleagues[137] involved the use of an Akt phosphorylation/activation inhibitor (perifosine) in a small group of patients who had incurable recurrent HNSCC, metastatic HNSCC, or both. Although the inhibitor had some preclinical antitumor activity in vivo, no objective clinical responses were appreciated, with 18 of 19 patients having disease that progressed at 8 weeks' follow-up.[137] Akt activation, however, has also been associated with resistance to EGFR inhibition in a non–small cell lung cancer model,[138] and therefore, benefits from combined targeted molecular therapy are still of potential interest. The potential clinical usefulness of the PI3-K/Akt pathway as a therapeutic target and a prognostic marker in HNSCC is promising.

Mammalian Target of Rapamycin

One of the downstream cell-growth regulators associated with the PI3-K/Akt pathway is an atypical serine/threonine kinase named mTOR. Although Akt helps control cellular proliferation and growth through the coordination of mitogenic signaling with energy- and nutrient-sensing pathways that control protein synthesis, it requires mTOR to fully exert these effects.[139] mTOR is involved in modulation of the cell cycle and ribosomal function to subsequently participate in cell growth and apoptosis.[140] When activated through Akt, mTOR phosphorylates the translation regulator p70-S6 kinase, which in turn activates the ribosomal S6 protein, a protein involved in translation and one of the most downstream targets of the PI3-K/Akt/mTOR pathway. This activation of S6 ribosomal protein thus adds to the control of cell growth through increased manipulation of mRNA translation.[141]

Amornphimoltham and colleagues[139] found that in clinical specimens from patients who had HNSCC and from HNSCC-derived cell lines, aberrant accumulation of activated S6 (p-S6) was a frequent occurrence in early dysplastic lesions and carcinomas. These investigators also showed that the activated ribosomal protein was decreased when HNSCC cell lines were treated with rapamycin, a macrolide antibiotic and a known inhibitor of mTOR.[139] Similar findings were seen when rapamycin was used in an HNSCC xenograft model. In vivo, rapamycin's effects included induction of apoptosis and inhibition of cellular growth of the HNSCC cells, with subsequent tumor regression.[139] It has also been shown that rapamycin sensitivity of tumor cells is at least partially dependent on the dysregulation of the tumor suppressor gene *PTEN*, the well-known inhibitor of the PI3-K/Akt pathway.[142,143] In some of the HNSCC cell lines, EGFR inhibition had no effect on the activity of the mTOR pathway, indicating a potential clinical and therapeutic benefit when EGFR inhibitors and mTOR inhibitors are used in combination.[139] The study revealed the Akt/mTOR pathway to be a potential therapeutic target for the treatment of HNSCC, particularly in terms of development of analogs to rapamycin.

Nathan and colleagues[144] showed that one of the main downstream effectors of the Akt/mTOR pathway, eIF4E, was overexpressed in histologically "tumor-free" surgical margins of resected HNSCC samples and was an independent predictor of tumor recurrence. In a later study, the same group used an eIF4E-overexpressing, PTEN-mutant HNSCC cell line, FaDu, in a minimal residual disease murine model, and showed that the rapamycin analog temsirolimus (CCI-779) was effective in prolonging survival, including improved tumor-free survival.[145] It was concluded that CCI-779 represented a new potential targeted therapy for the treatment of HNSCC, because overexpression and activation of mTOR occurs in many of these tumors.[139,146]

Nuclear Factor–Kappa B

NF-κB transcription factors are the final downstream mediators of many of the earlier-mentioned pathways and therefore play a key role in head and neck cancers. It has become clear that NF-κB–mediated inflammatory signaling is overexpressed in many HNSCCs. Expression has also been shown to be associated with tumorigenesis and metastasis.[147,148] Constitutive NF-κB activation has been shown to be common when induced by carcinogen exposure or stimulation with oncogenic viruses, with induced levels of activation being seen in tissue specimens of HNSCC.[149–151] Increases in nuclear localization of NF-κB have been detected in roughly 85% of patients who have HNSCC, with increased immunostaining correlating with worse prognosis of the disease.[151]

NF-kB is known to be an important factor in regulating the expression of genes associated with angiogenesis (interleukin [IL]-8), apoptosis (Bcl-xL), cellular proliferation (cyclin D1), and proinflammatory cytokine cascades (IL-6, IL-1α).[148,150,152–156] In terms of cell survival and apoptosis, NF-κB, in close association with STAT3 and *p53*, has been found to directly affect the balance of proapoptotic and antiapoptotic proteins in SCC cell lines.[157] NF-κB is also known be involved in attenuated sensitivity to cytotoxic anticancer therapy.[155,158] Similarly, the reactive oxygen species that ionizing radiation creates in the body have been shown to induce NF-κB as a cytoprotective mechanism within tumor cells, rendering the radiation therapy less effective.[159] There is even evidence that NF-κB has direct carcinogenic effects that give tumor cells the ability to evade the regulatory functions of the immune system.[148] It has also been shown that tobacco smoke condensate and betel nut extract activate NF-κB indirectly by way of degradation of inhibitor κB (IκB) proteins.[160,161]

With its constitutive activation and proven role in radiation therapy resistance, its inhibition is a logical target for therapy. Salicylates, antioxidants, nonsteroidal anti-inflammatory drugs, prostaglandins, and glucocorticoids have shown effectiveness in various settings to inhibit NF-κB.[162] IκB kinase beta inhibitors have also shown some effectiveness in preclinical studies in various carcinomas, yet no head and neck carcinoma studies are currently underway.[163] Further development of these novel therapies continues in the hopes that through inhibition of NF-κB, a decrease in tumor invasion, aggressiveness, and metastasis will be realized.

Heat Shock Protein 90

Heat shock protein 90 (Hsp90) is a molecular chaperone that induces conformational changes in numerous protein substrates including transcription factors and protein kinases.[164,165] Hsp90 has been shown to be involved with proteins in many signaling pathways important for tumor cell survival, proliferation, and metastasis. Specifically, Hsp90 is associated with the EGFR pathway, IGF-R, Akt, ERK, Ikβ kinases, *p53*, and STAT3.[165] It has been shown to be constitutively expressed at up to 10 times higher levels in tumor cells compared with normal cells.[166] Therefore, therapeutic inhibition of Hsp90 offers the potential to simultaneously disrupt numerous pathways known to be involved in the progression toward malignant phenotypes.

A geldanamycin derivative and semisynthetic analog, 17-AAG (Tanespimycin), became the first Hsp90 inhibitor to enter clinical testing.[167] Recently, Shintani and colleagues[168] investigated the effects of 17-AAG on radiation sensitivity on oral SCC cell lines in vitro. They found that the radiation response was enhanced in 17-AAG–treated cells, but only in cell lines with wild-type *p53* expression. Yin and colleagues[169] recently used a novel Hsp90 inhibitor, EC5, in their study of eight HNSCC cell lines. EC5, a benzoquinone ansamycin antibiotic derivative, was shown to have antitumor effects in xenograft models.[169] These investigators also compared these results with 17-AAG, and it was shown that EC5 caused more potent antitumor effects in these models.[169]

PROGNOSTIC AND DIAGNOSTIC MARKERS, GENETIC PROFILING

With the advent of increasingly sophisticated molecular detection techniques and technologies such as DNA microarrays, large numbers of genetic markers are able to be tested with greater ease. In a study by Roepman and colleagues,[170] predictor gene sets were found to have greater predictive power in the detection of local nodal metastases from primary tumor samples than the current clinical diagnosis and staging systems. Although this technology offers excellent opportunities to further dissect the molecular and genetic interactions that participate in carcinogenesis, it is clear that conflicting data and findings will persist as continued improvement in analysis and interpretation occurs.

Early in the molecular study of head and neck cancer, several studies demonstrated an association between *p53* abnormalities and poor outcome. Yet, other large follow-up studies failed to demonstrate such an association.[78] The prognostic significance of p16 aberrations has also been variable. Most studies conducted on the significance of EGFR and cyclin D1 overexpression have shown them to be associated with a worse prognosis in patients who have HNSCC.[78] Similarly, genetic alterations of Cox-2, p27, *p53*, CCDN1, and vascular endothelial growth factor, among others, have been shown in various studies to be associated with an increased risk of metastasis, disease recurrence, or overall worse prognosis.[78,171] Like many other markers, however, there have been other studies that have failed to confirm these significant findings.

As single molecular markers, most that have been studied to date have failed to show sufficient predictive potential in terms of the course of disease, prognosis, and survival. Although single markers may not prove to have the clinical applicability that many had hoped for, combinations of different molecular markers and genetic expression patterns may offer more promising diagnostic and prognostic value. Using cDNA microarray technology, Chung and colleagues[172] looked at 60 HNSCC tumor samples and categorized them into four distinct subtypes of HNSCC, each showing clinically unique behavior. Not only did they show that these subtypes showed distinct behavior clinically but they also concluded that the status of possible regional metastases could be predicted by genetic microarray analysis of the primary lesion.[172] Other combinatorial approaches using biomarkers and traditional clinical markers have been proposed and will likely gain increasing interest.[173] Selection from among the competing markers and their incorporation into clinical practice will be one of the major challenges on the horizon for physicians.

SUMMARY

Although cancer is generally thought of as a disease of DNA, the risk for any individual of developing a tumor based on his or her genomic makeup cannot be explicitly determined given our current scope of knowledge. The risk, however, is certainly a function of germline DNA composition, interaction with the environment (especially toxins and infections), and perhaps an arbitrary component of statistical probability applied over the years of a normal lifespan. The types of genetic damage incurred are probably primarily to DNA in the form of deletions, amplifications, or focal damaging mutations, although other mechanisms are increasingly noted to be important, including epigenetic changes to chromatin. No matter what the mechanism, the ultimate event is a perturbation of normal cellular biomolecules and homeostasis leading to the hallmark processes of cancer characterized by pathways such as those described in the preceding sections.

Certainly, most scientists and clinicians emphasize models of carcinogenesis similar to the ones just described—heavily focused on molecular events and cancer pathways. Yet, even though our research colleagues rely heavily on an increasingly sophisticated set of molecular assays and reagents, the clinical care of the head and neck cancer patient is currently almost devoid of any molecular diagnostic. Likewise, the set of targeted cancer therapies for our patients remains limited, and prognosis or response to therapy has rarely if ever been assigned based on molecular testing. The landscape, however, appears likely to change in the near future. One has only to look at the therapies listed in **Table 2** to witness the increasing need to identify which specific genes and pathways are altered in a particular tumor. It is likely that patients at differential risk of developing cancer are increasingly likely to be identified from germline DNA, in the form of mutations or SNPs. Tumors that are primarily attributable to viral etiologies are likely to be identified with potentially altered treatment paradigms, or perhaps averted entirely through vaccines. The integration of molecular diagnostics and the molecular risk–based approach to cancer treatment that is pathway driven is likely to be not only a major success but also a major challenge that our generation faces over the coming years.

REFERENCES

1. Brennan JA, Boyle JO, Koch WM, et al. Association between cigarette smoking and mutation of the *p53* gene in squamous-cell carcinoma of the head and neck. N Engl J Med 1995;332(11):712–7.
2. Zain RB, Gupta PC, Warnakulasuriya S, et al. Oral lesions associated with betel quid and tobacco chewing habits. Oral Dis 1997;3(3):204–5.
3. Norton SA. Betel: consumption and consequences. J Am Acad Dermatol 1998; 38(1):81–8.
4. Warnakulasuriya S, Trivedy C, Peters TJ. Areca nut use: an independent risk factor for oral cancer. BMJ 2002;324(7341):799–800.
5. Lu CT, Yen YY, Ho CS, et al. A case-control study of oral cancer in Changhua County, Taiwan. J Oral Pathol Med 1996;25(5):245–8.
6. Denissenko MF, Pao A, Tang M, et al. Preferential formation of benzo[a]pyrene adducts at lung cancer mutational hotspots in P53. Science 1996;274(5286): 430–2.
7. Wilson DM 3rd, Bohr VA. The mechanics of base excision repair, and its relationship to aging and disease. DNA Repair (Amst) 2007;6(4):544–59.
8. Hung RJ, Hall J, Brennan P, et al. Genetic polymorphisms in the base excision repair pathway and cancer risk: a HuGE review. Am J Epidemiol 2005; 162(10):925–42.
9. Li C, Hu Z, Lu J, et al. Genetic polymorphisms in DNA base-excision repair genes ADPRT, XRCC1, and APE1 and the risk of squamous cell carcinoma of the head and neck. Cancer 2007;110(4):867–75.
10. Cheng L, Sturgis EM, Eicher SA, et al. Expression of nucleotide excision repair genes and the risk for squamous cell carcinoma of the head and neck. Cancer 2002;94(2):393–7.
11. Handra-Luca A, Hernandez J, Mountzios G, et al. Excision repair cross complementation group 1 immunohistochemical expression predicts objective response and cancer-specific survival in patients treated by cisplatin-based induction chemotherapy for locally advanced head and neck squamous cell carcinoma. Clin Cancer Res 2007;13(13):3855–9.
12. Shen MR, Jones IM, Mohrenweiser H. Nonconservative amino acid substitution variants exist at polymorphic frequency in DNA repair genes in healthy humans. Cancer Res 1998;58(4):604–8.
13. Lunn RM, Helzlsouer KJ, Parshad R, et al. XPD polymorphisms: effects on DNA repair proficiency. Carcinogenesis 2000;21(4):551–5.
14. Duell EJ, Wiencke JK, Cheng TJ, et al. Polymorphisms in the DNA repair genes XRCC1 and ERCC2 and biomarkers of DNA damage in human blood mononuclear cells. Carcinogenesis 2000;21(5):965–71.

15. Lunn RM, Langlois RG, Hsieh LL, et al. XRCC1 polymorphisms: effects on afla-toxin B1-DNA adducts and glycophorin A variant frequency. Cancer Res 1999; 59(11):2557–61.
16. Lei YC, Hwang SJ, Chang CC, et al. Effects on sister chromatid exchange fre-quency of polymorphisms in DNA repair gene XRCC1 in smokers. Mutat Res 2002;519(1–2):93–101.
17. Johnston LD, O'Malley PM. The recanting of earlier reported drug use by young adults. NIDA Res Monogr 1997;167:59–80.
18. Tashkin DP. Pulmonary complications of smoked substance abuse. West J Med 1990;152(5):525–30.
19. Tashkin DP. Is frequent marijuana smoking harmful to health? West J Med 1993; 158(6):635–7.
20. Hashibe M, Ford DE, Zhang ZF. Marijuana smoking and head and neck cancer. J Clin Pharmacol 2002;42(11 Suppl):103S–7S.
21. Zhang ZF, Morgenstern H, Spitz MR, et al. Marijuana use and increased risk of squamous cell carcinoma of the head and neck. Cancer Epidemiol Biomarkers Prev 1999;8(12):1071–8.
22. Donald PJ. Marijuana smoking—possible cause of head and neck carcinoma in young patients. Otolaryngol Head Neck Surg 1986;94(4):517–21.
23. Zimmerman S, Zimmerman AM. Genetic effects of marijuana. Int J Addict 1990; 25(1A):19–33.
24. Rosenblatt KA, Daling JR, Chen C, et al. Marijuana use and risk of oral squa-mous cell carcinoma. Cancer Res 2004;64(11):4049–54.
25. Lustig JP, Lugassy G, Neder A, et al. Head and neck carcinoma in Fanconi's anaemia—report of a case and review of the literature. Eur J Cancer B Oral Oncol 1995;31B(1):68–72.
26. Prime SS, Thakker NS, Pring M, et al. A review of inherited cancer syndromes and their relevance to oral squamous cell carcinoma. Oral Oncol 2001;37(1): 1–16.
27. Hecht F, Hecht BK. Cancer in ataxia-telangiectasia patients. Cancer Genet Cytogenet 1990;46(1):9–19.
28. Keukens F, van Voorst Vader PC, Panders AK, et al. Xeroderma pigmentosum: squamous cell carcinoma of the tongue. Acta Derm Venereol 1989;69(6):530–1.
29. Cohen EE, Rosen LS, Vokes EE, et al. Axitinib is an active treatment for all his-tologic subtypes of advanced thyroid cancer: results from a phase II study. J Clin Oncol 2008.
30. Wells SA Jr, GJ, Gagel RF, et al. Vandetanib in metastatic hereditary medullary thyroid cancer: follow-up results of an open-label phase II trial. J Clin Oncol 2007;25:303s.
31. Gillison ML. Current topics in the epidemiology of oral cavity and oropharyngeal cancers. Head Neck 2007;29(8):779–92.
32. Canto MT, Devesa SS. Oral cavity and pharynx cancer incidence rates in the United States, 1975–1998. Oral Oncol 2002;38(6):610–7.
33. Shiboski CH, Schmidt BL, Jordan RC. Tongue and tonsil carcinoma: increasing trends in the U.S. population ages 20-44 years. Cancer 2005;103(9):1843–9.
34. Schantz SP, Yu GP. Head and neck cancer incidence trends in young Ameri-cans, 1973–1997, with a special analysis for tongue cancer. Arch Otolaryngol Head Neck Surg 2002;128(3):268–74.
35. Chaturvedi AK, Engels EA, Anderson WF, et al. Incidence trends for human pap-illomavirus-related and -unrelated oral squamous cell carcinomas in the United States. J Clin Oncol 2008;26(4):612–9.

36. Syrjanen S. HPV infections and tonsillar carcinoma. J Clin Pathol 2004;57(5): 449–55.
37. Woods KV, Shillitoe EJ, Spitz MR, et al. Analysis of human papillomavirus DNA in oral squamous cell carcinomas. J Oral Pathol Med 1993;22(3):101–8.
38. Mork J, Lie AK, Glattre E, et al. Human papillomavirus infection as a risk factor for squamous-cell carcinoma of the head and neck. N Engl J Med 2001;344(15): 1125–31.
39. Miller CS, Johnstone BM. Human papillomavirus as a risk factor for oral squamous cell carcinoma: a meta-analysis, 1982–1997. Oral Surg Oral Med Oral Pathol Oral Radiol Endod 2001;91(6):622–35.
40. Luo CW, Roan CH, Liu CJ. Human papillomaviruses in oral squamous cell carcinoma and pre-cancerous lesions detected by PCR-based gene-chip array. Int J Oral Maxillofac Surg 2007;36(2):153–8.
41. Herrero R, Castellsague X, Pawlita M, et al. Human papillomavirus and oral cancer: the International agency for research on cancer multicenter study. J Natl Cancer Inst 2003;95(23):1772–83.
42. Gillison ML, Koch WM, Capone RB, et al. Evidence for a causal association between human papillomavirus and a subset of head and neck cancers. J Natl Cancer Inst 2000;92(9):709–20.
43. El-Mofty SK, Patil S. Human papillomavirus (HPV)-related oropharyngeal nonkeratinizing squamous cell carcinoma: characterization of a distinct phenotype. Oral Surg Oral Med Oral Pathol Oral Radiol Endod 2006;101(3):339–45.
44. Ragin CC, Modugno F, Gollin SM. The epidemiology and risk factors of head and neck cancer: a focus on human papillomavirus. J Dent Res 2007;86(2):104–14.
45. Kreimer AR, Clifford GM, Snijders PJ, et al. HPV16 semiquantitative viral load and serologic biomarkers in oral and oropharyngeal squamous cell carcinomas. Int J Cancer 2005;115(2):329–32.
46. Klussmann JP, Weissenborn SJ, Wieland U, et al. Prevalence, distribution, and viral load of human papillomavirus 16 DNA in tonsillar carcinomas. Cancer 2001;92(11):2875–84.
47. D'Souza G, Kreimer AR, Viscidi R, et al. Case-control study of human papillomavirus and oropharyngeal cancer. N Engl J Med 2007;356(19):1944–56.
48. Gillison ML, D'Souza G, Westra W, et al. Distinct risk factor profiles for human papillomavirus type 16-positive and human papillomavirus type 16-negative head and neck cancers. J Natl Cancer Inst 2008;100(6):407–20.
49. Califano J, van der Riet P, Westra W, et al. Genetic progression model for head and neck cancer: implications for field cancerization. Cancer Res 1996;56(11): 2488–92.
50. Tran N, Rose BR, O'Brien CJ. Role of human papillomavirus in the etiology of head and neck cancer. Head Neck 2007;29(1):64–70.
51. Slebos RJ, Yi Y, Ely K, et al. Gene expression differences associated with human papillomavirus status in head and neck squamous cell carcinoma. Clin Cancer Res 2006;12(3 Pt 1):701–9.
52. Ansari-Lari MA, Staebler A, Zaino RJ, et al. Distinction of endocervical and endometrial adenocarcinomas: immunohistochemical p16 expression correlated with human papillomavirus (HPV) DNA detection. Am J Surg Pathol 2004;28(2):160–7.
53. Zhang MQ, El-Mofty SK, Davila RM. Detection of human papillomavirus-related squamous cell carcinoma cytologically and by in situ hybridization in fine-needle aspiration biopsies of cervical metastasis: a tool for identifying the site of an occult head and neck primary. Cancer 2008;114(2):118–23.

54. Kreimer AR, Clifford GM, Boyle P, et al. Human papillomavirus types in head and neck squamous cell carcinomas worldwide: a systematic review. Cancer Epidemiol Biomarkers Prev 2005;14(2):467–75.
55. Fakhry C, Gillison ML. Clinical implications of human papillomavirus in head and neck cancers. J Clin Oncol 2006;24(17):2606–11.
56. Fearon ER, Vogelstein B. A genetic model for colorectal tumorigenesis. Cell 1990;61(5):759–67.
57. Weinberg R. Oncogenes, antioncogenes, and the molecular bases of multistep carcinogenesis. Cancer Res 1989;49:3713–21.
58. Argiris A, Karamouzis MV, Raben D, et al. Head and neck cancer. Lancet 2008; 371(9625):1695–709.
59. Hanahan D, Weinberg RA. The hallmarks of cancer. Cell 2000;100(1):57–70.
60. Slaughter DP, Southwick HW, Smejkal W. Field cancerization in oral stratified squamous epithelium; clinical implications of multicentric origin. Cancer 1953; 6(5):963–8.
61. Sidransky D, Mikkelsen T, Schwechheimer K, et al. Clonal expansion of p53 mutant cells is associated with brain tumour progression. Nature 1992;355(6363):846–7.
62. Bedi GC, Westra WH, Gabrielson E, et al. Multiple head and neck tumors: evidence for a common clonal origin. Cancer Res 1996;56(11):2484–7.
63. Hugo H, Ackland ML, Blick T, et al. Epithelial–mesenchymal and mesenchymal–epithelial transitions in carcinoma progression. J Cell Physiol 2007;213(2): 374–83.
64. Moustakas A, Heldin CH. Signaling networks guiding epithelial-mesenchymal transitions during embryogenesis and cancer progression. Cancer Sci 2007; 98(10):1512–20.
65. Mani SA, Guo W, Liao MJ, et al. The epithelial-mesenchymal transition generates cells with properties of stem cells. Cell 2008;133(4):704–15.
66. Chung CH, Parker JS, Ely K, et al. Gene expression profiles identify epithelial-to-mesenchymal transition and activation of nuclear factor-kappaB signaling as characteristics of a high-risk head and neck squamous cell carcinoma. Cancer Res 2006;66(16):8210–8.
67. Worsham MJ, Chen KM, Meduri V, et al. Epigenetic events of disease progression in head and neck squamous cell carcinoma. Arch Otolaryngol Head Neck Surg 2006; 132(6):668–77.
68. Thariat J, Milas L, Ang KK. Integrating radiotherapy with epidermal growth factor receptor antagonists and other molecular therapeutics for the treatment of head and neck cancer. Int J Radiat Oncol Biol Phys 2007;69(4):974–84.
69. Citri A, Yarden Y. EGF-ERBB signalling: towards the systems level. Nat Rev Mol Cell Biol 2006;7(7):505–16.
70. Kalyankrishna S, Grandis JR. Epidermal growth factor receptor biology in head and neck cancer. J Clin Oncol 2006;24(17):2666–72.
71. Ciardiello F, Tortora G. EGFR antagonists in cancer treatment. N Engl J Med 2008;358(11):1160–74.
72. Herbst RS, Giaccone G, Schiller JH, et al. Gefitinib in combination with paclitaxel and carboplatin in advanced non-small-cell lung cancer: a phase III trial—INTACT 2. J Clin Oncol 2004;22(5):785–94.
73. Grandis JR, Tweardy DJ. TGF-alpha and EGFR in head and neck cancer. J Cell Biochem Suppl 1993;17F:188–91.
74. Takes RP, Baatenburg de Jong RJ, Schuuring E, et al. Differences in expression of oncogenes and tumor suppressor genes in different sites of head and neck squamous cell. Anticancer Res 1998;18(6B):4793–800.

75. Ang KK, Berkey BA, Tu X, et al. Impact of epidermal growth factor receptor expression on survival and pattern of relapse in patients with advanced head and neck carcinoma. Cancer Res 2002;62(24):7350–6.
76. Kim S, Grandis JR, Rinaldo A, et al. Emerging perspectives in epidermal growth factor receptor targeting in head and neck cancer. Head Neck 2008;30(5): 667–74.
77. Ford AC, Grandis JR. Targeting epidermal growth factor receptor in head and neck cancer. Head Neck 2003;25(1):67–73.
78. Lothaire P, de Azambiya E, Dequanter D, et al. Molecular markers of head and neck squamous cell carcinoma: promising signs in need of prospective evaluation Head Neck 2006;28(3):256–69.
79. Reuter CW, Morgan MA, Eckardt A. Targeting EGF-receptor-signalling in squamous cell carcinomas of the head and neck. Br J Cancer 2007;96(3):408–16.
80. Sok JC, Coppeti FM, Thomas SM, et al. Mutant epidermal growth factor receptor (EGFRvIII) contributes to head and neck cancer growth and resistance to EGFR targeting. Clin Cancer Res 2006;12(17):5064–73.
81. Karamouzis MV, Grandis JR, Argiris A. Therapies directed against epidermal growth factor receptor in aerodigestive carcinomas. J Am Med Assoc 2007; 298(1):70–82.
82. Akimoto T, Hunter NR, Buchmiller L, et al. Inverse relationship between epidermal growth factor receptor expression and radiocurability of murine carcinomas. Clin Cancer Res 1999;5(10):2884–90.
83. Liang K, Ang KK, Milas L, et al. The epidermal growth factor receptor mediates radioresistance. Int J Radiat Oncol Biol Phys 2003;57(1):246–54.
84. Schmidt-Ullrich RK, Valerie KC, Chan W, et al. Altered expression of epidermal growth factor receptor and estrogen receptor in MCF-7 cells after single and repeated radiation exposures. Int J Radiat Oncol Biol Phys 1994;29(4):813–9.
85. Schmidt-Ullrich RK, Contessa JN, Lammering G, et al. ERBB receptor tyrosine kinases and cellular radiation responses. Oncogene 2003;22(37):5855–65.
86. Bonner JA, Harari PM, Giralt J, et al. Radiotherapy plus cetuximab for squamous-cell carcinoma of the head and neck. N Engl J Med 2006;354(6):567–78.
87. Clinical trials.gov [cited 2007 September 21]. Available at: http://www.clinical trials.gov/. Accessed April 28, 2008.
88. Burtness B, Goldwasser MA, Flood W, et al. Phase III randomized trial of cisplatin plus placebo compared with cisplatin plus cetuximab in metastatic/recurrent head and neck cancer: an eastern cooperative oncology group study. J Clin Oncol 2005;23(34):8646–54.
89. Soulieres D, Senzer NN, Vokes EE, et al. Multicenter phase II study of erlotinib, an oral epidermal growth factor receptor tyrosine kinase inhibitor, in patients with recurrent or metastatic squamous cell cancer of the head and neck. J Clin Oncol 2004;22(1):77–85.
90. Eriksen JG, Steiniche T, Askaa J, et al. The prognostic value of epidermal growth factor receptor is related to tumor differentiation and the overall treatment time of radiotherapy in squamous cell carcinomas of the head and neck. Int J Radiat Oncol Biol Phys 2004;58(2):561–6.
91. Bentzen SM, Atasoy BM, Daley FM, et al. Epidermal growth factor receptor expression in pretreatment biopsies from head and neck squamous cell carcinoma as a predictive factor for a benefit from accelerated radiation therapy in a randomized controlled trial. J Clin Oncol 2005;23(24):5560–7.
92. Pollak MN, Schernhammer ES, Hankinson SE. Insulin-like growth factors and neoplasia. Nat Rev Cancer 2004;4(7):505–18.

93. Mitsiades CS, Mitsiades N. Treatment of hematologic malignancies and solid tumors by inhibiting IGF receptor signaling. Expert Rev Anticancer Ther 2005; 5(3):487–99.

94. Larsson O, Girnita A, Girnita L. Role of insulin-like growth factor 1 receptor signalling in cancer. Br J Cancer 2005;92(12):2097–101.

95. Khandwala HM, McCutcheon IE, Flyvbjerg A, et al. The effects of insulin-like growth factors on tumorigenesis and neoplastic growth. Endocr Rev 2000; 21(3):215–44.

96. Baxter RC. The role of insulin-like growth factors and their binding proteins in tumor hypoglycemia. Horm Res 1996;46(4–5):195–201.

97. Resnicoff M, Abraham D, Yutanawiboonchai W, et al. The insulin-like growth factor I receptor protects tumor cells from apoptosis in vivo. Cancer Res 1995; 55(11):2463–9.

98. DeAngelis T, Ferber A, Baserga R. Insulin-like growth factor I receptor is required for the mitogenic and transforming activities of the platelet-derived growth factor receptor. J Cell Physiol 1995;164(1):214–21.

99. Sell C, Dumenil G, Deveaud C, et al. Effect of a null mutation of the insulin-like growth factor I receptor gene on growth and transformation of mouse embryo fibroblasts. Mol Cell Biol 1994;14(6):3604–12.

100. Resnicoff M, Ambrose D, Coppola D, et al. Insulin-like growth factor-1 and its receptor mediate the autocrine proliferation of human ovarian carcinoma cell lines. Lab Invest 1993;69(6):756–60.

101. Trojan J, Johnson TR, Rudin SD, et al. Treatment and prevention of rat glioblastoma by immunogenic C6 cells expressing antisense insulin-like growth factor I RNA. Science 1993;259(5091):94–7.

102. Sell C, Rubini M, Rubin R, et al. Simian virus 40 large tumor antigen is unable to transform mouse embryonic fibroblasts lacking type 1 insulin-like growth factor receptor. Proc Natl Acad Sci U S A 1993;90(23):11217–21.

103. Reinmuth N, Fan F, Liu W, et al. Impact of insulin-like growth factor receptor-I function on angiogenesis, growth, and metastasis of colon cancer. Lab Invest 2002;82(10):1377–89.

104. Zeng H, Datta K, Neid M, et al. Requirement of different signaling pathways mediated by insulin-like growth factor-I receptor for proliferation, invasion, and VPF/VEGF expression in a pancreatic carcinoma cell line. Biochem Biophys Res Commun 2003;302(1):46–55.

105. Zhang X, Lin M, van Golen KL, et al. Multiple signaling pathways are activated during insulin-like growth factor-I (IGF-I) stimulated breast cancer cell migration. Breast Cancer Res Treat 2005;93(2):159–68.

106. Long L, Rubin R, Baserga R, et al. Loss of the metastatic phenotype in murine carcinoma cells expressing an antisense RNA to the insulin-like growth factor receptor. Cancer Res 1995;55(5):1006–9.

107. Zeigler ME, Dutcheshen NT, Gibbs DF, et al. Growth factor-induced epidermal invasion of the dermis in human skin organ culture: expression and role of matrix metalloproteinases. Invasion Metastasis 1996;16(1):11–8.

108. Goel HL, Breen M, Zhang J, et al. Beta1A integrin expression is required for type 1 insulin-like growth factor receptor mitogenic and transforming activities and localization to focal contacts. Cancer Res 2005;65(15):6692–700.

109. Abe S, Funato T, Takahashi S, et al. Increased expression of insulin-like growth factor I is associated with Ara-C resistance in leukemia. Tohoku J Exp Med 2006; 209(3):217–28.

110. Allen GW, Saba C, Armstrong EA, et al. Insulin-like growth factor-I receptor signaling blockade combined with radiation. Cancer Res 2007;67(3):1155–62.
111. Camirand A, Lu Y, Pollak M. Co-targeting HER2/ErbB2 and insulin-like growth factor-1 receptors causes synergistic inhibition of growth in HER2-overexpressing breast cancer cells. Med Sci Monit 2002;8(12):BR521–6.
112. Desbois-Mouthon C, Cacheux W, Blivet-Van Eggelpoel MJ, et al. Impact of IGF-1R/EGFR cross-talks on hepatoma cell sensitivity to gefitinib. Int J Cancer 2006; 119(11):2557–66.
113. Gee JM, Robertson JF, Gutteridge E, et al. Epidermal growth factor receptor/HER2/insulin-like growth factor receptor signalling and oestrogen receptor activity in clinical breast cancer. Endocr Relat Cancer 2005;12(Suppl 1):S99–111.
114. Knowlden JM, Hutcheson IR, Barrow D, et al. Insulin-like growth factor-I receptor signaling in tamoxifen-resistant breast cancer: a supporting role to the epidermal growth factor receptor. Endocrinology 2005;146(11):4609–18.
115. Wan X, Helman LJ. Effect of insulin-like growth factor II on protecting myoblast cells against cisplatin-induced apoptosis through p70 S6 kinase pathway. Neoplasia 2002;4(5):400–8.
116. Wiseman LR, Johnson MD, Wakeling AE, et al. Type I IGF receptor and acquired tamoxifen resistance in oestrogen-responsive human breast cancer cells. Eur J Cancer 1993;29A(16):2256–64.
117. Yin D, Tamaki N, Parent AD, et al. Insulin-like growth factor-I decreased etoposide-induced apoptosis in glioma cells by increasing bcl-2 expression and decreasing CPP32 activity. Neurol Res 2005;27(1):27–35.
118. Ouban A, Muraca P, Yeatman T, et al. Expression and distribution of insulin-like growth factor-1 receptor in human carcinomas. Hum Pathol 2003;34(8):803–8.
119. Jones HE, Goddard L, Gee JM, et al. Insulin-like growth factor-I receptor signalling and acquired resistance to gefitinib (ZD1839; Iressa) in human breast and prostate cancer cells. Endocr Relat Cancer 2004;11(4):793–814.
120. Ueda S, Hatsuse K, Tsuda H, et al. Potential crosstalk between insulin-like growth factor receptor type 1 and epidermal growth factor receptor in progression and metastasis of pancreatic cancer. Mod Pathol 2006;19(6):788–96.
121. Chakravarti A, Loeffler JS, Dyson NJ. Insulin-like growth factor receptor I mediates resistance to anti-epidermal growth factor receptor therapy in primary human glioblastoma cells through continued activation of phosphoinositide 3-kinase signaling. Cancer Res 2002;62(1):200–7.
122. Tao Y, Pinzi V, Bourhis J, et al. Mechanisms of disease: signaling of the insulin-like growth factor 1 receptor pathway—therapeutic perspectives in cancer. Nat Clin Pract Oncol 2007;4(10):591–602.
123. Barnes CJ, Ohshiro K, Rayala SK, et al. Insulin-like growth factor receptor as a therapeutic target in head and neck cancer. Clin Cancer Res 2007;13(14):4291–9.
124. Slomiany MG, Black LA, Kibbey MM, et al. Insulin-like growth factor-1 receptor and ligand targeting in head and neck squamous cell carcinoma. Cancer Lett 2007;248(2):269–79.
125. Riedemann J, Macaulay VM. IGF1R signalling and its inhibition. Endocr Relat Cancer 2006;13(Suppl. 1):S33–43.
126. Garcia-Echeverria C, Pearson MA, Marti A, et al. In vivo antitumor activity of NVP-AEW541—a novel, potent, and selective inhibitor of the IGF-IR kinase. Cancer Cell 2004;5(3):231–9.
127. Brazil DP, Yang ZZ, Hemmings BA. Advances in protein kinase B signalling: AKTion on multiple fronts. Trends Biochem Sci 2004;29(5):233–42.

128. Kada F, Saji M, Ringel MD. Akt: a potential target for thyroid cancer therapy. Curr Drug Targets Immune Endocr Metabol Disord 2004;4(3):181–5.
129. Bussink J, van der Kogel AJ, Kaanders JH. Activation of the PI3-K/AKT pathway and implications for radioresistance mechanisms in head and neck cancer. Lancet Oncol 2008;9(3):288–96.
130. P Oc, Rhys-Evans P, Modjtahedi H, et al. Vascular endothelial growth factor family members are differentially regulated by c-erbB signaling in head and neck squamous carcinoma cells. Clin Exp Metastasis 2000;18(2):155–61.
131. Vokes EE, Cohen EE, Mauer AM, et al. A phase I study of erlotinib and bevacizumab for recurrent or metastatic squamous cell carcinoma of the head and neck (HNC). J Clin Oncol 2005;23:5504.
132. Massarelli E, Liu DD, Lee JJ, et al. Akt activation correlates with adverse outcome in tongue cancer. Cancer 2005;104(11):2430–6.
133. Amornphimoltham P, Sriuranpong V, Patel V, et al. Persistent activation of the Akt pathway in head and neck squamous cell carcinoma: a potential target for UCN-01. Clin Cancer Res 2004;10(12 Pt 1):4029–37.
134. Molinolo AA, Hewitt SM, Amornphimoltham P, et al. Dissecting the Akt/mammalian target of rapamycin signaling network: emerging results from the head and neck cancer tissue array initiative. Clin Cancer Res 2007;13(17):4964–73.
135. Lim J, Kim JH, Paeng JY, et al. Prognostic value of activated Akt expression in oral squamous cell carcinoma. J Clin Pathol 2005;58(11):1199–205.
136. Kim D, Dan HC, Park S, et al. AKT/PKB signaling mechanisms in cancer and chemoresistance. Front Biosci 2005;10:975–87.
137. Karamouzis MV FD, Johnson R, et al. Phase II trial of pemetrexed (P) and bevacizumab (B) in patients with recurrent metastatic head and neck squamous cell carcinoma (HNSCC): an interim analysis [abstract]. J Clin Oncol 2007;25:6049.
138. Williamson Sk, Moon J, Huang CH, et al. A phase II trial of BAY 43-9006 in patients with recurrent and/or metastatic head and neck squamaous cell carcinoma (HNSCC): a Southwest Oncology Group (SWOG) trial. J Clin Oncol 2007;25:3766–73.
139. Amornphimoltham P, Sodhi A, Patel V, et al. Mammalian target of rapamycin, a molecular target in squamous cell carcinomas of the head and neck. Cancer Res 2005;65(21):9953–61.
140. Elser C, Siu LL, Winquist E, et al. Phase II trial of sorafenib in patients with recurrent or metastatic squamous cell carcinoma of the head and neck or nasopharyngeal carcinoma. J Clin Oncol 2007;25(24):3766–73.
141. Wendel HG, De Stanchina E, Fridman JS, et al. Survival signalling by Akt and eIF4E in oncogenesis and cancer therapy. Nature 2004;428(6980):332–7.
142. Neshat MS, Mellinghoff IK, Tran C, et al. Enhanced sensitivity of PTEN-deficient tumors to inhibition of FRAP/mTOR. Proc Natl Acad Sci U S A 2001;98(18):10314–9.
143. Sansal I, Sellers WR. The biology and clinical relevance of the PTEN tumor suppressor pathway. J Clin Oncol 2004;22(14):2954–63.
144. Nathan CO, Franklin S, Abreo FW, et al. Analysis of surgical margins with the molecular marker eIF4E: a prognostic factor in patients with head and neck cancer. J Clin Oncol 1999;17(9):2909–14.
145. Nathan CO, Amirghahari N, Rong X, et al. Mammalian target of rapamycin inhibitors as possible adjuvant therapy for microscopic residual disease in head and neck squamous cell cancer. Cancer Res 2007;67(5):2160–8.
146. Nathan CO, Amirghahari N, Abreo F, et al. Overexpressed eIF4E is functionally active in surgical margins of head and neck cancer patients via activation of the

Akt/mammalian target of rapamycin pathway. Clin Cancer Res 2004;10(17): 5820–7.

147. Dong G, Chen Z, Kato T, et al. The host environment promotes the constitutive activation of nuclear factor-kappaB and proinflammatory cytokine expression during metastatic tumor progression of murine squamous cell carcinoma. Cancer Res 1999;59(14):3495–504.

148. Loercher A, Lee TL, Ricker JL, et al. Nuclear factor-kappaB is an important modulator of the altered gene expression profile and malignant phenotype in squamous cell carcinoma. Cancer Res 2004;64(18):6511–23.

149. Chen Z, Malhotra PS, Thomas GR, et al. Expression of proinflammatory and proangiogenic cytokines in patients with head and neck cancer. Clin Cancer Res 1999;5(6):1369–79.

150. Ondrey FG, Dong G, Sunwoo J, et al. Constitutive activation of transcription factors NF-(kappa)B, AP-1, and NF-IL6 in human head and neck squamous cell carcinoma cell lines that express pro-inflammatory and pro-angiogenic cytokines. Mol Carcinog 1999;26(2):119–29.

151. Zhang PL, Pellitteri PK, Law A, et al. Overexpression of phosphorylated nuclear factor-kappa B in tonsillar squamous cell carcinoma and high-grade dysplasia is associated with poor prognosis. Mod Pathol 2005;18(7):924–32.

152. Dong G, Loukinova E, Chen Z, et al. Molecular profiling of transformed and metastatic murine squamous carcinoma cells by differential display and cDNA microarray reveals altered expression of multiple genes related to growth, apoptosis, angiogenesis, and the NF-kappaB signal pathway. Cancer Res 2001;61(12):4797–808.

153. Duan J, Friedman J, Nottingham L, et al. Nuclear factor-kappaB p65 small interfering RNA or proteasome inhibitor bortezomib sensitizes head and neck squamous cell carcinomas to classic histone deacetylase inhibitors and novel histone deacetylase inhibitor PXD101. Mol Cancer Ther 2007;6(1):37–50.

154. Duffey DC, Chen Z, Dong G, et al. Expression of a dominant-negative mutant inhibitor-kappaBalpha of nuclear factor-kappaB in human head and neck squamous cell carcinoma inhibits survival, proinflammatory cytokine expression, and tumor growth in vivo. Cancer Res 1999;59(14):3468–74.

155. Kato T, Duffey DC, Ondrey FG, et al. Cisplatin and radiation sensitivity in human head and neck squamous carcinomas are independently modulated by glutathione and transcription factor NF-kappaB. Head Neck 2000;22(8):748–59.

156. Van Waes C, Chang AA, Lebowitz PF, et al. Inhibition of nuclear factor-kappaB and target genes during combined therapy with proteasome inhibitor bortezomib and reirradiation in patients with recurrent head-and-neck squamous cell carcinoma. Int J Radiat Oncol Biol Phys 2005;63(5):1400–12.

157. Lee TL, Yeh J, Friedman J, et al. A signal network involving coactivated NF-kappaB and STAT3 and altered *p53* modulates BAX/BCL-XL expression and promotes cell survival of head and neck squamous cell carcinomas. Int J Cancer 2008;122(9):1987–98.

158. Wang CY, Cusack JC Jr, Liu R, et al. Control of inducible chemoresistance: enhanced anti-tumor therapy through increased apoptosis by inhibition of NF-kappaB. Nat Med 1999;5(4):412–7.

159. Li N, Karin M. Ionizing radiation and short wavelength UV activate NF-kappaB through two distinct mechanisms. Proc Natl Acad Sci U S A 1998;95(22): 13012–7.

160. Anto RJ, Mukhopadhyay A, Shishodia S, et al. Cigarette smoke condensate activates nuclear transcription factor-kappaB through phosphorylation and

degradation of IkappaB(alpha): correlation with induction of cyclooxygenase-2. Carcinogenesis 2002;23(9):1511–8.

161. Lin SC, Lu SY, Lee SY, et al. Areca (betel) nut extract activates mitogen-activated protein kinases and NF-kappaB in oral keratinocytes. Int J Cancer 2005;116(4):526–35.

162. Allen CT, Ricker JL, Chen Z, et al. Role of activated nuclear factor-kappaB in the pathogenesis and therapy of squamous cell carcinoma of the head and neck. Head Neck 2007;29(10):959–71.

163. Van Waes C. Nuclear factor-kappaB in development, prevention, and therapy of cancer. Clin Cancer Res 2007;13(4):1076–82.

164. Morimoto RI, Kline MP, Bimston DN, et al. The heat-shock response: regulation and function of heat-shock proteins and molecular chaperones. Essays Biochem 1997;32:17–29.

165. Stravopodis DJ, Margaritis LH, Voutsinas GE. Drug-mediated targeted disruption of multiple protein activities through functional inhibition of the Hsp90 chaperone complex. Curr Med Chem 2007;14(29):3122–38.

166. Ferrarini M, Heltai S, Zocchi MR, et al. Unusual expression and localization of heat-shock proteins in human tumor cells. Int J Cancer 1992;51(4):613–9.

167. Solit DB, Rosen N. Hsp90: a novel target for cancer therapy. Curr Top Med Chem 2006;6(11):1205–14.

168. Shintani S, Zhang T, Aslam A, et al. *p53*-dependent radiosensitizing effects of Hsp90 inhibitor 17-allylamino-17-demethoxygeldanamycin on human oral squamous cell carcinoma cell lines. Int J Oncol 2006;29(5):1111–7.

169. Yin X, Zhang H, Burrows F, et al. Potent activity of a novel dimeric heat shock protein 90 inhibitor against head and neck squamous cell carcinoma in vitro and in vivo. Clin Cancer Res 2005;11(10):3889–96.

170. Roepman P, Wessels LF, Kettelarij N, et al. An expression profile for diagnosis of lymph node metastases from primary head and neck squamous cell carcinomas. Nat Genet 2005;37(2):182–6.

171. Thomas GR, Nadiminti H, Regalado J. Molecular predictors of clinical outcome in patients with head and neck squamous cell carcinoma. Int J Exp Pathol 2005; 86(6):347–63.

172. Chung CH, Parker JS, Karaca G, et al. Molecular classification of head and neck squamous cell carcinomas using patterns of gene expression. Cancer Cell 2004;5(5):489–500.

173. Kumar B, Cordell KG, Lee JS, et al. EGFR, p16, HPV Titer, Bcl-xL and *p53*, sex, and smoking as indicators of response to therapy and survival in oropharyngeal cancer. J Clin Oncol 2008;26(19):3128–37.

Human Papillomavirus in HNSCC: Recognition of a Distinct Disease Type

Laura Vidal, MD[a], Maura L. Gillison, MD, PhD[b],*

KEYWORDS

• HPV • Papillomavirus • Oral • Cancer • Oropharynx

The overall incidence of head and neck cancer has declined over the past two decades in the United States, likely because of a decline in smoking rates.[1] Concomitantly, however, an increase in the incidence of oropharyngeal cancer has been observed in the United States and some European countries, particularly among young men, nonsmokers, and nondrinkers.[2–4] Human papillomavirus (HPV), a sexually transmitted infection, is now recognized as an etiologic factor for a subset of oral squamous cell carcinomas (OSCCs), in particular those that arise from the oropharynx.[5–8] A recent analysis of data from the Surveillance, Epidemiology, and End Results registry demonstrated that the proportion of OSCCs arising from anatomic sites potentially related to HPV significantly increased from 1973 to 2004 in the United States, particularly among white men aged 40 to 59 years.[9] Additionally, the age at diagnosis for HPV-related tumors declined during this time period. By contrast, the incidence for HPV-unrelated OSCCs sites decreased over time for both men and women over the age of 40. Although it has been estimated that 20% to 25% of head and neck cancers are attributable to HPV, the observed incidence trends may increase the HPV-attributable fraction over time. Mucosal HPVs are known to infect the upper aerodigestive tract.[10] The oncogenic types (eg, HPV-16) are able to induce malignant transformation of an infected cell. Two viral oncoproteins, E6 and E7, promote tumor growth by inactivating the tumor suppressor pathways p53 and Rb.[11–14] As a consequence of the viral oncoproteins, HPV-positive tumors have a specific molecular and genetic signature distinct from that of HPV-negative tumors. In addition, recent data indicate that patients with HPV-positive OSCC seem to have a better prognosis and clinical outcome when compared with those with HPV-negative disease.[5,15] All these

[a] Department of Medical Oncology, Princess Margaret Hospital, Toronto, Ontario, Canada
[b] Johns Hopkins Medical Institutions, 1650 Orleans Street, CRB-1 3M 54A, Baltimore, MD 21231, USA
* Corresponding author.
E-mail address: gillima@jhmi.edu (M.L. Gillison).

Hematol Oncol Clin N Am 22 (2008) 1125–1142
doi:10.1016/j.hoc.2008.08.006
hemonc.theclinics.com
0889-8588/08/$ – see front matter © 2008 Elsevier Inc. All rights reserved.

differential molecular, clinical, and pathologic characteristics indicate that HPV-positive head and neck squamous cell carcinoma (HNSCC) is a distinctive disease entity.

BIOLOGY OF HUMAN PAPILLOMAVIRUS

HPV belongs to the Papillomaviridae family, small DNA viruses that are widely distributed, having been detected in species from mammals to birds.[16] HPVs specifically infect humans. There are currently approximately 120 genotypes of HPVs based on the level of similarity among nucleotide sequences in specific genomic regions (ie, E6, E7, and L1).[16] HPVs infect exclusively epithelial cells. Each HPV type is preferentially associated with specific clinical lesions and has an anatomic site preference for either cutaneous or mucosal squamous epithelium.[17] The cutaneous types are commonly found in the general population and cause common warts. HPV-5 and -8 are associated with squamous cell carcinomas of the skin that arise in patients with epidermodysplasia verruciformis, a rare genodermatosis with a selective defect in cell-mediated immunity.[18,19] The mucosotropic types are further classified into nononcogenic or low-risk types or as oncogenic or high-risk types, those HPV types with strong epidemiologic associations with cervical cancer[20] and the potential to induce malignant transformation in vitro.[21,22] The most common low-risk types are HPV-6 and -11 and are mainly responsible for benign lesions, such as anogenital warts or oral papillomas. High-risk types (eg, HPV-16, -18, -31, -33, and -45) are predominantly found in squamous cell carcinomas of the cervix,[23] other anogenital malignancies,[24–26] and in a subset of head and neck cancers.[5]

The HPV genome is a small double-stranded circular DNA molecule of approximately 8000 base pairs. The genetic organization of all papillomaviruses is very similar.[27] The coding information for HPV exists on one strand, and is divided into three major regions. The early region (E1–8) consists of genes responsible for transcription, plasmid replication, and transformation. The late region codes for the major (L1) and minor (L2) capsid proteins. The long-control region contains the regulatory elements for transcription and replication (**Fig. 1**). The E1 and E2 proteins are required for replication and maintenance of the viral genome.[28] Although cooperation of E1 and E2 is required to initiate viral replication, E2 in addition plays an important role as a transcriptional repressor of both E6 and E7 oncogene expression.[29] E4 protein is encoded in the early region but expressed late in infection. The role of the E4 gene is still not known, but it is thought to promote the productive phase of the papilloma virus life cycle.[30,31] E5 activates specific growth factor receptors[32,33] and seems to be involved in the vegetative phase of the viral cycle.[34] E6 and E7 encode the papillomavirus major oncoproteins. The E6 protein of the high-risk papillomaviruses induces the degradation of p53, the gatekeeper of the cell cycle, by ubiquitin-mediated process.[35] In addition, E6 has been shown to activate telomerase in infected cells, prolonging the lifespan of the epithelial cells and enabling the production of viral progeny.[36] The E7

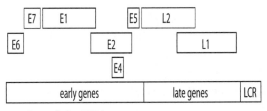

Fig. 1. Linear representation of the HPV genome.

protein binds the retinoblastoma tumor suppressor (pRB)[14] and other proteins, such as histone deacetylases, which control the activity of the essential transcription factor E2F.[37] E7 liberates active E2F from an inactive pRB-E2F complex by targeting pRB, allowing E2F to drive the cell into S phase and proliferation. E7 has also been demonstrated to disrupt normal cell cycle control through blockade of specific cyclin-dependent kinases inhibitors.[38,39] The late genes L1 and L2 encode viral capsid proteins used in the construction of new viruses. The L1 protein alone, or L1 coexpressed with L2, is able to self-assemble into virus-like particles that are morphologically and immunologically similar to native virions, but lack potentially oncogenic DNA.[40,41] Virus-like particles are the basis of prophylactic HPV vaccines designed to elicit virus-neutralizing antibodies to protect against initial HPV infection. L1 capsid proteins are firstly synthesized in the cytoplasm before being transported to the nucleus, to package viral chromatin. L2, the minor capsid component, seems to bind specific sites of DNA replication in the nucleus and recruit L1 for new viral particles to be assembled.[42,43]

The papillomavirus life cycle is closely tied to the epithelial differentiation program. Papillomaviruses replicate exclusively in keratinocytes. Keratinocyte stem cells are the initial target of papillomavirus infections.[44] Microtraumas (small wounds) in the skin or mucosal surface allow the virus to access the basal layer of the epithelium. No single receptor for HPV entry has been definitively identified to date. Some data support a role for α6 integrin, which is expressed primarily during wound healing, as a candidate receptor.[45] Additionally, a ubiquitous polysaccharide expressed on the cell surface, glycosaminoglycan heparan sulfate, may play a role in the initial attachment required for HPV infection.[46] HPV uses the host cell DNA machinery to perpetuate the production of viral progeny. Following infection, HPVs establish their DNA genome within the host cell nucleus, expressing early HPV proteins. In this phase, the HPV genome is maintained at a low copy number and provides a reservoir of viral DNA for further cell divisions. As basal cells and viral DNA divide, some daughter cells may persist in the basal layers, whereas other daughter cells move toward the upper layers of the epithelium and begin to differentiate. It is during this differentiation process (vegetative phase) that the viral genome replicates to a higher copy number and the capsid proteins are expressed and that virions are assembled and eventually shed.[44]

HUMAN PAPILLOMAVIRUS INFECTION AND MALIGNANT TRANSFORMATION

Mucosal HPVs are commonly transmitted by close contact, in particular sexual contact, although other routes of infection have been documented.[47–49] Most individuals (80%–85%) acquire an HPV infection at some stage in their lives, generally in childhood for cutaneous types (hand and plantar warts) and in early adulthood for mucosal types by sexual transmission. Like many other viral infections in healthy individuals, most (around 80%) HPV infections clear spontaneously:[50] progression to malignancy is relatively rare.[51] In a large follow-up study of approximately 600 women, it was observed that among HPV infections that persisted at least 12 months, the risk of cervical intraepithelial neoplasia (grade 2 or greater) diagnosed by 30 months was 21% and increased to 53% for women younger than 30 years old.[52]

Cervical cancer serves as a model for HPV-mediated pathogenesis. In cervical cancers, the HPV viral genome frequently integrates into the host-cell genome, preferentially, although not exclusively, at common fragile sites.[53] Viral integration may disrupt the E2 coding region, resulting in the loss of E2-mediated transcriptional control and dysregulated expression of the E6 and E7 oncoproteins. As for cervical cancer, the HPV genome may be episomal, integrated, or both in oropharyngeal carcinomas.[54,55]

Although some HNSCC, primarily tonsillar carcinomas,[55] do not contain integrated HPV DNA, expression of the viral oncogenes can still be detected, indicating viral integration is not a necessary step for carcinogenesis.

The mechanism of viral-induced cell growth is well established and analogous to other tumor viruses that deregulate cell growth.[56] Both E6 and E7 oncoproteins interfere with well-established tumor suppressor pathways, such as p53 and Rb, among others,[57,58] leading to a disturbance of cell cycle control and a deficiency in DNA repair (**Fig. 2**).[59] E7 also disrupts centrosome duplication resulting in genomic instability and aneuploidy, one of the hallmarks of a cancer cell.[60]

On the basis of epidemiologic and molecular evidence, in 1995 the International Agency for Research on Cancer recognized that the high-risk HPV types 16 and 18 were carcinogenic in humans.[61] The low-risk HPV E6 proteins do not seem to affect p53 levels,[62] whereas the low-risk HPV E7 proteins bind to the pRB proteins with much lower efficiency and are unable to induce genomic instability.[63]

Establishing the link between HPV and a subset of HNSCC was initially difficult because of the heterogeneity of HNSCC, and the fact that only a fraction of cases are HPV-associated. Syrjänen and colleagues[64] were the first to observe that some OSCC have morphologic and immunohistochemical features indicative of HPV infection. Since the first report of HPV DNA detection in HNSCC,[65] high-risk HPV (predominantly types 16, 31, and 33) have been repeatedly detected in a variable proportion of HNSCC and the viral genome has been specifically found localized to the tumor cells and transcriptionally active.[66,67] The transforming potential of HPVs in the upper

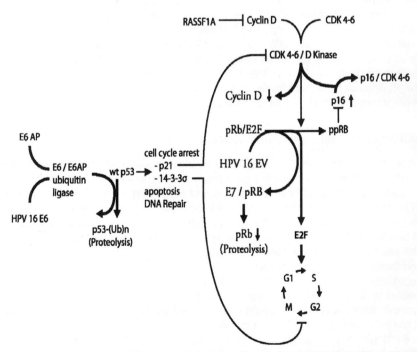

Fig. 2. HPV-mediated oncogenesis through inactivation of p53 and pRb by HPV oncoproteins E6/7. (*From* Gillison M. Human papillomavirus-associated head and neck cancer is a distinct epidemiologic, clinical, and molecular entity. Semin Oncol 2004;31:744–54; with permission.)

airway has been supported by in vitro studies demonstrating HPV immortalization of oral keratinocytes.[68-71] Additionally, E6 and E7 have been identified in vivo in a transgenic mouse model for HPV-associated HNSCC as the major transforming oncogenes,[72] as has been previously described for cervical cancer.[73]

Although expression of high-risk oncogenes can result in immortalization of an infected cell, their expression alone is not sufficient for transformation of human keratinocytes in culture.[74] For cervical cancers, other cofactors, such smoking[75,76] or long-term use of oral contraceptives, have been shown to modify the probability of HPV infection persistence and progression to cancer.[77] Immunosuppression is also associated with persistence of HPV infection at cervical and anal sites. Studies derived from immunocompromised patients suggest that a defective immune response may contribute to the progression of HPV-associated tumors.[78-80] Contrary to other viruses, HPV do not infect and replicate in antigen-presenting cells located in the epithelium, nor cause cell lysis, so there is no opportunity for antigen-presenting cells to present virion-derived antigens to the immune system. Furthermore, there is no bloodborne phase of infection, so the immune system outside the epithelium has little opportunity to detect the virus.[81] Although seroconversion occurs in 50% to 70%[50] of patients with HPV infection, the development of antibodies occurs late in infection, often months after the initial infection.[81]

HPV-induced cancers seem to retain viral oncogene expression for years or decades,[82] so strategies to target gene expression to prevent further tumor growth could be used even at later stages of disease. More importantly, because HPV-induced cancers seem to appear years after the initial infection,[8,83,84] it provides the excellent, but at this time theoretic, opportunity to implement adequate screening strategies to diagnose cancers at an earlier stage.

HUMAN PAPILLOMAVIRUS IN HEAD AND NECK CANCER
Prevalence of Human Papillomavirus in Head and Neck Cancers

Since the first description of a potential link between HPV infection and head and neck cancer,[64] several studies have strongly supported an etiologic role for HPV in cancers arising from specific mucosal sites within the head and neck.[5,8,85] Detection of HPV genomic DNA has been found in approximately 25% of all HNSCC using sensitive polymerase chain reaction–based methods.[86] The association is strongest for oropharynx cancers, with detection rates of 50% or more,[7,66,87,88] possibly because of a facilitated viral access to basal mucosal cells in the tonsillar crypts and an apparent predilection of this anatomic site to transformation by HPVs, analogous to the cervical transformation zone. In a meta-analysis, within the oropharyngeal subsite, the association between HPV-16 and cancer was strongest for tonsil (odds ratio, 15.1; 95% confidence interval [CI], 6.8–33.7). When the meta-analysis included data for the oropharynx as a whole, the odds ratio was 4.3 (95% CI, 2.1–8.9) compared with the oral cavity (odds ratio, 2; 95% CI, 1.2–3.4) and larynx (odds ratio, 2; 95% CI, 1.0–4.2).[89]

Prevalence rates of HPV in OSCC seem to vary within studies, however, depending on ethnic and geographic location,[85,86,90,91] tumor subsite,[85,87,91,92] and HPV detection methods.[86,92-99] Polymerase chain reaction has been widely used to identify and type the HPV DNA genome because of high sensitivity.[84,87,88,93,100] Polymerase chain reaction assay has been found to be subject to contamination, however, which can yield false-positives results, so careful sample acquisition and processing are required.[101] Recent studies[8,15,102] have shown that in situ hybridization, using a signal amplification system,[103] is very sensitive, relatively inexpensive, and permits visualization of single copies of HPV-16 in an infected cell. Moreover, it can be successfully used in clinical samples, including tumor cells from fine-needle aspirated neck masses, which makes this approach easily applicable to clinical practice.[104] Among all detected types, high-risk HPV-16 is the most common type identified in all head and neck cancers[5,84,105–108] and accounts for 90% to 95% of HPV-related oropharyngeal cancer.[68] A number of other high-risk types (18, 31, 33, and 35) account for the remaining 5% to 10% of HPV-positive HNSCC.

Despite the prevalence of HPV observed in a large number of epidemiology studies, to establish a pathogenic role for the HPV in HNSCC it is not sufficient to find HPV-DNA in cancer specimens, but identification of markers of viral oncogene expression within tumor cell nuclei is also required. For HPV-positive HNSCC there are some studies that have demonstrated the presence of viral characteristics that are considered major determinants of HPV-associated carcinogenesis, such as viral oncoprotein expression;[109–111] integration into cell genome;[5,55] and high (greater than or equal to one copy per cell) viral load.[66,112] In addition, the specific presence of antibodies to HPV-16 E6 and E7 in sera of HPV HNSCC patients has provided evidence for expression of these viral oncoproteins.[113] Several case-control studies have been able to correlate the presence of HPV-DNA in specimens of oropharyngeal cancers with high prevalence of antibodies for oncoproteins E6, E7, or both.[114,115] Furthermore, case-control studies have reported strong associations between HPV seropositivity and OSCC.[8,85,116,117] In particular, the prospective study by Mork and colleagues[84] demonstrated a 14-fold increased risk for subsequent development of oropharyngeal cancer among HPV-16 seropositive individuals.

MOLECULAR CHARACTERISTICS

Although inactivation of p53 and pRb are both common findings in most HNSCC, their disruption occurs by different mechanisms in HPV-positive and -negative tumors. The molecular-genetic alterations found in HPV-positive tumors reflect the oncogenic function of E6 and E7. E6 inactivates p53 function,[110] and several studies have found an inverse association between HPV-positive tumors and p53 mutations,[110,118] whereas others have noted a reduced but persistent prevalence of p53 mutations in HPV-positive tumors. A recent study demonstrated the presence of p53 mutations in both HPV-16–positive and HPV-16–negative HNSCCs (25% versus 52%). Disruptive p53 mutations were only identified, however, in HPV-16–negative carcinomas. Specifically, none of the HPV-16–positive tonsillar cancers had functionally disruptive p53 mutations, in contrast to the 57% prevalence found in HPV-negative tonsillar cancers (0% versus 57%; $P = .008$).[111] Because of the ability of protein E7 to down-regulate pRb expression, HPV-positive HNSCC express decreased cyclin D and pRb.[110] In addition, pRb negatively regulates the cyclin-dependent kinase inhibitor p16 (CDKN2A), which is often found up-regulated in HPV-positive HNSCC.[119,120] Interestingly, p16 protein expression is lost in tobacco- and alcohol-associated HNSCC because of mutation, deletion, or gene methylation.[121] Whereas HPV-positive HNSCC are associated with wild-type p53, down-regulation of cyclin D, pRb, and up-regulation of p16, HPV-negative HNSCC are characterized instead by p53 gene mutation, increased cyclin D, normal or increased levels of pRb, and decreased p16. These results support the existence of two distinct carcinogenetic pathways for the development of HNSCC: one driven by carcinogenic effects of tobacco, alcohol, or both and another by HPV-induced genomic instability.

Some studies have demonstrated an inverse correlation between HPV-positive tumors and epidermal growth factor receptor (EGFR) expression.[122,123] Other markers for cell proliferation and apoptosis have been shown to be expressed differently in

HPV-positive and -negative HNSCC: PCNA, MIB-1, and survivin expression were found to be higher in HPV-negative tumors than in HPV-positive tumors.[124]

RISK FACTORS

Emerging data indicate that risk factors for HPV-positive HNSCC are markedly different from those classically associated with HPV-negative HNSCC (eg, tobacco and alcohol). A recent case-control study showed that oral HPV infection was strongly associated with oropharyngeal cancers in cases with or without a history of significant exposure to tobacco and alcohol.[8] Additionally, sexual behavior, a surrogate for exposure to HPV, was strongly associated with risk. For example, a high lifetime number of vaginal-sex partners was associated with oropharyngeal cancer (odds ratio, 3.1; 95% CI, 1.5–6.5), as was a high lifetime number of oral-sex partners (odds ratio, 3.4; 95% CI, 1.3–8.8). Another study by the same investigators demonstrated that sexual behavior and marijuana use were associated with HPV-16–positive HNSCC, whereas tobacco, alcohol, and poor oral hygiene were associated primarily with HPV-negative HNSCC.[102] These results seem to contradict other studies, which showed an additive effect between oral HPV infection, tobacco or alcohol use, and oral cancer;[115,117] larger studies are needed to evaluate possible interactions among these exposures.

In addition, defects in the immune system response seem to place subjects at higher risk of HPV-positive HNSCC and other HPV-associated malignancies.[125,126] The recent observation that the use of marijuana, after adjusting for confounding factors, was strongly associated with HPV-16–positive OSCC, could be explained by an immunomodulatory effect of cannabinoids in HPV-mediated cancer.[102]

CLINICOPATHOLOGIC CHARACTERISTICS

HPV-positive HNSCC patients tend to present with different clinical and histopathologic characteristics than patients with HPV-negative HNSCC (**Table 1**). Most of the studies have found that patients with HPV-positive oropharyngeal tumors tend to be younger (40–60 years) by approximately 5 years, on average, when compared with HPV-negative patients (≥60 years).[6,8,15,117,127,128] Some studies support a predominance of HPV-positive HNSCC among men (3:1 ratio) as compared with women.[8,15,102] In the univariate analysis in the study by Gillison and colleagues,[102] patients with HPV-positive tumors tended to be predominantly white and to have a higher education and economical status than those with HPV-negative HNSCC.

Table 1
Distinctive clinicopathologic characteristics for HPV-positive and HPV-negative HNSCC

	HPV-Positive	HPV-Negative
Anatomic site	Tonsil Base of tongue	All sites
Histology	Basaloid	Keratinized
Age	Younger	Older
Gender	3:1 men	3:1 men
Social economic status	High	Low
Risk factors	Sexual behavior	Alcohol and tobacco
Survival	Improved	Worse
Incidence	Increasing	Decreasing

Multiple studies have demonstrated that HPV-positive HNSCC tend to arise mostly from the lingual and palatine tonsils compared with other sites in the oropharynx,[5,88,102,129,130] and frequently present with poorly differentiated nonkeratinizing, basaloid features[5,15,109,131] compared with HPV-negative HNSCC, which presents with more differentiated and keratinized morphology.

The presence of HPV has been found to correlate significantly with small tumor size and the presence of local metastases, and a more advanced AJCC TNM tumor stage (positive lymph nodes) at the time of diagnosis.[88,132,133] In a study by Fakhry and colleagues,[15] although nodal status and overall TNM stage did not differ by HPV status, HPV-positive tumors were more likely than HPV-negative tumors to have a tumor stage of T2 versus T3 to T4 ($P = .02$). In a study by Paz and colleagues,[88] evaluating 167 patients with upper aerodigestive tract cancer, only 4 of the 24 patients with HPV DNA in their tumors had negative lymph nodes (17%), whereas lymph nodes were negative in 73 of the 140 patients (56%) without HPV in their tumors. None of the HPV-positive HNSCC patients presented with early stage I disease, two presented with stage II, and the rest with stage III and IV (92%), whereas 50 (36%) of 141 of the HPV-negative patients were stage I or II. Other studies, however, have not found a correlation between nodal status, tumor stage, and HPV status.[5,134] Recently, the presence of cystic lymph node metastasis in neck dissection specimens was strongly associated with HPV-positive tonsillar cancers.[135]

PROGNOSTIC AND TREATMENT IMPLICATIONS

A recent meta-analysis of papers reporting analysis of the impact of tumor HPV status on survival outcomes conducted by investigators at the University of Pittsburgh demonstrated that patients with HPV-positive HNSCC had a lower risk of dying (meta HR, 0.85; 95% CI, 0.7–1.0), and a lower risk of recurrence (meta HR, 0.62; 95%CI, 0.5–0.8) than HPV-negative HNSCC patients.[136]

More recently, data from a new phase 2 prospective study conducted by the Eastern Cooperative Oncology Group (ECOG 2399) have confirmed that the presence of HPV infection actually heralds a better prognosis in patients with HPV-positive HNSCC. The ECOG 2399 trial assessed organ preservation, disease-free survival, and patterns of failure with taxane-based induction chemotherapy followed by taxane-based concurrent chemoradiation in 96 patients with resectable stage III and IV larynx and oropharyngeal cancer. HPV-positive tumors were detected in 40% of the patients by in situ hybridization and were oropharyngeal tumors. Tumor HPV status was statistically significantly associated with higher response rates after induction chemotherapy (82% versus 55%) and after chemoradiation treatment (84% versus 57%). Additionally, patients with HPV-positive tumors presented with improved 2-year overall survival (95% versus 62%) and a risk of disease progression that was 72% lower than that observed for the HPV-negative patients.[15]

A similar study by Worden and colleagues[137] that evaluated response to therapy and clinical outcomes in 66 patients with oropharyngeal cancer also found that the presence and titer of high-risk HPV-16 was associated with better response to chemotherapy ($P = .001$) and chemoradiotherapy ($P = .005$); better overall survival ($P = .007$); and better disease-specific survival ($P = .008$). The biologic reasons responsible for this survival difference remain unclear, but many hypotheses have been put forth and include the absence of field cancerization, immune surveillance to viral-specific tumor antigens, and an intact apoptotic response to radiation.[6,138–140]

The results of these studies seem to confirm HPV status as a biomarker of prognosis in head and neck cancer. These findings will likely have important therapeutic implications for treatment practices. Additionally, they may necessitate a reinterpretation of survival rates found in reported phase 3 trials. Are the improvements over time a result of therapeutics or the result of tumor HPV status? Data from the Surveillance, Epidemiology, and End Results registry demonstrated an absolute improvement of 23.1% during the period from 1973 to 2004 in 2-year overall survival for regional stage HPV-related tumors treated with radiation compared with a 3.1% improvement for HPV-unrelated OSCCs. Although these results could in part be attributable to better use of radiation and concomitant chemotherapy,[141] the significant improvement in survival over time could also be explained in part by the increasing proportion of HPV-positive tumors over time and their better response to radiation.[138,142]

In a study of 100 patients with HPV-positive oropharyngeal tumors those patients coexpressing both HPV and p16 had a significantly better overall survival when compared with both tumors that were HPV-negative or HPV-positive but not expressing p16.[143] A more recent study by Kumar and colleagues[144] examined the expression of several biomarkers (eg, EGFR, p16, Bcl-xl, and p53) in the pretreatment biopsies of 50 patients with locally advanced oropharyngeal cancer and their association with high-risk HPV, response to induction chemotherapy, chemotherapy-radiation, and survival. HPV DNA detection and p16 expression were strongly correlated. When EGFR and p16 expression were combined, the clinical benefit was better for patients with tumors expressing high p16 and low EGFR. Instead, high EGFR expression, low HPV titer, and low p53/high Bcl-xL were associated with a significantly worse clinical outcome. Interestingly, in patients with tumors with higher EGFR and p16 expression (or HPV titers), the survival probability was improved when compared with those without HPV DNA detection or p16 expression. Given that p16 and tumor HPV status are highly correlated, it is not possible to evaluate the independent effects of either.

There is clearly the need to implement a reliable and easy diagnostic test to detect HPV in paraffin-embedded tumor specimens of patients with HNSCC. In the absence of direct measures of HPV, such as in situ hybridization, p16 expression is a reasonable surrogate biomarker for HPV-associated oropharyngeal tumors.[104,133,144,145] The expression of p16 has been shown to correlate strongly with in situ hybridization and HPV gene expression and to distinguish polymerase chain reaction false-positives from true-positives.[146]

SUMMARY

The incidence of tonsillar cancer has increased in the United States, and recent data suggest that this increase may be explained by HPV infection. In contrast to the once-traditional profile of the elderly patient with head and neck cancer with a long history of smoking and drinking, HPV infection is changing the demographic to include young, nonsmoking, and nondrinking patients. Data indicate that patients with HPV-positive HNSCC have a better prognosis and treatment responses to current standard of care therapies compared with patients with HPV-negative HPV HNSCC. HPV-associated disease may be having profound effects on past, current, and future clinical trial results. Pretreatment screening for HPV disease should be implemented in future clinical trial designs for HNSCC.

HPV status should now be considered a biomarker for prognosis in head and neck cancer patients. Furthermore, the TNM classification may need to take into account these biologic and molecular parameters to better identify patients who are more likely to benefit from standard treatment; molecular targeted agents; and HPV-targeted strategies, such as therapeutic vaccines currently undergoing clinical trials. Tailoring individual treatment in tonsillar cancer may be of critical importance to increase patient survival while at the same time attempting to reduce the long-term toxicities in a young patient population largely expected to survive their cancer.

REFERENCES

1. Ries LAG, Melbert D, Krapcho M, et al. SEER Cancer Statistics Review. Bethesda: National Cancer Institute; 2006. 1975–2004.
2. Shiboski CH, Schmidt BL, Jordan RC, et al. Tongue and tonsil carcinoma: increasing trends in the US population ages 20–44 years. Cancer 2005;103: 1843–9.
3. Canto MT, Devesa SS. Oral cavity and pharynx cancer incidences rates in the United States, 1975–1998. Oral Oncol 2002;38:610–7.
4. Frisch M, Hjalgrim H, Jaeger AB, et al. Changing patterns of tonsillar squamous cell carcinoma in the United States. Cancer Causes Control 2000;11:489–95.
5. Gillison ML, Koch WM, Capone RB. Evidence for a casual association between human papillomavirus and a subset of head and neck cancers. J Natl Cancer Inst 2000;92:709–20.
6. Mellin H, Friesland S, Lewensohn R, et al. Human papillomavirus (HPV) DNA in tonsillar cancer: clinical correlates, risk of relapse, and survival. Int J Cancer 2000;89:300–4.
7. Hammarstead L, Lindquist D, Dahlstrand H, et al. Human papillomavirus as a risk factor for the increase in incidence of tonsillar cancer. Int J Cancer 2006;119:2620–3.
8. D'Souza G, Kreimer AR, Viscidi R, et al. Case-control study of human papillomavirus and oropharyngeal cancer. N Engl J Med 2007;356:1944–56.
9. Chaturvedi AK, Engels EA, Anderson WF, et al. Incidence trends for human papillomavirus-related and -unrelated oral squamous cell carcinomas in the United States. J Clin Oncol 2008;26:612–9.
10. Franceschi S, Munoz N, Bosch XF, et al. Human papillomavirus and cancers of the upper aerodigestive tract: a review of epidemiological and experimental evidence. Cancer Epidemiol Biomarkers Prev 1996;5:567–75.
11. Werness BA, Levine AJ, Howley PM. Human papillomavirus types 16 and 18 E6 proteins with p53. Science 1990;248:76–9.
12. Huibregtse JM, Scheffner M, Howley PM. A cellular protein mediates association of p53 with the E6 oncoprotein of human papillomavirus types 16 or 18. EMBO J 1991;10:4129–35.
13. Boyer SN, Wazer DE, Band V. E7 protein of human papilloma virus-16 induces degradation of retinoblastoma protein through the ubiquitin-proteasome pathway. Cancer Res 1996;56:4620–4.
14. Dyson N, Howley PM, Munger K, et al. The human papilloma virus-16 E7 oncoprotein is able to bind to the retinoblastoma gene product. Science 1989;243: 934–7.
15. Fakhry C, Westra W, Li S, et al. Improved survival of patients with human papillomavirus-positive head and neck squamous cell carcinoma in a prospective clinical trial. J Natl Cancer Inst 2008;100:261–9.
16. de Villiers EM, Fauquet C, Broker TR, et al. Classification of papillomaviruses. Virology 2004;324:17–27.
17. Hazard K, Andersson K, Dillner J, et al. Human papillomavirus subtypes are not uncommon. Virology 2007;362:6–9.

18. Adachi A, Kiyono T, Hayashi Y, et al. Detection of human papillomavirus (HPV) type 47 DNA in malignant lesions from epidermodysplasia verruciformis by protocols for precise typing of related HPV DNAs. J Clin Microbiol 1996;34:369–75.
19. Majewski S, Jablonska S, Orth G. Epidermodysplasia verruciformis; immunological and nonimmunological surveillance mechanisms; role in tumor progression. Clin Dermatol 1997;15:321–34.
20. Munoz M, Bosch FX, de Sanjose S, et al. Epidemiologic classification of human papillomavirus types associated with cervical cancer. N Engl J Med 2003;348:518–27.
21. Zur Hausen H, de Villiers EM. Human papillomaviruses. Annu Rev Microbiol 1994;48:427–47.
22. Howley PM. Role of human papillomavirus in human cancer. Cancer Res 1991;51:5019s–22s.
23. Bosch FX, Manos MM, Munoz N, et al. Prevalence of human papillomavirus in cervical cancer: a world perspective. J Natl Cancer Inst 1995;87:796–802.
24. Bloss JD, Liao S-Y, Wilczynski SP, et al. Clinical and histologic features of vulvar carcinomas analyzed for human papillomavirus status: evidence that squamous cell carcinoma de la vulva has more than one etiology. Human Pathol 1991;22:711–8.
25. Wiener JS, Effert PJ, Humphrey PA, et al. Prevalence of human papillomavirus type 16 and 18 in squamous cell carcinoma of the penis: a retrospective analysis of primary and metastatic lesions by differential polymerase chain reaction. Int J Cancer 1992;50:694–701.
26. Zaki SR, Judd R, Coffield LM, et al. Human papillomavirus infection and anal carcinoma: retrospective analysis by in situ hybridization and polymerase chain reaction. Am J Pathol 1992;140:1345–55.
27. Howley PM, Lowy DR. Papillomaviruses. In: Knipe DM, Howley PM, editors. Fields virology 2. 5th edition. Philadelphia: Lippincott, Williams & Wilkins, Wolters Kluwer; 2007. p. 2299–354.
28. Wu X, Xiao W, Brandsma JL. Papilloma formation by cottontail rabbit papillomavirus requires E1 and E2 regulatory genes in addition to E6 and E7 transforming genes. J Virol 1994;68:6097–102.
29. Thierry F, Yaniv M. The BPV1-E2-trans-acting protein can be either an activator or repressor of the HPV18 regulatory region. EMBO J 1987;6:3391–7.
30. Nakahara T, Nishimura A, Tanaka M, et al. Modulation of the cell division cycle by human papillomavirus type 18 E4. J Virol. 2002;76:10914–20.
31. Nakahara T, Peh WL, Doorbar J, et al. Human papillomavirus type 16 E1 circumflex E4 contributes to multiple facets of the papillomavirus life cycle. J Virol. 2005;79:13150–65.
32. Straight SW, Hinkle PM, Jewers RJ, et al. The E5 oncoprotein of human papillomavirus type 16 transforms fibroblasts and effects the downregulation of the epidermal growth factor receptor in keratinocytes. J Virol 1993;67:4521–32.
33. Crusius K, Auvinen A, Alonso A. Enhancement of EGF and PMA-mediated MAP kinase activation in cells expressing the human papillomavirus type 16 E5 protein. Oncogene 1997;15:1437–44.
34. Genther SM, Sterling S, Duensing S, et al. Quantitative role of the human papillomavirus type 16 E5 gene during the productive stage of the viral life cycle. J Virol 2003;22:2832–42.
35. Scheffner M, Werness BA, Huibregtse JM, et al. The E6 oncoprotein encoded by human papillomavirus types 16 and 18 promotes the degradation of p53. Cell 1990;63:1129–36.

36. Klingelhutz AJ, Foster SA, McDougall JK. Telomerase activation by the E6 gene product of human papillomavirus type 16. Nature 1996;380:79–82.
37. Longworth MS, Wilson R, Laimins LA. HPV31 E7 facilitates replication by activating E2F2 transcription through its interaction with HDACs. EMBO J 2005;24: 1821–30.
38. Zerfass-Thome K, Zwerschke W, Mannhardt B, et al. Inactivation of the cdk inhibitor p27KIP1 by the human papillomavirus type 16 E7 oncoprotein. Oncogene 1996;13:2323–30.
39. Funk JO, Waga S, Harry JB, et al. Inhibition of CDK activity and PCNA-dependent DNA replication by p21 is blocked by interaction with the HPV-16 E7 oncoprotein. Genes Dev 1997;11:2090–100.
40. Kirnbauer R. Papillomavirus-like particles for serology and vaccine development. Intervirology 1996;39:54–61.
41. Hagensee ME, Yaegashi N, Galloway DA. Self-assembly of human papillomavirus type 1 capsids by expression of the L1 protein alone or by coexpression of the L1 and L2 capsid proteins. J Virol 1993;67:315–22.
42. Florin L, Schäfer F, Sotlar K, et al. Reorganization of nuclear domain 10 induced by papillomavirus capsid protein 12. Virology 2002;295:97–107.
43. Darshan MS, Lucchi J, Harding E, et al. The L2 minor capsid protein of human papillomavirus type 16 interacts with a network of nuclear import receptors. J Virol 2004;78:12179–88.
44. Stubenrauch F, Laimins LA. Human papillomavirus life cycle: active and latent phases. Semin Cancer Biol 1999;9:379–86.
45. Evander M, Frazer IH, Payne E, et al. Identification of the alpha6 integrin as a candidate receptor for papillomaviruses. J Virol 1997;71:2449–56.
46. Giroglou T, Florin L, Schafer F, et al. Human papillomavirus infection requires cell surface heparan sulfate. J. Virol. 2001;75:1565–70.
47. Cason J, Kaye J, Pakarin F, et al. HPV-16 transmission. Lancet 1995;345:197–8.
48. Smith EM, Ritchie JM, Yankowitz J, et al. Human papillomavirus prevalence and types in newborns and parents: concordance and modes of transmission. Sex Transm Dis 2004;31:57–62.
49. Rintala MA, Grenman SE, Puranen MH, et al. Transmission of high-risk human papillomavirus (HPV) between parents and infants: a prospective study of HPV in families in Finland. J Clin Microbiol 2005;43:376–81.
50. Jenson AB, Kurman RJ, Lancaster WD. Tissue effects of and host response to human papillomavirus infection. Dermatol Clin 1991;9:203–9.
51. Schiffman M, Castle PE, Jeronimo J, et al. Human papillomavirus and cervical cancer. The Lancet 2007;370:890–907.
52. Rodriguez AC, Schiffman M, Herrero R, et al. Rapid clearance of human papillomavirus and implications for clinical focus on persistent infections. J Natl Cancer Inst 2008;100:513–7.
53. Wentzensen N, Vinokurova S, von Knebel Doeberitz M. Systematic review of genomic integration sites of human papillomavirus genomes in epithelial dysplasia and invasive cancer of the female lower genital tract. Cancer Res 2004;64: 3878–84.
54. Jeon S, Allen-Hoffman B, Lambert P. Integration of HPV 16 into the human genome correlates with a selective growth advantage for the cell. J Virol 1995; 69:2989–97.
55. Mellin H, Dahlgren L, Munck-Wikland E, et al. Human papillomavirus type 16 is episomal and a high viral load may be correlated to better prognosis in tonsillar cancer. Int J Cancer 2002;102:152–8.

56. Hebner CM, Laimins LA. Human papillomaviruses: basic mechanisms of pathogenesis and oncogenicity. Rev Med Virol 2006;16:83–97.
57. Lechner MS, Laimins LA. Inhibition of p53 DNA binding by human papillomavirus E6 proteins. J Virol 1994;68:4262–73.
58. Munger K, Werness BA, Dyson N, et al. Complex formation of human papillomavirus E7 proteins with the retinoblastoma tumor suppression gene product. EMBO 1989;13:4099–105.
59. Munger K,, Baldwin A, Edwards KM, et al. Mechanisms of human papillomavirus-induced oncogenesis. J Virol 2004;78:11451–60.
60. Duensing A, Crum CP, Munger K, et al. Centrosome abnormalities, genomic instability and carcinogenic progression. Can Res 2001;61:1356–2360.
61. IARC Working group on the Evaluation of Carcinogenic Risks to Humans. Human papillomaviruses. IARC Monogr Eval Carcinog Risks Hum 1995;64:1–378.
62. Gage JR, Meyers C, Wettstein FO. The E7 proteins of the nononcogenic human papillomavirus type 6b (HPV-6b) and of the oncogenic HPV-16 differ in retinoblastoma protein binding and other properties. J. Virol 1990;64:723–30.
63. Crook T, Tidy JA, Vousden KH. Degradation of p53 can be targeted by HPV E6 sequences distinct from those required for p53 binding and trans-activation. Cell 1991;67(3):547–56.
64. Syrjanen K, et al. Morphological and immunohistochemical evidence suggesting human papillomavirus (HPV) involvement in oral squamous cell carcinogenesis. Int J Oral Surg 1983;12:418–24.
65. de Villiers EM, Weidhauer H, Otto H, et al. Papillomavirus DNA in human tongue carcinomas. Int J Cancer 1985;36:575–8.
66. Klussmann J, Weissenborn S, Wieland U, et al. Prevalence, distribution, and viral load of human papillomavirus 16 DNA in tonsillar carcinomas. Cancer 2001; 92:2875–84.
67. van Houten VM, Snijders PJ, van den Brekel MW, et al. Biological evidence that human papillomaviruses are etiologically involved in a subgroup of head and neck squamous cell carcinomas. Int J Cancer 2001;93:232–5.
68. Snijders PJ, Scholes AG, Hart CA, et al. Prevalence of mucosotropic human papillomaviruses in squamous-cell carcinoma of the head and neck. Int J Cancer 1996;66:464–9.
69. Wazer DE, Liu X-L, Chu Q, et al. Immortalization of distinct human mammary epithelial cell types by human papilloma virus 16 E6 or E7. Proc Natl Acad Sci U S A 1995;92:3687–91.
70. Halbert CL, Demers GW, Galloway DA. The E7 gene of human papillomavirus type 16 is sufficient for immortalization of human epithelial cells. J Virol 1991; 65:473–8.
71. Park NH, Min BM, Li SL, et al. Immortalization of normal human oral keratinocytes with type 16 human papillomavirus. Carcinogenesis 1991;12:1627–31.
72. Strati K, Lambert PF. Role of Rb-dependent and Rb-independent functions of papillomavirus E7 oncogene in head and neck cancer. Cancer Res 2007;67: 11585–93.
73. Riley RR, Duensing S, Brake T, et al. Dissection of human papillomavirus E6 and E7 function in transgenic mouse models of cervical carcinogenesis. Cancer Res 2003;63:4862–71.
74. Hawley-Nelson P, Vousden KH, Hubbert NL, et al. HPV16 E6 and E7 proteins cooperate to immortalize human foreskin keratinocytes. EMBO J 1989;8:3905–10.
75. International Collaboration of Studies of Cervical Cancer. Carcinoma of the cervix and tobacco smoking: collaborative reanalysis of individual data on 13,541

women with carcinoma of the cervix and 23,017 women without carcinoma of the cervix from 23 epidemiological studies. Int J Cancer 2006;118:1481–95.

76. Vaccarella S, Herrero R, Snijders PJ. Smoking and human papillomavirus infection: pooled analysis of the International agency for research on cancer HPV prevalence surveys. Int J Epidemiol 2008;37:536–46.

77. Castle PE. Beyond human papillomavirus: the cervix, exogenous secondary factors and the development of cervical precancer and cancer. J Low Genit Tract Dis 2004;8:224–30.

78. Melbye M, Palefsky J, Gonzales J, et al. Immune status as a determinant of human papillomavirus detection and its association with anal epithelial abnormalities. Int J Cancer 1990;46:203–6.

79. Caussy D, Goedert JJ, Palefsky J, et al. Interaction of human immunodeficiency and papilloma viruses: association with anal epithelial abnormality in homosexual men. Int J Cancer 1990;46:214–9.

80. Johnson JC, Burnett AF, Willet GD, et al. High frequency of latent and clinical human papillomavirus cervical infections in immunocompromised human immunodeficiency virus-infected women. Obstet Gynecol 1992;79:321–7.

81. Tindle R. Immune evasion in human papillomavirus-associated cervical cancer. Nature Rev 2002;2:1–7.

82. Crook T, Morgenstern JP, Crawford L, et al. Continued expression of HPV-16 E7 protein is required for maintenance of the transformed phenotype of cells co-transformed by HPV-16 plus EJ-ras. EMBO J 1989;8(2):513–9.

83. Goldie SJ, Grima D, Kohli M, et al. A comprehensive natural history model of HPV infection and cervical cancer to estimate the clinical impact of a prophylactic HPV-16/18 vaccine. Int J Cancer 2003;106:896–904.

84. Mork L, Lie AK, Glattre E, et al. Human papillomavirus infection as a risk factor for squamous-cell carcinoma of the head and neck. N Engl J Med 2001;344:1125–31.

85. Herrero R, Castellsague X, Pawlita M, et al. Human papillomavirus and oral cancer: the International Agency for Research on cancer multicenter study. J Natl Cancer Inst 2003;95:1772–83.

86. Kreimer AR, Clifford GM, Boyle P, et al. Human papillomavirus types in head and neck squamous cell carcinomas worldwide: a systematic review. Cancer Epidemiol Biomarkers Prev 2005;14:467–75.

87. Venuti A, Badaracco G, Rizzo C, et al. Presence of HPV in head and neck tumours: high prevalence in tonsillar localization. J Exp Clin Cancer Res 2004;23:561–6.

88. Paz IB, Cook N, Odom-Maryon T, et al. Human papillomavirus (HPV) in head and neck cancer: an association of HPV with squamous cell carcinoma of Waldeyer's tonsillar ring. Cancer 1997;79:595–604.

89. Hobbs CG, Sterne JA, Bailey M, et al. Human papillomavirus and head and neck cancer: a systematic review and meta-analysis. Clin Otolaryngol 2006;31:259–66.

90. Li W, Thompson CH, Xin D, et al. Absence of human papillomavirus in tonsillar squamous cell carcinomas from Chinese patients. Am J Pathol 2003;163:2185–9.

91. Li W, Thompson CH, Cossart YE, et al. The site of infection and ethnicity of the patient influence the biological pathways to HPV-induced mucosal cancer. Mod Pathol 2004;17:1031–7.

92. Miller CS, White DK. Human papillomavirus expression in oral mucosa, premalignant conditions, and squamous cell carcinoma; a retrospective review of the literature. Oral Surg Oral Med Oral Pathol Oral Radiol Endod 1996;91:622–35.

93. Remmerbach TW, Brinckmann UG, Hemprich A, et al. PCR detection of human papillomavirus of the mucosa: comparisation between MY09/11 and GP5+/6+ primer sets. J Clin Virol 2004;30:302–8.

94. Miller CS, Johnstone BM. Human papillomavirus as a risk factor for oral squamous cell carcinoma: a meta-analysis, 1982-1997. Oral Surg Oral Med Oral Pathol Oral Radiol Endod 2001;91:622–35.

95. Ostwald C, Muller P, Barten M, et al. Human papillomavirus DNA in oral squamous cell carcinomas and normal mucosa. J Oral Pathol Med 1994;23: 220–5.

96. Balaram P, Nalinkumari KR, Abraham E, et al. Human papillomaviruses in 91 oral cancers from India betel quid chewers: high prevalence and multiplicity of infections. Int J Cancer 1995;61:450–4.

97. Greer RO Jr, Douglas JM Jr, Breese P, et al. Evaluation of oral and laryngeal specimens for human papillomavirus DNA by dot blot hybridization. J Oral Pathol 1990;19:35–8.

98. Garcia-Millan R, Hernandez H, Panade L, et al. Detection and typing of human papillomavirus DNA in benign and malignant tumors of laryngeal epithelium. Acta Otolaryngol 1998;118:754–8.

99. Smith EM, Summersgill KF, Allen J, et al. Human papillomavirus and risk of laryngeal cancer. Ann Otol Rhinol Laryngol 2000;109:1069–76.

100. McKaig RG, Baric RS, Olshan AF. Human papillomavirus and head and neck cancer: epidemiology and molecular biology. Head and Neck 1998;20:250–65.

101. Roman A, Fife KH. Human papillomaviruses: are we ready to type? Clin Microbiol Rev 1989;2:166–90.

102. Gillison ML, D'Souza G, Westra W, et al. Distinct risk factor profiles for human papillomavirus type 16-positive and human papillomavirus type 16-negative head and neck cancers. J Natl Cancer Inst 2008;100:407–20.

103. Lizard G, Démares-Poulet MJ, Roignot P. In situ hybridization detection of single-copy human papillomavirus on isolated cells, using a catalyzed signal amplification system: GenPoint. Diagn Cytopathol 2001;24(2):112–6.

104. Begum S, Gillison ML, Nicol TL, et al. Detection of human papillomavirus-16 in fine-needle aspirates to determine tumor origin in patients with metastatic squamous cell carcinoma of the head and neck. Clin Cancer Res 2007;13(4): 1186–91.

105. Niedobitek G, Pitteroff S, Herbst S, et al. Detection of human papillomavirus type 16 DNA in carcinomas of the palatine tonsil. J Clin Pathol 1990;43:918–21.

106. Adams V, Schmid S, Zariwala M, et al. prevalence of human papillomavirus DNA in head and neck cancer carrying wild type or mutant p53 tumor suppressor genes. Anticancer Res 1999;19:1–6.

107. Venuti A, Manni V, Morello R, et al. Physical state and expression of human papillomavirus in laryngeal carcinoma and surrounding normal mucosa. J Med Virol 2000;60:396–402.

108. Zang ZY, Sdek P, Cao J, et al. Human papillomavirus type 16 and 18 DNA in oral squamous cell carcinoma and normal mucosa. Int J Oral Maxillofac Surg 2004; 33:71–4.

109. Wilczynski SP, Lin BT, Xie Y, et al. Detection of human papillomavirus DNA and oncoprotein overexpression is associated with distinct morphological patterns of tonsilar squamous cell carcinoma. Am J Pathol 1998;152:145–56.

110. Wiest T, Schwartz E, Enders C, et al. Involvement of intact HPV 16 E6/E7 gene expression in head and neck cancers with unaltered p53 status and perturbed pRb cell cycle control. Oncogene 2002;21:1510–7.

111. Westra WH, Taube JM, Poeta ML, et al. Inverse relationship between human papillomavirus-16 infection and disruptive p53 gene mutations in squamous cell carcinoma of the head and neck. Clin Cancer Res 2008;14(2):366–9.

112. Badaracco G, Rizzo C, Mafera B, et al. Molecular analyses and prognostic relevance of HPV in head and neck tumours. Oncol Rep 2007;17:931–9.

113. Ragin CC, Modugno F, Gollin SM. The epidemiology and risk factors of head and neck cancer; a focus on human papillomavirus. J Dent Res 2007;86:101–14.

114. Zumbach K, Hoffmann M, Kahn T, et al. Antibodies against oncoproteins E6 and E7 of human papillomavirus types 16 and 18 in patients with head and neck squamous cell carcinoma. Int J Cancer 2000;85:815–8.

115. Schwartz SM, Daling JR, Dr Doody, et al. Oral cancer risk in relation to sexual history and evidence of human papillomavirus infection. J Natl Cancer Inst 1998;90:1626–36.

116. Hansson BG, Rosenquist K, Antonsson A, et al. Strong association between infection with human papillomavirus and oral and oropharyngeal squamous cell carcinoma: a population-based case-control study in southern Sweden. Acta Otolaryngol 2005;125:1337–44.

117. Smith EM, Ritchie JM, Summersgill KF, et al. Age, sexual behavior and human papillomavirus infection in oral cavity and oropharyngeal cancers. Int J Cancer 2004;108:766–72.

118. Balz V, Scheckenbach K, Gotte K, et al. Is the p53 inactivation frequency in squamous cell carcinomas of the head and neck underestimated? Analysis of p53 exons 2–11 and human papillomavirus 16/18 E6 transcripts in 123 unselected tumor specimens. Cancer Res 2003;63:1188–91.

119. Hafkamp HC, Speel EJ, Haesevoets A, et al. A subset of head and neck squamous cell carcinomas exhibits integration of HPV16/18 DNA and overexpression of p16INK4A and p53 in the absence of mutations in p53 exons 5–8. Int J Cancer 2003;107:394–400.

120. Li Y, Nichols MA, Shay JW, et al. Transcriptional repression of the D-type cyclin-dependent kinase inhibitor p16 by the retinoblastoma susceptibility gene product pRb. Cancer Res 1994;54:6078–82.

121. Olshan AF, Weisller MC, Pei H. Alterations of the p16 gene in head and neck cancer: frequency and association with p53, PRAD-1 and HPV. Oncogene 1997;14:811–8.

122. Reimers N, Kasper HU, Weiisenborn SJ, et al. Combined analysis of HPV-DNA, p16 and EGFR expression to predict prognosis in oropharyngeal cancer. Int J Cancer 2007;120:1731–8.

123. Kumar B, Cordell KG, Lee JS, et al. Response to therapy and outcomes in oropharyngeal cancer are associated with biomarkers including human papillomavirus, epidermal growth factor receptor, gender and smoking. Int J Radiat Oncol Biol Phys 2001;69:S109–11.

124. Lo Muzio L, Angelo M, Procaccini M, et al. Expression of cell cycle markers and human papillomavirus infection in oral squamous cell carcinoma: use of fuzzy neural networks. Int J Cancer 2005;115:717–23.

125. Lowy D, Gillison ML. New link between Fanconi anemia and human papillomavirus associated malignancies. J Natl Cancer Inst 2003;95:1648–50.

126. Frisch M, Biggar RJ, Goedert JJ. Human papillomavirus-associated cancers in patients with human immunodeficiency virus infection and acquired immunodeficiency syndrome. J Natl Cancer Inst 2000;92:1500–10.

127. Strome SE, Savva A, Brissett AE, et al. Squamous cell carcinoma of the tonsils: a molecular analysis of HPV associations. Clin Cancer Res 2002;8:1093–100.

128. Cruz IB, Snijders PJ, Steenbergen RD, et al. Age-dependence of human papillomavirus DNA presence in oral squamous cell carcinomas. Eur J Cancer B Oral Oncol 1996;32:55–62.
129. Ritchie JM, Smith EM, Summersgill KF, et al. Human papillomavirus infection as a prognostic factor in carcinomas of the oral cavity and oropharynx. Int J Cancer 2003;104:336–44.
130. Ringstrom E, Peters E, Hasegawa M, et al. Human papillomavirus type 16 and squamous cell carcinoma of the head and neck. Clin Cancer Res 2002;8: 3187–92.
131. Poetsch M, Lorenz G, Banku A, et al. Basaloid in contrast to non-basaloid head and neck squamous cell carcinomas display aberrations especially in cell cycle control genes. Head and Neck 2003;25:904–10.
132. Haraf D, Nodzenski E, Brackman D, et al. Human papilloma virus and p53 in head and neck cancer: clinical correlates and survival. Clin Cancer Res 1996; 2:755–62.
133. Hafkamp HC, Manni J, Haesevoets A, et al. Marked differences in survival rate between smokers and nonsmokers with HPV 16-associated tonsillar carcinomas. Int J Cancer 2008;122:2656–64.
134. Fouret P, Martin F, Flahaut A, et al. Human papillomavirus infection in the malignant and premalignant head and neck epithelium. Diagn Mol Pathol 1995;4: 122–7.
135. Goldenberg D, Begum S, Westra WH. Cystic lymph node metastasis in patients with head and neck cancer: an HPV-associated phenomenon. Head Neck 2008; 30:898–903.
136. Ragin CC, Taioli E. Survival of squamous cell carcinoma of the head and neck in relation to human papillomavirus infection: review and meta-analysis. Int J Cancer 2007;121:1813–20.
137. Worden FP, Kumar B, Lee JS, et al. Chemoselection as a strategy for organ preservation in advanced oropharynx cancer: response and survival positively associated with HPV-16 copy number. J Clin Oncol 2008 [Epub ahead of print].
138. Lindel K, Beer KT, Laissue J, et al. Human papillomavirus positive squamous cell carcinoma of the oropharynx: a radiosensitive subgroup of head and neck carcinoma. Cancer 2001;92:805–13.
139. DeWeese TL, Walsh JC, Dillehay LE, et al. Human papillomavirus E6 and E7 oncoproteins alter cell cycle progression but not radiosensitivity of carcinoma cells treated with low-does-rate radiation. Int J Radiat Oncol Biol Phys 1997;37: 145–54.
140. Ferris RL, Martinez I, Sirianni N, et al. Human papillomavirus-16 associated squamous cell carcinoma of the head and neck (SSCHN): a natural disease model provides insight into viral carcinogenesis. Eur J cancer 2005;41:807–15.
141. Bourhis J, Guigay J, Temam S, et al. Chemo-radiotherapy in head and neck cancer. Ann Oncol 2006;17:39–41.
142. Li W, Thompson CM, O'Brien CJ, et al. Human papillomavirus positivity predicts favourable outcome for squamous carcinoma of the tonsil. Int J Cancer 2003; 106:553–8.
143. Weinberger PM, Yu Z, Haffty BG, et al. Molecular classification identifies a subset of human papillomavirus- associated oropharyngeal cancer with favourable prognosis. Clin Oncol 2006;24:736–47.
144. Kumar B, Cordell K, Lee J, et al. EGFR, p16, HPV titer, bcl-xL and p53, sex, and smoking as indicators of response to therapy and survival in oropharyngeal cancer. J Clin Oncol 2008;26:3128–37.

145. Kim SH, Koo BS, Kang S, et al. HPV integration begins in the tonsillar crypt and leads to the alteration of p16,EGFR and c-myc during tumor formation. Int J Cancer 2007;120:1418–25.
146. Smeets SJ, Hesselink AT, Speel EJ. A novel algorithm for reliable detection of human papillomavirus in paraffin embedded head and neck cancer specimen. Int J Cancer 2007;121:2465–72.

Human Papillomavirus in HNSCC: A European Epidemiologic Perspective

Lisa Licitra, MD[a],*, Giulia Zigon, PhD[b], Gemma Gatta, MD[b],
Maria-José Sánchez, MD, PhD[c], Franco Berrino, MD[b],
EUROCARE Working Group[d]

KEYWORDS

- Human papillomavirus • Head and neck cancer
- European incidence trends • Survival trends

Head and neck squamous cell carcinomas (HNSCC) arise from the mucosa of the upper digestive tract. Taken together, they have an annual, world-standardized incidence of 25/100,000 and 4/100,000 in European men and women, respectively, with significant variations among the European regions.[1]

Head and neck cancers are subcategorized according to their site of origin because of different etiology, management, and outcome. Strong carcinogenic and epidemiologic evidence supports an etiopathogenetic role of tobacco and alcohol; approximately 90% of cases are caused by them. Recently, oncogenic human papillomaviruses (HPV), probably sexually transmitted, have been associated with a subset of HNSCC.[2] HPV DNA is present in the tumors, more frequently in those that arise in the oropharynx, although it has been detected rarely in oral cavity, larynx,

This research was supported by the Compagnia di San Paolo, Torino, Italy.

[a] Head and Neck Medical Oncology Unit, Fondazione IRCCS, Istituto Nazionale dei Tumori, Via Venezian 1, 20133 Milan, Italy

[b] Department of Preventive and Predictive Medicine, Fondazione IRCCS, Istituto Nazionale dei Tumori, Via Venezian 1, 20133 Milan, Italy

[c] Andalusian School of Public Health-Granada, CIBER Epidemiología y Salud Pública (CIBERESP, Spain), Granada 18080, Spain

[d] **Austria,** M Hackl (Austrian National Cancer Registry); **Germany,** H Ziegler (Saarland Cancer Registry); **Italy,** M Federico (Modena Cancer Registry); V De Lisi (Parma Cancer Registry); R Tumino (Cancer Registry Azienda Ospedaliera, Civile M.P.Arezzo, Ragusa, Italy); F Falcini, (Romagna Cancer Registry, I.R.S.T); E Paci (Tuscan Cancer Registry); **Poland,** J Rachtan (Cracow Cancer Registry); **Slovenia,** M Primic-Žakelj (Cancer Registry of Slovenia); **Sweden** Å Klint (Cancer Registry of Sweden); **Switzerland** M Usel (Geneva Cancer Registry); SM Ess (St. Gall Cancer Registry); **The Netherlands,** O Visser (Amsterdam Cancer Registry); **UK (Scotland),** DH Brewster (Scottish Cancer Registry); **UK (Wales),** JA Steward (Welsh Cancer Intelligence and Surveillance Unit)

* Corresponding author.

E-mail address: lisa.licitra@istitutotumori.mi.it (L. Licitra).

Hematol Oncol Clin N Am 22 (2008) 1143–1153

doi:10.1016/j.hoc.2008.10.002

hemonc.theclinics.com

and hyopharynx cancers. HPV-positive testing varies across countries in different series, ranging from 20% to 72% depending on the detection techniques.[3] More recent studies tend to report an increase in HPV tumor positivity.[4] Patients who have HPV-positive tumors display an epidemiologic, biologic, and outcome profile that has paved the way for considering it a separate tumor entity that deserves special attention and care.

Recently, a rising number of oropharyngeal cancers together with a declining incidence of oral cavity, larynx, and hypopharyngeal cancer has been reported in the United States.[5,6] Similar rising numbers were seen in Sweden for cases of tonsil cancer.[7] Prognosis varies according to different sites, and oropharynx and hypopharynx cancer survival rates significantly increased over the period from 1973 to 1999, whereas rates of laryngeal cancer survival significantly decreased.[5] Recently, a site-specific incidence and survival analysis of HPV-related tumor sites (including oropharyngeal subsites) as opposed to HPV-unrelated sites (including oral cavity subsites) offered the opportunity to study the impact of HPV on the epidemiology of HNSCC.[8] The analysis demonstrated that the proportion of potentially HPV-related cases of HNSCC increased in the United States from 1973 to 2004, particularly in the most recent birth cohorts. It also demonstrated that 2-year survival rates were particularly improved in HPV-related tumor sites.

Because incidence and survival figures in Europe differ from those reported in the United States, we explored the potential impact of HPV on the epidemiology of HNSCC in Europe using data from some population-based cancer registries that have been involved in the EUROCARE (EUROpean CAncer REgistries based study on cancer patients survival) project. The aim of this study was to assess incidence and survival of HPV-related and -unrelated HNSCC sites from 15 European population-based cancer registries.

PATIENTS AND METHODS
Data Sources

This analysis was performed on 29,265 adult (aged ≥ 15 years) cancer cases diagnosed in the period from 1988 to 2002 in ten European countries (15 population-based cancer registries). The registries were selected according to their complete coverage for the diagnosis period from 1988 to 2002. The data on cancer incidence and survival were derived from the EUROCARE-4 dataset providing incidence information for patients diagnosed from January 1, 1988 to December 31, 2002 and followed up to December 31, 2003. Five of the 15 registries were national with 100% of population coverage (Sweden, Austria, Slovenia, Scotland, and Wales), and the other 10 were regional, representing 5 European countries (Poland, Germany, Netherlands, Switzerland, Italy).

We classified the cancers into two groups according to their anatomic site specificity and the etiologic relationship with HPV: (1) sites that were HPV-related ($n = 11,183$) and (2) sites that were HPV-unrelated ($n = 18,082$). The HPV-related cancer sites included the following International Classification of Disease for Oncology version-3 (ICD-O-3) topography codes:[9] base of tongue (C019, $n = 2566$), lingual tonsil (C024, $n = 120$), palatine tonsil (C090–099, $n = 4863$), oropharynx (C100–109, $n = 3631$), and Waldeyer's ring (C142, $n = 3$). The HPV-unrelated sites included cancers of the tongue (C020–023, C025–029, $n = 6396$), gum (C030–039, $n = 1642$), floor of mouth (C040–049, $n = 4924$), palate (C050–059, $n = 1655$), and other unspecified parts of the mouth (C060–069, $n = 3465$). Only the squamous cell carcinomas were considered for the analysis (ICD-O-3 histology codes: 8050–8076, 8078, 8083, 8084, and 8094). Cancers of the lip, nasopharynx, larynx, and hypopharynx were excluded from the analysis.

Table 1 lists the countries and the population-based cancer registries included in the analysis, the percentage national coverage, and the number of cancer patients diagnosed in the period from 1988 to 2002 for the HPV-related and -unrelated HNSCC.

Statistical Analysis

Differences in patient characteristics (age at diagnosis and sex) between HPV-related and HPV-unrelated sites were assessed using the Student's *t*-test and the chi-square

Table 1

Characteristics of HPV-related and HPV-unrelated head and neck squamous cell carcinomas from 1988 to 2002 and national coverage of the cancer registries considered in the study

Characteristic	HPV-Related[a]		HPV-Unrelated[b]		National
	No.	%	No.	%	Coverage (%)
Age at diagnosis (years)[c]					
Mean	60.0		63.3		
Standard deviation	11.2		13.1		
Sex[d]					
Male	8696	77.8	12,173	67.3	
Female	2487	22.2	5909	32.7	
Registry					
Sweden	1797	16.1	3708	20.5	99.8
Poland					
Cracow	116	1.0	248	1.4	1.9
Austria	3054	27.3	3335	18.4	100
Germany					
Saarland	698	6.2	1113	6.2	1.3
The Netherlands					
Amsterdam	829	7.4	1401	7.7	17.6
Switzerland					
Geneva	366	3.3	377	2.1	5.6
St Gallen	189	1.7	216	1.2	7.2
Italy					
Firenze	264	2.4	539	3.0	2
Modena	139	1.2	260	1.4	1.1
Parma	144	1.3	259	1.4	0.7
Ragusa	19	0.2	56	0.3	0.5
Romagna	212	1.9	337	1.9	1.7
Slovenia	1385	12.4	1305	7.2	100
Scotland	1363	12.2	3732	20.6	100
Wales	608	5.4	1196	6.6	100
Total	11,183	100.0	18,082	100.0	

Countries with national coverage are listed in upper case.
 [a] HPV-related sites include base of tongue (C01.9), lingual tonsil (C02.4), tonsil (C09), oropharynx (C10), and Waldeyer's ring (C14.2).
 [b] HPV-unrelated sites include tongue (C02), gum (C03), floor of mouth (C04), and palate and other and unspecified parts of mouth (C05,C06).
 [c] Student's *t* test P < .001.
 [d] Chi-squared test P < .001.

test. Incidence rates were calculated by calendar year of diagnosis and were age standardized using the European standard population. The time trends age-standardized incidence rates for HPV-related and HPV-unrelated groups were analyzed by calendar year of cancer diagnosis and across sex and age (30–39 years, 40–49 years, 50–59 years, 60+ years) using the log-linear joinpoint regression, implemented in the Joinpoint Regression program.[10] Incidence data trends were characterized in terms of an annual percent change (APC), assuming the change at a constant percentage of the rate of the previous year.

Three years' cumulative relative survival (RS) was calculated for the HPV-related and the HPV-unrelated stratified by calendar period of diagnosis (1988–1992, 1993–1997, 1998–2002) and sex, by applying actuarial methods implemented in the software SEER*Stat.[11] RS was computed as the ratio between observed survival of patients diagnosed with cancer and survival expected in a group of individuals of the corresponding sex and age belonging to the general population.[12,13] Expected survival was estimated according to the Hakulinen method by using the official mortality data.[14] To account for differences in the age structure of the populations studied, RS was adjusted for age using the international standard for cancer survival analysis.[15]

RESULTS

Patients with HPV-related HNSCC were diagnosed at younger ages than patients with HPV-unrelated HNSCC (mean age at diagnosis, 60.0 years and 63.3 years, respectively; $P<.001$). Cases involving men were approximately 80% in the HPV-related cancer sites and decreased to 67% in the HPV-unrelated cancer sites (**Table 1**).

Incidence Trends

The HPV-unrelated cancer sites had an age-standardized incidence higher than the HPV-related cancer cases (3.8 versus 2.5/100,000 year). Incidence of the HPV-related cases significantly increased by an APC of 3.37% from 1988 to 2002 (CI 2.8–3.9) (**Fig. 1**). Age-adjusted incidence rates of HPV-unrelated HNSCC increased

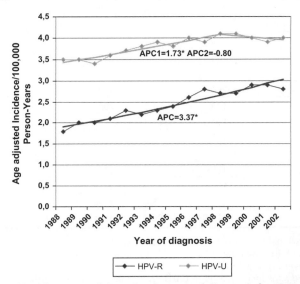

Fig. 1. Age-adjusted incidence trends by calendar year of diagnosis for HPV-related and–unrelated sites. The asterisk for the annual percentage change (APC) in incidence denotes statistical significance ($P<.05$).

significantly from 1988 to 1998 (APC = 1.73%; CI 1.2–2.3), and incidence rates became stable from 1998 to 2002 (APC = −0.80%; CI −3.0–1.5) (**Fig. 1**).

Age-adjusted incidence rates of HPV-related and HPV-unrelated HNSCC were higher among men than women; for HPV-related HNSCC, the incidence rates increased significantly from 1988 to 2002 in women (APC =4.95; CI 3.9–6.0) and men (APC = 2.73; CI 2.1–3.4) (**Fig. 2**A). For HPV-unrelated HNSCC, the incidence rates increased significantly only in women (APC = 2.80; CI 2.2–3.4), whereas the incidence trend was stable among men (APC = 0.36; CI −0.2–0.9) (**Fig. 2**B).

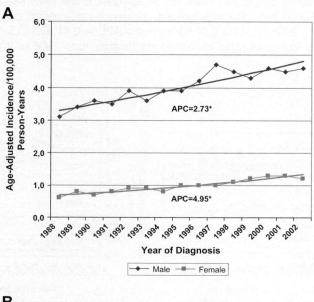

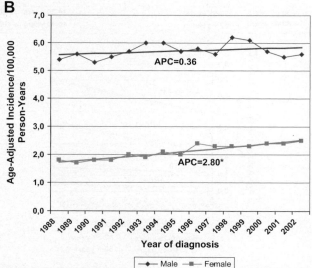

Fig. 2. Age-adjusted incidence trends by calendar year of diagnosis stratified by sex. The asterisk for the annual percentage change (APC) in incidence denotes statistical significance at (*P*<.05). (*A*) HPV related. (*B*) HPV unrelated.

The HPV-related cancer cases showed different incidence trends by age. The age-adjusted incidence rates increased significantly from 1988 to 2002 in the older age groups of patients (50–59 years, APC = 3.99; CI 3.2–4.7; 60+ years, APC = 3.25; CI 2.6–3.9) and were stable in younger patients (30–39 years, APC = 1.11; CI −1.7 –4.0). For patients aged 40 to 49 years, incidence rates increased significantly from 1988 to 1997 (APC = 5.10; CI 2.5–7.7) and then they decreased not significantly (APC = −3.54; CI −8.5–1.7) (**Fig. 3**A). Incidence trend by age for the HPV-related cancers did not differ by sex (data not shown). The HPV-unrelated incidence rates in men increased slightly in the oldest population (60+ years, APC = 0.62; CI 0.1– 1.2) and decreased significantly in the 30- to 39-year-old age class (APC = −1.80; CI −3.2––0.3). For all the other age groups, incidence rates remained stable (40–49 years, APC = −0.22; C.I −1.3–0.9; 50–59 years, APC = 0.41; CI −0.5–1.3) (**Fig. 3**B). In women, the incidence rates increased significantly from 1988 to 2002 for all the age groups

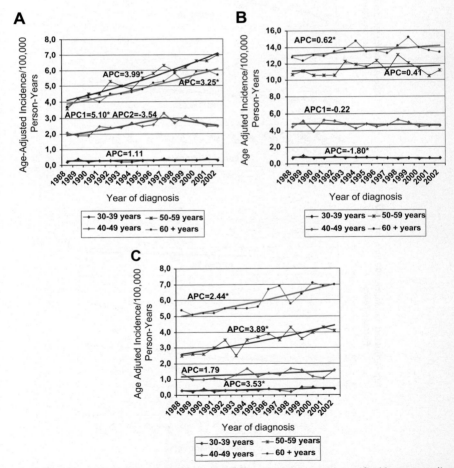

Fig. 3. Age-adjusted incidence trends by calendar year of diagnosis stratified by age at diagnosis and sex (only for the HPV-unrelated sites). The asterisk for the annual percentage change (APC) in incidence for each age category denotes statistical significance (*P*<.05). (*A*) HPV related. (*B*) HPV-unrelated man. (*C*) HPV-unrelated woman.

(30–39 years, APC = 3.53; CI 0.6–6.6; 50–59 years, APC = 3.89; CI 2.5–5.2; 60+ years, APC = 2.44; CI 1.6–3.3), with the exception of the women between 40 and 49 years (APC = 1.79; CI −0.6–4.2) (**Fig. 3C**).

Survival Trends

Three-year age-standardized RS figures were lower in patients who had HPV-related HNSCC than patients who had HPV-unrelated cancer (**Fig. 4**). Survival improved in HPV-related cases (1988–1992, RS = 40.8% SE = 2.61; 1993–1997, RS = 42.6% SE = 2.33; 1998–2002, RS = 49.4% SE = 2.50) and in HPV-unrelated cases (1988–1992, RS = 50.2% SE = 1.740; 1993–1997, RS = 54.7% SE = 1.69; 1998–2002 RS = 56.6% SE = 1.74). For both types of cancers, 3-year age-standardized RS figures were higher in women than men. The men with HPV-related cancer experienced the most pronounced increase during the last period from 1998 to 2002 (1988–1992, RS = 38.1% SE = 3.02; 1993–1997, RS = 39.2% SE = 2.73; 1998–2002, RS = 47.4% SE = 3.01), whereas the RS for women with HPV-related cancer improved gradually (1988–1992, RS = 50.0% SE=5.20; 1993–1997, RS = 52.7% SE = 4.44; 1998–2002, RS = 55.5% SE = 4.47) (**Fig. 5**).

DISCUSSION

During the period from 1988 to 2002, incidence rates of head and neck squamous cell carcinomas increased more for HPV-related than HPV-unrelated cancer sites in the European populations analyzed in this study. For HPV-related and -unrelated cases, incidence rates were higher in men than women. Conversely, incidence rates increased linearly more in women than men. Age of diagnosis was significantly lower for related subsites. Three-year survival rates improved more in HPV-related than -unrelated cancer sites, and women had better rates of survival than men. Our results were similar to those described in the article by Chaturvedi and colleagues[8] for the United States. The authors attributed the changing epidemiology of oral squamous cell carcinomas to HPV diffusion.

Tobacco and alcohol consumption are known risk factors for head and neck cancer. Incidence trends of HPV-unrelated cases increased in women, whereas they remained stable in men. These trends are consistent with rates observed for lung cancer in the

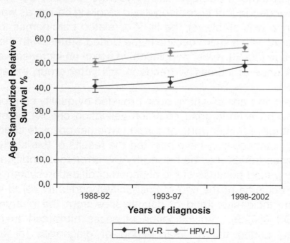

Fig. 4. Three-year age-standardized relative survival for HPV-related sites and HPV-unrelated sites stratified by calendar period.

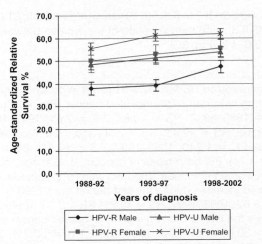

Fig. 5. Three-year age-standardized relative survival for HPV-related sites and HPV-unrelated sites by calendar period and sex.

European countries included in this study, with increasing and sharply decreasing mortality and incidence in women and men, respectively.[16] Because smoking and alcohol are also established risk factors for the subsites we classified as HPV-related, we could hypothesize that the incidence increase in the latter could be caused by increasing exposure to HPV. Similar to studies in the United States, recent studies suggested that in Europe the number of sexual partners is increasing and that the age of initiation for sexual activity is falling.[17]

Differently from the SEER-based study, in which the incidence of HPV-related carcinoma increased during the study period only for patients aged 40 to 49 and 50 to 59 years, we observed an increase for the age group 50+, indicating that in European Union the risk of developing an HPV-related tumor seems to be delayed as compared with that observed in the United States. It has been suggested that younger patients are less likely to have smoked and used alcohol excessively to corroborate the hypothesis of a viral tumor's pathogenesis in younger people. Our results imply that the risk might be independent from alcohol and smoking habits, as was suggested recently.[18] Incidence was stable for the HPV-unrelated carcinomas in the same age group as compared with a sharp decline in the United States, with the only exception for the younger age (30–39 years) population, in which an increase was seen. We did not find any evidence of increasing trends in this latter group except for unrelated tumors in women.

The data used in this analysis have been provided by quality controlled cancer registries. They also have undergone common validation checks before their pooling into a unique database.[19] It is worth assessing whether possible changes in registration and coding practices may have affected the results of this study, however. The observed incidence trends may be biased by the erroneous codification of subsites during the study period because of the changed codification system—from ICD-9 to the ICD-10—or because of the use of unspecified codes (NOS) in some registries. We analyzed the incidence trend of cancer sites from the pharynx NOS (C14.0) and tongue NOS (C02.9). The incidence of cases attributed to both categories slightly changed during the 15-year period of diagnosis: for tongue NOS, it decreased from 0.8 to 0.6 per 100,000, whereas pharynx NOS increased from 0.1 to 0.2.

The incidence of HPV-related and -unrelated cancers varied during the same period by an order of magnitude higher and could not be affected by changing attribution of cases to not specified categories. Another possible cause of bias is the use of unspecified morphology codes. We analyzed the incidence rates of unspecified morphologies codes 8000–8004 (cancer NOS) and 8010–8011 (carcinoma NOS). The overall annual incidence rates of unspecified morphologic cases were 0.2 and 0.3 per 100,000 in HPV-related and -unrelated sites, respectively. Although for the HPV-related sites the rates were stable, for the HPV-unrelated sites they were slightly reduced from 0.4 to 0.2 per 100,000. We also believe that in this case a misclassification bias could not have influenced the observed pattern of results.

The survival results were consistent with survival data already published for Europe for the oral cavity (52.2%), tongue (39.6%), and oropharynx (43.9%) for the diagnosis period from 1990 to 94.[20] The HPV-related cancer sites had poorer prognosis than the unrelated ones, and women survived longer than men. The best improvement was seen in men with HPV-related carcinoma between 1993 and 2002. We speculated that a greater number of patients with HPV-related carcinoma underwent more effective treatment, including radiotherapy and chemotherapy, either because of treatment improvements or because of an intrinsic higher chemotherapy and radiotherapy sensitivity, such as that associated with the presence of HPV in the tumor.[21–23] Because HPV-negative cancers benefit less from both treatments and no major therapeutic advances have been achieved during the considered period, observed improved survival trends might suggest that the number of HPV-positive tumors is increasing, particularly in men. In the SEER-based analysis, HPV-related tumors were more often diagnosed at an advanced stage than HPV-unrelated tumor sites. Unfortunately, we were not able to provide survival trends according to tumor stage, which possibly limited the value of our observation.

Because incidence and mortality rates of lung cancers and most cancers caused by tobacco smoking are becoming stable or decreasing in Europe, at least for men, we expected to observe the same for oral cavity and oropharynx squamous cell carcinomas examined in this paper. Our study showed that this is true only for men younger than age 60. By contrast, we found an increasing incidence of HPV-related cancer sites in men. In women, incidence increased for HPV-related and -unrelated sites. We think that this phenomenon has to be monitored in the future and expand the European-observed population for future analyses. Tobacco and alcohol are well known as the two most important factors related to head and neck cancers, but effective strategies still must be identified and applied in the female populations of different European countries. HPV infection is sexually transmitted, and high-risk sexual behavior is associated with oral HPV infection.[24] We believe that even in the absence of clear knowledge of the relationship between HPV infection and oral tumors, as that achieved for cervical cancer, strategies of primary prevention to reduce high-risk sexual behavior among adolescents and the young population must be considered in public health. Vaccination of adolescents and young adults to hasten the reduction of HPV-16 prevalence has been recommended; however, the effect has not been demonstrated at population level.

REFERENCES

1. Ferlay J, Bray F, Pisani P, et al. GLOBOCAN 2002 cancer incidence, mortality and prevalence worldwide. IARC CancerBase No. 5, version 2.0. Lyon (France): IARCPress; 2004.

22. Engeland S, Mellin H, Munck-Wikland E, et al. Human papilloma virus (HPV) and p53 immunostaining in advanced tonsillar carcinoma, relation to radiotherapy response and survival. Anticancer Res 2001;21(3):335-34.

23. Lindel K, Beer KT, Laissue J, et al. Human papillomavirus positive squamous cell carcinoma of the oropharynx, a radiosensitive subgroup of head and neck carcinoma. Cancer 2001;92(4):805-13.

24. D'Souza G, Kreimer AR, Viscidi R, et al. Case-control study of human papillomavirus and oropharyngeal cancer. N Engl J Med 2007;356(19):1944-56.

Induction Chemotherapy in Locally Advanced Head and Neck Cancer: A New Standard of Care?

Jochen H. Lorch, MD*, Marshall R. Posner, MD, Lori J. Wirth, MD,
Robert I. Haddad, MD

KEYWORDS

- Head and neck cancer • Induction chemotherapy
- Neoadjuvant therapy • Targeted therapy

Squamous cell cancer of the head and neck (SCCHN) accounts for approximately 5% of newly diagnosed cancers and accounts for 644,000 cases and over 350,000 cancer deaths worldwide each year.[1] Most cases present with potentially curable locally advanced disease. Despite advances in the treatment of these patients, long-term disease-free survival and overall survival remain poor. Approximately 40% to 60% of patients develop local recurrences, and 20% to 30% will be diagnosed with distant metastatic disease.[2]

In recent years, chemotherapy has emerged as an integral component in the management of locally advanced SCCHN. It has been incorporated as induction or neoadjuvant chemotherapy, which is delivered before definitive locoregional treatment, concurrently with radiation as chemoradiotherapy (CRT) or as adjuvant chemotherapy after conclusion of definitive local therapy. A large meta-analysis using data from 63 trials and a total of over 10,000 patients treated with various chemotherapy and radiation regimens has helped to establish the role of concomitant chemotherapy in locally advanced SCCHN.[3] This analysis identified an 8% improvement in 5-year survival when chemotherapy was part of the CRT treatment regimen and a 5% improvement with cisplatin and 5FU (PF) induction chemotherapy (**Table 1**). A follow-up analysis that included an additional 23 trials for a total of over 16 000 patients confirmed a 5% benefit at 5 years in patients who had received PF induction chemotherapy as part of their regimen.[4] Other randomized trials have solidified

Dana Farber Cancer Institute, SW430, 44 Binney Street, Boston, MA 02115, USA
* Corresponding author.
E-mail address: jochen_lorch@dfci.harvard.edu (J.H. Lorch).

Hematol Oncol Clin N Am 22 (2008) 1155–1163
doi:10.1016/j.hoc.2008.08.004
0889-8588/08/$ – see front matter © 2008 Elsevier Inc. All rights reserved.

hemonc.theclinics.com

Table 1
Effects of chemotherapy on survival at 5 years: from the meta-analysis

Trial Category	Number of Trials	Number of Patients	Difference (%)	P Value
All trials	65	10,850	+4	<0.0001
Adjuvant	8	1854	+1	0.74
Induction	31	5269	+2	0.10
Cisplatin and 5FU	15	2487	+5	0.01
Other chemotherapy	16	2782	0	0.91
Concomitant	26	3727	+8	<0.0001

Data from Monnerat C, Faivre S, Ternam S, et al. End points of new agents in induction chemotherapy for locally advanced head and neck cancers. Ann Oncol 2002;13:995–1006.

evidence that the addition of chemotherapy before or during radiation treatment with curative intent results in benefits in terms of organ preservation,[5–7] longer time to disease progression,[5–10] better locoregional control,[11] fewer distant metastases,[7,9] and longer overall survival times.[8–13]

Induction chemotherapy is an attractive treatment option, as it allows the assessment of tumor response and the selection of appropriate patients for organ preservation, and improves local control while reducing the rate of distant metastases.[14] Data from randomized trials in patients with stage 3 and 4 locally advanced laryngeal cancer have demonstrated that induction chemotherapy with PF followed by radiation in cases when a response to the chemotherapy regimen can be achieved is equivalent to surgery and resulted in a 64% rate of organ preservation.[5] Furthermore, data from European trials in the 1990s demonstrated promising results, with high response rates to PF induction chemotherapy, a high rate of organ preservation, and at least a trend toward improved survival, particularly in patients who had unresectable tumors.[9,15] Some clinicians, however, felt discouraged by the only modest 2% increase in survival demonstrated in the meta-analysis in patients who received neoadjuvant chemotherapy.[3] A closer look at the data, however, led to further insight, and there was some reason for optimism. Beyond the obvious limitations of a meta-analysis, this study included various chemotherapy regimens with numerous drug regimens and schedules that would be considered suboptimal by today's standards, limiting the applicability of the results to today's situation. Furthermore, the response to chemotherapy was not taken into account in this study. Subset analysis of cases in which the combination of a platinum with PF had been used was associated with an overall 16% lower risk of death and a significant 5% survival benefit at 5 years. It also has been argued that this analysis may have underestimated the actual benefit, because the study included patients who underwent inappropriately timed surgical interventions between chemotherapy and radiation.

A randomized phase 3 organ preservation trial conducted by the European Organization for Research and Treatment of Cancer (EORTC) evaluated PF induction chemotherapy with definitive radiation vs. standard surgery and radiation in patients who had operable pyriform sinus cancer.[6] Preservation of the larynx was possible in 42% of cases, and there was a lower rate of distant failures without a significant difference in survival. More recently, the Intergroup 91-11 study compared induction chemotherapy, concurrent CRT, and radiation alone in patients who had intermediate stage laryngeal cancer. The rate of larynx preservation favored concurrent CRT over induction chemotherapy. A recent long-term analysis from this trial, however, reported that the long-term laryngectomy-free survival was equivalent in the CRT and the induction chemotherapy arms, and both were significantly superior to radiotherapy alone.[16] Interestingly, the long-term survival data suggested a trend toward superior survival in the PF induction chemotherapy arm compared with CRT or radiotherapy alone. One of the issues of concern is the high rate of larynx preservation compared with laryngectomy-free survival, suggesting an increased rate of death from toxicity—with preserved larynx—in the CRT arm.

Recently, results from another randomized organ preservation trial were reported, in which PF induction chemotherapy and radiotherapy were compared with alternating PF-based CRT in patient who had resectable larynx and hypopharynx cancer.[16] As in prior trials, induction chemotherapy with PF was equivalent for survival and organ preservation compared with CRT.

TAXANES

Definitive concomitant CRT has been the standard of care for patients with stage 3 and 4 SCCHN who do not undergo surgical resection. Induction chemotherapy, particularly in the United States, has remained the exception and largely has been restricted to research protocols. In recent years, the remarkable antitumor effect of taxanes in SCCHN has revived interest in induction chemotherapy. It was thought that by adding a taxane to the induction chemotherapy regimen, the already 60% to 90% overall response rate and 35% complete response rate seen with PF could be increased further, resulting in more substantial clinical benefit. Several groups have tried to improve outcomes by incorporating taxanes in PF induction chemotherapy regimens. Data from phase 1 and 2 trials suggest that the combination of docetaxel with cisplatin and 5FU (TPF) is safe and has a high rate of complete clinical and pathologic responses. Haddad and colleagues[17,18] reported a response rate of 80% to 100% with TPF induction chemotherapy followed by aggressive twice-daily fractionated radiotherapy. The local failure rate was 31%, and distant recurrences occurred at a remarkably low 6% rate. All the distant recurrences were associated with locoregional failures. Thus, there was a 37% rate of local and distant failures with TPF, suggesting perhaps that induction chemotherapy followed by CRT further reduce local recurrences could and result in a lower risk for local and distant recurrent disease.

Based on the extensive phase 2 data on induction TPF, three large randomized phase 3 trials were designed to explore whether the addition of docetaxel to PF induction chemotherapy could improve outcomes compared with induction of chemotherapy with PF alone (**Table 2**). In the TAX323 study (**Table 3**), the regimen used in the experimental arm was based on studies conducted by Schrijvers and colleagues[19,20] (Docetaxel 75 mg/m^2 day 1, Cisplatin 75 mg/m^2 on day 1, 5FU 750 mg/m^2 by continuous infusion for 5 days), which had demonstrated good safety and promising efficacy. The PF regimen consisted of the original Wayne State treatment plan, which included Cisplatin 100 mg/m^2 and 5FU 1000 mg/m^2 administered by continuous infusion days 1 through 5. Three hundred fifty-eight patients who had unresectable, locally advanced SCCHN were enrolled, and 177 were randomized to receive TPF followed by RT; 181 underwent PF followed by radiation therapy. The endpoint of this trial was progression-free survival (PFS). With a median follow-up of 32.5 months, the median progression-free survival was 11 months in the TPF group vs. 8.2 months in the control arm (hazard ratio [HR] 0.72, $P = .007$). Treatment with TPF resulted in a reduction in the risk of death by 27% ($P = .02$), with a median overall survival of 18.8 months, as compared with 14.5 months in the PF group. TPF was tolerated better with less grade 3 and 4 nausea (0.6% vs. 6.6%), vomiting (0.6% vs. 4.5%), mucositis (4.6% vs. 11.2%), grade 3 hearing loss (0% vs. 2.8%), and grade 3 and 4 thrombocytopenia

Table 2
Experience with docetaxel-based induction in locally advanced squamous cell cancer of the head and neck

Study	N (Criteria)	Primary Endpoint	Regimens	Result
Vermorken, 2007 (European Organization for Research and Treatment of Cancer 24791/ TAX 323)	358 (unresectable)	PFS	Cisplatin and 5FU (PF) → RT vs. taxane docetaxel + cisplatin and 5FU (TPF) TPF → RT	TPF led to higher PFS and OS (P<.05)
Posner, 2007 (TAX 324)	501 (advanced)	OS	PF → chemoradiotherapy (CRT) vs. TPF → CRT	TPF improved OS at 3 years (P<.01)
Calais 2006[a] (GORTEC 2000–01)	213 (resectable)	Larynx preservation	PF vs. TPF	TPF led to higher LxP, CR

[a] Preliminary results.

(5.2% vs. 17.9%). There was a higher incidence of febrile neutropenia in patients on the TPF arm (76.9% vs. 52.5%), while the number of treatment-related deaths was lower compared with the controls (2.3% vs. 5.5%).

A second phase 3 trial, the TAX 324 trial (**Table 4**), randomized 501 patients who had resectable and unresectable SCCHN to TPF or PF followed by CRT with weekly carboplatin and daily radiotherapy.[21] In this study, the primary endpoint was overall survival. The TPF regimen used was slightly more dose-dense than the one tested in TAX 323, with a higher per cycle dose of PF (TPF: docetaxel 75 mg/m^2 day 1, cisplatin 100

Table 3
Survival results of TAX 323

	Taxane Docetaxel + Cisplatin and 5FU (TPF)-177	Cisplatin and 5FU (PF)-181
Progression-free survival		
Median duration (months)	11.0	8.2
Hazard ratio	0.72 (CI 0.57–0.91)	
Median survival (months)	18.8	14.5
Hazard ratio	0.73 (CI 0.56–0.94)	
Kaplan-Meir survival		
1-year	72%	55%
2-year	43%	32%
3-year	37%	26%
Response to induction chemotherapy/induction plus chemoradiotherapy (%)		
Overall	68/72	54/59
Complete	15/59	12/36
Partial	105/69	85/70

Table 4
Survival results of TAX 324

	Taxane Docetaxel + Cisplatin and 5FU (TPF)-255	Cisplatin and 5FU (PF)-246
Median survival (months)	70.6+	30.1
95% CI	49–NR	20.9–51.5
Died	41%	53%
Kaplan-Meir survival		
1-year	80% [75.0–84.9]	69% [64.1–75.7]
2-year	67% [61.5–73.2]	54% [48.2–60.8]
3-year	62% [55.9–68.2]	48% [41.7–54.5]
Hazard ratio TPF:PF (95% CI_	0.70 [0.54–0.90]	
Log–rank p value	.0058	

mg/m^2 day 1 and 5FU 1000 mg/m^2 by continuous infusion for 4 days, and PF: cisplatin 100 mg/m^2 day 1, 5FU 1000 mg/m^2 as a continuous infusion for 5 days) for three cycles as opposed to the four cycles in TAX 323. With a minimum follow-up of 2 years, the risk of death was reduced by 30% in patients who had received TPF compared with the PF group (HR 0.70, P = .006). Overall survival at 3 years was 62% in the TPF group and 48% with PF. Interestingly, the rate of loco-regional recurrences with TPF was significantly better compared with induction treatment with PF, while distant metastatic failures were reduced only slightly and nonsignificantly (5% vs. 9%, P = .14). It is worth noting, however, that the rate of distant metastases was remarkably low in both arms. Subgroup analysis of patients with hypopharyngeal (n = 89) and laryngeal (n = 77) primarily revealed that with 41 months median follow-up, median overall survival was 59 (31 not reached) vs. 24 (13 to 42) months, and the HR for mortality was 0.62 (0.41 to 0.94, P = .02). The median PFS was 21 (12 to 58) vs. 11 (8 to 14) months, and the HR was 0.66 (0.45 to 0.97, P = .03) for TPF and PF, respectively. Among 67 and 56 operable patients in the TPF and PF arms, respectively, laryngectomy-free survival was significantly greater with TPF; the HR was 0.59 (0.37 to 0.95, P = .03). The 3-year laryngectomy-free survival was 52% (39% to 65%) vs. 32% (19% to 45%), favoring TPF.[22] With the results of previous phase 3 trials showing equivalence for laryngectomy-free survival and overall survival with PF or CRT, these results support the use induction chemotherapy with TPF and carboplatin/CRT as another acceptable treatment option for organ preservation in laryngeal and hypopharyngeal cancer. As expected, TPF was associated with a higher rate of neutropenia and neutropenic fever than PF (83% vs. 56% and 12% vs. 7%), but there was no difference in the rate of documented neutropenic infections. In addition, there were significantly fewer dose delays in the TPF arm and fewer dose reductions, which were caused entirely by prolonged neutropenia in the PF arm (39% vs. 1%, P<.001).

The French-based Groupe d'Oncologie Radiothérapie Téte et Cou study 2000-01 was designed to determine if the addition of docetaxel to PF induction chemotherapy results in a higher rate of organ preservation in patients who have operable locally advanced laryngeal and hypopharyngeal cancer.[23] Treatment-naive patients were randomized to receive three cycles of PF or TPF. Responding patients who had tumor regression greater than 50% and recovery of normal laryngeal mobility then received 70 Gy RT. The major endpoint of this trial, as with the EORTC 24954 study, was functional larynx preservation, which was defined as patients who are alive with an intact larynx without tracheostomy, tracheotomy, or gastrostomy. As of this time, the results of this study have been presented as an abstract only. The overall response rate was significantly higher in the TPF arm (82.8% vs. 60.8%, P = .0013), and a statistically significant increase in the number of patients proceeding to laryngeal preserving treatment was observed (80% vs. 58%). Total laryngectomy was performed on fewer patients in the TPF arm (16% vs. 32%). Overall, the functional laryngeal preservation was 63% in the TPF arm and 41% in the PF arm (P = .03).

Recently, data from an interim analysis of an ongoing Italian study were presented in abstract form. In this trial, 101 patients who had locally advanced stage 3 to 4 SCCHN were randomized to CRT using two cycles of cisplatin 20 mg/m^2 days 1 to 4, 5FU 800 mg/m^2 as a 96-hour CI weeks 1 and 6 during RT (66 to 70 Gy) (arm A), or TPF induction chemotherapy for three cycles (docetaxel 75 mg/m^2 and P 80 mg/m^2 on day 1, F 800 mg/m^2 96 hours CI) every 3 weeks followed by the same CT/RT (arm B). Radiological evaluation of responses 6 to 8 weeks from the end of CT/RT showed a complete response of 21.2% (CI: 64 to 89) in arm A and 50.0% (CI: 34 to 65) in arm B. Radiological CRs at 8 months for unresected patients were 40.0% in arm A and 57.1% in arm B. A trend toward superior survival was observed, with the median OS and 1-year OS respectively 33.3 months and 77.6% in arm A, while median OS was not reached in arm B, and one year OS was 86.0%.[24]

OTHER INDUCTION CHEMOTHERAPY REGIMENS

The arrival of targeted agents has expanded treatment options in patients with SCCHN in recent years. Because of their distinct mechanism of action and therefore different adverse effect profile, new combination regimens with acceptable toxicity profiles have become available. The EGF-receptor (EGF-R) antagonists, especially have been tested extensively since the late 1990s in patients with HNSCC. Emerging data suggest that the combination of the monoclonal antibody cetuximab with platinum plus 5FU is safe and results in a survival advantage in patients who have incurable head and neck cancer.[25] The results of a trial conducted at MD Anderson Cancer Center (Houston, TX) using the induction regimen consisting of six weekly cycles of paclitaxel 135 mg/m^2, carboplatin area under curve 2 and cetuximab 400 mg/m^2 week 1 then 250 mg/m^2 weekly (PC^2). Patients were treatment-naïve, and had locally advanced SCCHN with any primary site. The endpoint was clinico–radiographic complete response (CR). All 41 evaluable patients achieved a response in the primary site, 7 (17%) partial response, and 34 (83%) CR. Forty-three of 44 evaluable patients achieved a nodal response, 31 (70%) PR, and 12 (27%) CR. Overall, 11 of 45 (24%) patients were disease-free after CT. Toxicity was acceptable with grade 3/4 leukopenia in 34%, grade 3 folliculitis in 47% and serious hypersensitivity reactions in 4%. The Eastern Cooperative Group (ECOG) is testing a similar regimen using induction therapy with cetuximab, weekly carboplatin, and paclitaxel followed by combined CRT with weekly cetuximab, carboplatin, and paclitaxel plus radiotherapy.[26] Preliminary data suggest a high number of complete responses at the end of induction and after completion of chemoradiation. Survival data—the primary endpoint—are maturing. Recently, results from a phase 1 trial combining TPF with cetuximab were presented, suggesting that the combination is safe in combination with a lower 5FU dose to reduce gastrointestinal toxicity. Preliminary data on efficacy were encouraging. All patients achieved at least a partial response, and 14 out of 19 patients had a radiographic complete response. Among these, 12 patients had no evidence of disease on a rebiopsy after conclusion of induction therapy.[27]

SUMMARY

After 30 years of clinical trials, chemotherapy is an established part in the treatment of patients who have locally advanced SCCHN. In patients who are candidates for induction chemotherapy, TPF is the new standard of care on the basis of three studies positive for improved survival or organ preservation and reduced toxicity with TPF compared with PF. TPF induction therapy can be delivered safely with the appropriate supportive measures. Patient selection is crucial and close monitoring is important. It is also imperative that radiation therapy is not delayed after induction therapy. Early involvement of the radiation oncologist is crucial to assure a smooth and rapid transition from induction to radiotherapy or CRT. Most investigators using TPF in trials have abandoned radiation without concomitant chemotherapy after induction TPF and have adopted CRT in the sequential therapy approach as it is used in TAX 324. Weekly therapy with carboplatin as a radiation sensitizer is supported by a randomized trial in nasopharynx cancer, which proved equivalent efficacy and significantly less toxicity compared with bolus cisplatin.[28] Finally, randomized trials demonstrate that PF is equivalent to CRT for survival or organ preservation. If TPF is significantly better than PF, then it is possible but definitely not proven that TPF is better then CRT alone with cisplatin. Currently, trials are underway to explore whether TPF induction chemotherapy can improve outcomes compared with standard CRT alone, and results are awaited. While these trials are ongoing physicians can recommend that TPF sequential therapy and CRT both may be considered acceptable regimens for treatment of patients who have locally advanced disease. Given the excellent efficacy and good tolerability of this regimen, the activity of TPF may be enhanced further by the addition of targeted therapies. Ongoing phase 1 and 2 studies are addressing this question.

REFERENCES

1. Jemal A, Siegel R, Ward E, et al. Cancer statistics. CA Cancer J Clin 2007;57: 43–66.
2. Seiwert TY, Cohen EE. State-of-the-art management of locally advanced head and neck cancer. Br J Cancer 2005;92:1341–8.
3. Pignon JP, Bourhis J, Domenge C, et al. Chemotherapy added to locoregional treatment for head and neck squamous cell carcinoma: three meta-analyses of updated individual data. MACH-NC collaborative group. Meta-analysis of chemotherapy on head and neck cancer. Lancet 2000;355:949–55.
4. Monnerat C, Faivre S, Temam S, et al. End points for new agents in induction chemotherapy for locally advanced head and neck cancers. Ann Oncol 2002;13: 995–1006.
5. The Department of Veterans Affairs Laryngeal Cancer Study Group. Induction chemotherapy plus radiation compared with surgery plus radiation in patients with advanced laryngeal cancer. N Engl J Med 1991;324:1685–90.
6. Lefebvre JL, Chevalier D, Luboinski B, et al. Larynx preservation in pyriform sinus cancer: preliminary results of a European Organization for Research and Treatment of Cancer phase III trial. EORTC head and neck cancer cooperative group. J Natl Cancer Inst 1996;88:890–9.
7. Forastiere AA, Goepfert H, Maor M, et al. Concurrent chemotherapy and radiotherapy for organ preservation in advanced laryngeal cancer. N Engl J Med 2003;349:2091–8.

8. Zorat PL, Paccagnella A, Cavaniglia G, et al. Randomized phase III trial of neoadjuvant chemotherapy in head and neck cancer: 10-year follow-up. J Natl Cancer Inst 2004;96:1714–7.

9. Paccagnella A, Orlando A, Marchiori C, et al. Phase III trial of initial chemotherapy in stage III or IV head and neck cancers: a study by the Gruppo di Studio sui Tumori della Testa e del Collo. J Natl Cancer Inst 1994;86:265–72.

10. Al-Sarraf M, LeBlanc M, Giri PG, et al. Chemoradiotherapy versus radiotherapy in patients with advanced nasopharyngeal cancer: phase III randomized intergroup study 0099. J Clin Oncol 1998;16:1310–7.

11. Denis F, Garaud P, Bardet E, et al. Final results of the 94-01 French head and neck oncology and radiotherapy group randomized trial comparing radiotherapy alone with concomitant radiochemotherapy in advanced-stage oropharynx carcinoma. J Clin Oncol 2004;22:69–76.

12. Calais G, Alfonsi M, Bardet E, et al. Randomized trial of radiation therapy versus concomitant chemotherapy and radiation therapy for advanced-stage oropharynx carcinoma. J Natl Cancer Inst 1999;91:2081–6.

13. Jeremic B, Shibamoto Y, Milicic B, et al. Elective ipsilateral neck irradiation of patients with locally advanced maxillary sinus carcinoma. Cancer 2000;88: 2246–51.

14. Vermorken JB. Medical treatment in head and neck cancer. Ann Oncol 2005; 16(Suppl 2:ii):258–64.

15. Domenge C, Hill C, Lefebvre JL, et al. Randomized trial of neoadjuvant chemotherapy in oropharyngeal carcinoma. French Groupe d'Etude des Tumeurs de la Tete et du Cou (GETTEC). Br J Cancer 2000;83:1594–8.

16. Lefebvre J, Horiot J, Rolland F, et al. Phase III study on larynx preservation comparing induction chemotherapy and radiotherapy versus alternating chemoradiotherapy in resectable hypopharynx and larynx cancers. EORTC protocol 24954-22950. Proceedings of the American Society of Clinical Oncology 2007;25:Abstract # LBA6016.

17. Haddad R, Colevas AD, Tishler R, et al. Docetaxel, cisplatin, and 5-fluorouracil-based induction chemotherapy in patients with locally advanced squamous cell carcinoma of the head and neck: the Dana Farber Cancer Institute experience. Cancer 2003;97:412–8.

18. Haddad R, Tishler R, Wirth L, et al. Rate of pathologic complete responses to docetaxel, cisplatin, and fluorouracil induction chemotherapy in patients with squamous cell carcinoma of the head and neck. Arch Otolaryngol Head Neck Surg 2006;132:678–81.

19. Schrijvers D, Van Herpen C, Kerger J, et al. Docetaxel, cisplatin, and 5-fluorouracil in patients with locally advanced unresectable head and neck cancer: a phase I–II feasibility study. Ann Oncol 2004;15:638–45.

20. Vermorken JB, Remenar E, van Herpen C, et al. Cisplatin, fluorouracil, and docetaxel in unresectable head and neck cancer. N Engl J Med 2007;357:1695–704.

21. Posner MR, Hershock DM, Blajman CR, et al. Cisplatin and fluorouracil alone or with docetaxel in head and neck cancer. N Engl J Med 2007;357:1705–15.

22. Posner MR, Norris CM, Tishler R, et al. Sequential therapy for locally advanced larynx and hypopharynx cancer: subgroup analysis from the TAX 324 study. Proceedings of the American Society of Clinical Oncology 2008;26:Abstract # 6031.

23. Calais G, Pontreau Y, Alfonsi M, et al. Randomized phase III trial comparing induction chemotherapy using cisplatin (P) fluorouracil (F) with or without docetaxel (T) for organ preservation in hypopharynx and larynx cancer. Preliminary results

of GORTEC 2000-01. Proceedings of the American Society of Clinical Oncology 2006;24:5506.

24. Paccagnella A, Buffoli A, Koussis H, et al. Concomitant chemoradiotherapy (CT/RT) vs neoadjuvant chemotherapy with docetaxel/cisplatin/5-fluorouracil (TPF) followed by CT/RT in locally advanced head and neck cancer. Final results of a phase II randomized study. Proceedings of the American Society of Clinical Oncology 2008;26:Abstract # 6000.

25. Vermorken JB, Mesia R, Vega V, et al. Cetuximab extends survival of patients with recurrent or metastatic SCCHN when added to first line platinum based therapy—results of a randomized phase III (extreme) study. Proceedings of the American Society of Clinical Oncology 2007;24:abstract # 6091.

26. Wanebo HJ, Ghebremichael M, Burtness B, et al. Phase II evaluation of cetuximab (C225) combined with induction paclitaxel and carboplatin followed by C225, paclitaxel, carboplatin, and radiation for stage III/IV operable squamous cancer of the head and neck (ECOG, E2303). Proceedings of the American Society of Clinical Oncology 2007;25:Abstract # 6015.

27. Tishler RB, Posner M, Wirth L, et al. Cetuximab added to docetaxel, cisplatin, 5-fluorouracil induction chemotherapy (C-TPF) in patients with newly diagnosed locally advanced head and neck cancer: a phase I study. Proceedings of the American Society of Clinical Oncology 2008;26:Abstract # 6001.

28. Chitapanarux I, Lorvidhaya V, Kamnerdsupaphon P, et al. Chemoradiation comparing cisplatin versus carboplatin in locally advanced nasopharyngeal cancer: randomised, noninferiority, open trial. Eur J Cancer 2007;43:1399–406.

New Advances in High-Technology Radiotherapy for Head and Neck Cancer

Gregory J. Kubicek, MD[a,b,c], Mitchell Machtay, MD[a,b],*

KEYWORDS

• Radiotherapy • New technology • IMRT • IGRT • Cone-beam

Although advances in the treatment of head and neck cancer have come from incorporation of chemotherapy and targeted therapy,[1,2] radiotherapy remains the cornerstone of treatment in the definitive nonsurgical setting and is also widely used in postoperative patients with high-risk features.[3,4] Because head and neck cancer can be very aggressive with a tendency to recur locally, it is important to adequately irradiate all local-regional cancer cells (both gross disease and microscopic disease) to doses sufficient for tumor control. At the same time, many of the normal tissues in the head and neck area are very sensitive to radiation; such anatomic structures as the salivary glands, larynx, and constrictor muscles can be particularly damaged by treatment resulting in long-term sequelae.[5–10] This places the radiation oncologist in the difficult situation of attempting to provide high doses of radiation to tumor and target volumes and minimal doses of radiation to normal structures. New technologies along with increased clinical familiarity and experience with these technologies have allowed the practice of radiotherapy to increase the distance between tumor dose and normal tissue dose, which in turn improves the ratio of cancer cure to treatment morbidity.

INTENSITY-MODULATED RADIOTHERAPY

Intensity-modulated radiotherapy (IMRT) is similar to classic or traditional radiotherapy in that it uses photon (x-ray) -based radiotherapy to target certain structures (ie, tumor

[a] Department of Radiation Oncology, Jefferson Medical College, Thomas Jefferson University, Philadelphia, PA 19107, USA
[b] Kimmel Cancer Center, Thomas Jefferson University, Philadelphia, PA 19107, USA
[c] Bodine Center for Cancer Treatment, Thomas Jefferson University, 111 South 11th Street, Philadelphia, PA 19107, USA
* Corresponding author. Bodine Center for Cancer Treatment, Thomas Jefferson University, 111 South 11th Street, Philadelphia, PA 19107.
E-mail address: mitchell.machtay@jeffersonhospital.org (M. Machtay).

Hematol Oncol Clin N Am 22 (2008) 1165–1180
doi:10.1016/j.hoc.2008.08.014
0889-8588/08/$ – see front matter © 2008 Elsevier Inc. All rights reserved.

volume) and avoid others (ie, spinal cord). IMRT takes advantage of sophisticated computer algorithms and treatment planning, however, to heterogeneously distribute (modulate) the radiation beam intensity to allow differential dose to tumor versus normal structures. Traditional radiotherapy fields used relatively simple anteroposterior or lateral fields that could be slightly modified to allow exclusion of the spinal cord from the treatment field, but little else (**Fig. 1**A). IMRT creates a complex heterogenous dose pattern that can shape the radiation isodose curves around certain structures to decrease the relative dose (**Fig. 1**B).

IMRT begins with CT-based treatment planning in which anatomic structures (gross tumor, suspected microscopic local extensions of tumor, lymph node volumes, spinal cord, parotid, and so forth) are contoured (outlined) on the CT scan with incorporation of clinical information fully to define high-cancer risk areas. The next step is to assign treatment prioritization values (rank) and dose limits to these normal structures (eg, in a patient with a left-sided tumor the prioritization value assigned to the left parotid is low, whereas the value assigned to the right parotid is high); in this way, the computer program places more emphasis (modulation) on radiation beams that avoid the right parotid gland. This process is highly individualized in every patient and incorporates sites of disease and the doses to be used in the treatment. **Fig. 2** shows a typical physician-generated IMRT planning prescription, highlighting the differences in IMRT planning based on different tumor sites. Trained radiation dosimetrists using sophisticated computer planning algorithms adjust multiple aspects of the radiotherapy plan including the number of radiation beams, strength of the radiation beam segments, and direction of the beams to meet the criteria outlined in the IMRT script. The final plan is approved by the attending radiation oncologist before actual treatment. The end result is that the radiation dose can be sculpted as seen in **Fig. 1**B.

IMRT uses standard linear accelerators found in most radiotherapy practices; the major differences between IMRT and more traditional radiotherapy delivery techniques are the computer planning software and Linac hardware additions (usually micro-leaf collimators) that allow for the intensity modulation of the various radiotherapy

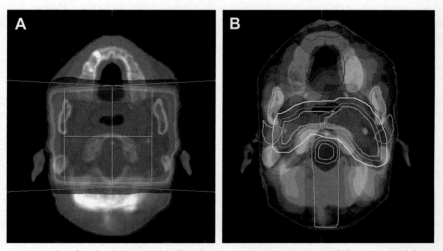

Fig. 1. Example of radiotherapy dose distribution using conventional (*A*) and IMRT (*B*) treatment plans. Conventional and IMRT dose plans for the same patient show the decreased area of high doses (red and orange) with the IMRT plan, but also the increased volume to tissue receiving lower doses (blue and green) of radiation.

B

TARGET	Fraction Size "x" number	GOAL	%VOL BELOW	MIN. DOSE	Rank*
CTV64	2 Gy x 32	6400	2.5	6300	100
PTV64	2 Gy x 32	6400	5	6200	100
CTV55	~1.72 Gy x32	5500	5	5400	100
PTV55	~1.72 Gy x32	5500	5	5400	90

OARs	Dose Limit	% vol above Dose Limit	MAX. DOSE	Rank*
CORD	3800	20%	4600	100
PRVCORD	4000	20%	5000	100
BRAINSTEM	4000	20%	5400	90
PRVBRAINSTEM	4500	10%	5600	90
OARpharynx	4600	33%	6600	70
Esophagus	4000	33%	5500	70
RtParotid	2600	50%	6600	60
LtParotid	2600	50%	6600	60
Lips	2400	25%	5000	60
Oral Cavity	3500	33%	6600	50
Mandible	5500	33%	6600	50

A

TARGET	Fraction Size "x" number	GOAL	%VOL BELOW	MIN. DOSE	Rank*
CTV63	2.1 Gy x 30	6300	2.5	6200	100
PTV63	2.1 Gy x 30	6300	5	6100	100
CTV58	1.93 Gy x 30	5800	5	5700	100
PTV58	1.93 Gy x 30	5800	5	5600	90

OARs	Previous Dose	Dose Limit	%vol above Dose Limit	MAX. DOSE	Rank*
CORD	N/A	3800	20%	4600	100
PRVCORD		4000	20%	5000	100
BRAINSTEM		4000	20%	5400	90
PRVBRAINSTEM		4500	10%	5600	90
Cerebellum		3000	25%	6000	70
right eye		2000	25%	2500	70
right optic n		4500	10%	5400	70
left optic n		3500	10%	4500	70
left eye		500	25%	1000	70
OARpharynx		3000	33%	6000	70
LtParotid		500	33%	1000	70
rt parotid		500			ref
Lt Submandibular		500	33%	1500	70
Lips		2400	25%	5000	60
Oral Cavity		3500	33%	6600	50
Mandible		5600	33%	7000	50

Fig. 2. Notice the different dose limits and ranking for several structures in these two IMRT forms. The first patient (A) has a right-sided tumor, and thus, the right-sided parotid is not being spared; while in the second patient (B), extra importance is placed on sparing the left-sided parotid gland (as seen by the lower dose limit and higher ranking).

beamlets. Because of the relative ease of incorporation of this technology (eg, compared with proton beam irradiation) and the obvious theoretic benefits, IMRT has quickly become standard for many cancers, including prostate and head and neck.

The available level I evidence (two randomized prospective trials) to document the efficacy of IMRT involves nasopharyngeal cancer (NPC). Similar in design, each trial randomized patients between conventional radiation and IMRT along with concurrent chemotherapy.[11,12] The results were that salivary gland (parotid) function was significantly and dramatically improved in both studies. Kam and coworkers[11] found a reduction in observer-rated xerostomia from 82.1% with conventional radiotherapy to 39.3% with IMRT along with improvements in measured parotid flow rates. Similarly, Pow and coworkers[12] found an improvement in stimulated saliva flow with IMRT and also found that patients treated with IMRT had an improvement in patient-reported quality of life scores. The primary end point for both studies was parotid function; neither trial was powered or intended to examine the role of IMRT in disease control or overall survival.

Although there is no level I evidence proving that IMRT is equal to or superior to conventional radiation therapy in terms of disease control, several large retrospective series have been reported.[13–17] As seen in **Table 1**, the outcomes seem very comparable with historical controls; in this case, comparison is to the best arm of the Intergroup study,[18] which randomized patients to radiation alone versus chemoradiothearpy. Based on the significant improvement in overall survival from the combination arm of this intergroup study, chemoradiotherapy is now the established standard of care for this disease site.

From the data reported thus far for NPC, it seems that IMRT has a significant improvement in maintaining parotid function and based on multiple retrospective reviews and prospective nonrandomized data, has equal or perhaps slightly improved local-regional tumor control. There are no randomized data in using IMRT for non-NPC disease sites, but published data from multiple institutions[19–31] using IMRT in the treatment of non-NPC head and neck cancer have been impressive (**Table 2**). IMRT may even outperform conventional treatment in tumor sites that have been traditionally hard to target safely and adequately with conventional therapy, such as paranasal sinus cancer[32] and recurrent tumors.[33,34]

Data are also available on favorable toxicity profiles in non-NPC patients treated with IMRT technology. Several authors have reported on parotid sparing[5–8] with IMRT. The benefit from IMRT parotid sparing has translated in some studies into improved quality of life; patients reported improvement in ability to swallow and communication.[35] In addition to the established ability for IMRT to spare the parotid glands and preserve parotid gland function, IMRT has also shown decreased toxicity versus

Table 1
Intensity-modulated radiotherapy treatment outcome in nasopharyngeal cancer

Study	Number of Patients	Stage	Median Follow-up (Months)	Local Control (%)	Overall Survival (%)
MSKCC[13]	74	I–IV	35	91	83
Hong Kong[14]	64	I–IV	29	92	90
UCSF[15]	67	I–IV	31	97	73
Hong Kong[16]	33	T1N0–1	24	100	100
Intergroup[18,a]	78	Stage III–IV	32	NR	76 (3 y)

[a] Arm B (chemoradiotherapy): patients in this study were treated with conventional (non-IMRT) radiotherapy, presented for historical comparison.

Table 2
Intensity-modulated radiotherapy treatment outcome in non-nasopharyngeal cancer disease sites

Study	Patient Number	Disease Site	Stage	Median Follow-up (Months)	Local Control (%)	Overall Survival (%)
Malinkrodt[19]	126	OPC, OC, larynx, HPC	I–IV	24	85	NR
MDACC[20]	80	OPC	T1–2, N+	17	94 (2 y)	NR
UCSF[21]	41	OPC	T1–4, N0–3	14	94	89
MSKCC[22]	50	OPC	I–IV	18	98	98
University of Iowa[23]	150	OPC, NPC, larynx, OC, HPC, sinus	I–IV	18	94 (2 y)	85 (2 y)
University of Michigan[24]	58	OPC, larynx, HPC	II–IV	27	79	NR
University of Nebraska[25]	158	NR	NR (85% III or IV)	17	94	80 (3 y)
MDACC[26]	51	OPC	T1–2, N0–3	45	94 (2 y)	94 (2 y)

Abbreviations: HPC, hypopharyngeal cancer; NPC, nasopharyngeal cancer; NR, not reported; OC, oral cavity; OPC, oropharynx.

historical norms with sparing other normal structures, such as the constrictor muscles,[36] and optic structures.[37] The general acceptance of IMRT technology has led to its inclusion in RTOG trials; RTOG 0234 and 0522 are the first major United States cooperative group studies incorporating IMRT into radiotherapy planning.

Although the benefits of IMRT warrant its widespread use, there are some potential downfalls to this technology. First, the planning for IMRT is much more intensive and expensive than traditional radiotherapy planning; this places a higher time commitment on both the physician and the dosimetrist. This prolonged treatment planning time can occasionally delay treatment initiation, which has been shown to be detrimental in the setting of head and neck cancer.[38] Second, because the total radiation dose is the same with either conventional treatment or with IMRT and because the IMRT plan uses only certain sections of each radiation beam, with unwanted beam segments being blocked out, the total time for each treatment is increased versus conventional radiotherapy, requiring the patient to remain on the treatment table for longer periods of time and again increasing cost. IMRT also places an increased mechanical strain on the linear accelerator because the output of radiation is increased secondary to the blocked segments.

Third, as with any new technology, there is a learning curve associated with IMRT: too tight of dose constraints on normal structures or too tight of dose sculpting can result in inadequate treatment of the cancer. A recent report[39] describes three cases in which patients had a recurrence near the parotid gland, which was spared using IMRT technology. It is possible that these recurrences may have been avoided with conventional radiotherapy that did not attempt to reduce the radiation dose to the parotid glands.

Fourth, it is also possible that IMRT may increase the incidence and severity of certain toxicities. The increased number of beams in combination with high-priority avoidance structures increases the potential for an increased dose to other normal structures. A recent report by Rosenthal and coworkers[40] describes the increased dose to several normal structures, such as brainstem, cochlea, and occipital scalp, which would have received less radiation with conventional radiation fields. This can cause patient toxicities, such as headaches and scalp alopecia, to an extent not expected with conventional treatment. Other authors have reported on increased acute skin and mucus membrane toxicity from IMRT.[41] It behooves the radiation oncologist using IMRT to perform careful anatomic contouring. If, for example, the lips, eyes, or brainstem (structures that infrequently receive radiation in conventional treatment) are not adequately contoured, the IMRT computer algorithm does not recognize these as important structures and instead views them as a "free path" by which to insert radiation beams.

Finally, some of the long-term effects of IMRT are not known. The increased radiation output from IMRT results in a slightly increased total body dose of irradiation to the patient; this is unavoidable because of radiation that leaks out from the linear accelerator head during long treatment times. In addition to this increased scatter radiation, IMRT exposes a larger volume of normal tissue to low-dose radiation in an effort to avoid high doses of radiation to one or more critical structures. The combined effects of increased scatter and low-dose radiation have a theoretic risk of increased secondary malignancies. It is well established that radiation has a small but finite risk of causing cancer. Despite IMRT being used for over a decade, the long time course and the relative infrequency of secondary malignancies means that it could be many years before the true incidence of IMRT-induced secondary cancers is known.

In summary, the clinical evidence including two randomized trials and multiple retrospective and prospective nonrandomized (level III evidence) reports with comparisons with historical norms do point to a benefit of IMRT technology in the treatment of head and neck cancer, both in terms of target coverage and sparing of normal tissues. Additional prospective data are eagerly awaited; a relatively large European study is currently randomizing patients with stage III and IV head and neck cancer to standard radiotherapy versus IMRT. Outside of carefully controlled clinical trials, it is imperative that the radiation oncologist implementing IMRT be highly experienced in the anatomic contouring and IMRT planning processes. There are potential concerns and potential (at least theoretic) disadvantages to IMRT; these need to be carefully studied. It is important to recognize goals, advantages, and limitations of IMRT and continue to gain experience as to which patients truly benefit the most from this exciting technology.

IMAGE-GUIDED RADIATION THERAPY

Image-guided radiotherapy (IGRT) is a broad term that is meant to convey the incorporation of multidimensional imaging (through various means) into the planning and implementation of radiotherapy. The concept of IGRT is nothing new; imaging has always been used in the design of radiotherapy fields, previously in the form of fluoroscopy, two-dimensional planning films, and more recently the routine use of CT simulation. With the vast improvements in diagnostic radiology that have occurred over the last decades, however, the level of complexity and volume of information is unprecedented. Improvements in three-dimensional imaging, such as positron emission tomography (PET) and MRI, are now readily available as is the ability to obtain daily CT scans and four-dimensional imaging (with time as the fourth dimension) that allows even greater precision and accuracy for radiotherapy treatments.

IGRT can be divided into three separate areas. The first is the use of IGRT in treatment planning including the integration of diagnostic radiology information into treatment field design before the patient starts treatment. Second is the use of various technologies (eg, Linac-mounted cone-beam CT [CBCT] scan devices) for improved treatment precision and correction of daily set-up variables. The third form of IGRT combines the first two and uses available technology to replan and adjust the radiotherapy throughout the course of treatment: adaptive radiotherapy.

Use of Diagnostic Radiology

One form of IGRT is in using diagnostic technology to better define treatment volumes. 18-F-Flurodeoxyglucose (FDG) PET scans, especially with incorporation of a diagnostic CT scan (PET-CT scans), are increasingly used in radiotherapy planning. FDG-PET scans use a radioactive glucose that is taken up at a higher rate by tumor and involved lymph nodes than by normal tissues; this can allow differentiation between tumor volume and normal structures. PET scans can also help discover tumors areas that appear normal on CT scan but have significantly increased metabolic activity (and likely contain malignancy) as shown in **Fig. 3**. Clinical experience is growing regarding the ability of PET scans better to define gross disease and nodal volumes.[42–47] For example, Heron and coworkers[42] reported on the use of integrated PET-CT radiotherapy planning versus conventional CT planning and found that the CT-based planning overestimated the tumor volume by 150% compared with PET-CT–based planning.

Clinical outcomes of PET-CT–based radiotherapy planning have shown impressive tumor control and toxicity when compared with historical norms,[45,47] but to date there has not been any prospective randomized trials examining the role of PET scans in radiotherapy planning.

Some new advances within PET scanning include radiotracers other than FDG. It is well known that hypoxic areas within tumor volumes are less sensitive to radiation than areas that are well oxygenated. It is unknown if hypoxic areas also have decreased FDG-PET avidity, which may result in undertreatment of hypoxic areas based on these PET scans. PET scans showing increased uptake with the radiotracer fluorine-18-labeled fluoromisonidazole (18F-FMISO) have been shown to correlate with hypoxic areas within tumor cells.[48] Lee and coworkers[49] performed FMISO-PET and FDG-PET scans on 10 patients and used the information from the FMISO-PET scans

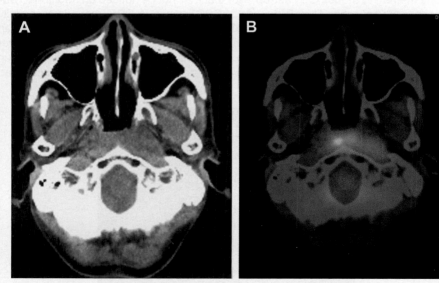

Fig. 3. Example of using PET scan information in better defining areas at risk of containing tumor. Although the CT scan (*A*) does not clearly show disease, the PET scan (*B*) demonstrates obvious areas of increased uptake representative of disease.

(presumed to represent hypoxic areas within the tumor volume) for an IMRT boost, increasing the dose to the hypoxic areas to a total dose of 84 Gy (approximately 20% higher radiotherapy dose than standard radiotherapy IMRT). Although more data are needed to demonstrate usefulness for this technique, it offers promise of further improvement on being able to treat aggressive or radioresistant cancers.

Technology to Improve Daily Set-Up Variation

Elaborate IMRT plans can be created in hopes of achieving the ideal situation of maximal tumor-target coverage while sparing critical normal anatomic structures. These plans often have very narrow distances between high- and low-dose regions so that even small changes, on the order of 5 to 8 mm, can result in 50% to 70% changes in radiation dose. Even the best IMRT plans fail if the patient anatomy and position that is used to create the plan does not consistently represent the patient anatomy and position at the time of daily radiotherapy delivery. Organ motion and patient positioning errors can result in excessive irradiation of organs at risk or inadequate dose to the target.

The classic method for patient set-up is to immobilize the patient using a face mask (**Fig. 4**). Markings are made on this mask and before the daily radiotherapy treatments; radiation therapy technologists use the mask marks to position the patient. The positioning is typically confirmed by taking a two-dimensional radiograph (portal film) before the first radiation treatment and then periodically (different institutions have different policies on how often these verification films are taken; once per week is a commonly accepted standard). If the verification films show an obvious displacement, the patient is repositioned before treatment. These two-dimensional verification films are capable of detecting most large errors (>5–10 mm), but have limitations because they only use two dimensions and can lead to missing potential set-up inaccuracy. They are also highly dependent on bony rather than soft tissue and tumor geometry.

One method to reduce daily set-up error that may not be noticed on traditional two-dimensional verification films is the use of CBCT scans. A CBCT scan is essentially a CT scanner built into the linear accelerator. The CBCT is used to obtain a CT scan of the patient in the anatomic area of interest (eg, the head and neck region) after the patient has been positioned on the treatment table. After the CBCT has been taken, a computer algorithm aligns the CBCT to the initial planning CT scan and

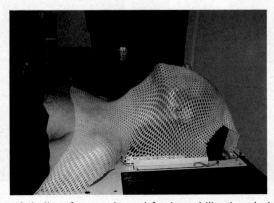

Fig. 4. Picture of head shell or face mask used for immobilization during radiotherapy in treating a head and neck malignancy.

adjustments, if required, can be made before the start of treatment. The use of CBCT has been well described in the treatment of prostate cancer[50] and several authors have reported on the use of CBCT in head and neck radiotherapy.[51,52] Hong and co-workers[51] analyzed the magnitude of difference between two- and three-dimensional patient set-ups, finding that substantial set-up errors could be discovered when all six degrees of freedom were registered. This set-up error was then used to calculate do-simetric consequences of not correcting these errors, finding that the planning tumor volume could be underdosed by as much as 20% to 30%. Others[53,54] have found re-ductions in the parotid and spinal cord dose with the use of daily imaging for position verification.

CBCTs have the potential to increase set-up accuracy, and this could allow reduc-tion in the tumor margins that would increase the distance from the high-dose radia-tion areas to the normal structures. Even small changes in margin can have significant effects on normal tissue doses and outcomes. Van Asselen and coworkers[55] found that dose to the parotid gland increases 1.3 Gy/mm of extra margin around the target volume and that reducing the margin around the tumor from 6 to 3 mm results in a re-duction in long-term parotid dysfunction of 20%.

The extra patient-received radiation dose that is associated with CBCT is about 3 cGy with most CBCT systems,[56,57] whereas the typical daily radiation treatment dose is 180 to 200 cGy. The daily CBCT represents 1% to 1.5% of the daily radiation dose. It should be mentioned, however, that unlike the daily radiation dose, the dose from the CBCT involves significantly more normal tissue and has higher skin dose. Several authors[58,59] have attempted to ascertain the degree of risk from secondary cancers associated with the radiation dose from a CT scan, and although these data remain highly speculative the potential for risk should be kept in mind.

Adaptive Radiation Therapy

A third way that IGRT can be used in radiotherapy is in replanning radiotherapy during the course of treatment; this is in essence adapting the initial radiotherapy plan to changes that occur during the radiotherapy treatments. Over the course of radiother-apy, which can last 8 weeks, there is often significant weight loss and anatomic var-iation; certain anatomic structures do not have the same size and volume they occupied before radiation. Several authors have reported on the changes that can oc-cur over the course of radiotherapy[54,60,61] and have found changes in the parotid glands as much as 53.6% and that the tumor can decrease by more than 90%, result-ing in potential shifts of up to several centimeters for the tumors and about 1 cm for the parotid glands.

Radiation planning has traditionally been implemented solely on the patient's initial (pretreatment) anatomy. This contrasts with the significant changes that occur throughout a radiotherapy course; daily doses may not be the same as the doses dur-ing the beginning of radiotherapy. As seen in **Fig. 5**, the patient's initial anatomy (and initial radiotherapy plan) is significantly different from the plan during the middle of treatment. By repeating a CT-simulation scan at one or more time points during the course of therapy, a second treatment plan, using the patient's altered anatomy, can be used to increase the accuracy of the radiotherapy. Realization of the anatomic changes and subsequent radiotherapy replanning can result in improved dose to both tumor and normal structures. Several authors[60,62,63] found that without replanning, tumor coverage and dosimetry decreases (despite the typical decrease in tumor vol-ume size during therapy), whereas at the same time spinal cord dose is increased by up to 10%.

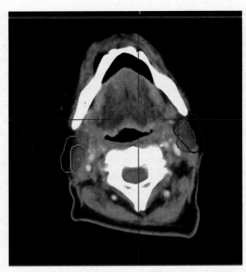

Fig. 5. Example of changes in parotid volume and location during radiotherapy. Repeat CT scan taken mid-way through course of radiotherapy showing decreased size and altered location of parotids on repeat scan (pink and blue) versus parotid size and location before initiating radiotherapy (green and red).

To date, there have not been any randomized trials examining the role and potential benefit for IGRT. This is caused in part by the recent development and continued evolution of IGRT technology and also by the inherent difficulty in randomizing patients to conventional versus cutting edge techniques. Continued practice and well-designed studies will accumulate data as to which patients are most likely to benefit from IGRT and the degree of this benefit.

PROTON THERAPY

Most radiotherapy is delivered using photons (or electron beams), but radiotherapy can also be implemented using particles, such as neutrons, protons, or heavy ions (eg, carbon). Proton therapy is especially attractive because of its theoretic dose distribution in normal tissue. Photons have a gradual intensity decay as they transverse tissue, whereas protons have a lower steady decline in intensity until a certain depth at which the intensity increases rapidly and then decreases equally rapidly. This sudden peak in dose is known as the "Bragg peak" and can allow the proton beam to be targeted on the tumor and have very little dose to normal structures on the other side (very little exit dose). Protons are currently only available in a limited number of centers and experience is limited, especially in the treatment of head and neck cancer. The only reported results of proton therapy in head and neck cancer involve several rare and difficult to treat tumors, such as chordomas[64] and other skull-based tumors.[65]

Theoretic plans have been created testing conventional IMRT versus intensity-modulated proton therapy, showing a significant advantage in tumor coverage and normal tissue sparing with the intensity-modulated proton therapy plans.[66,67] It should be emphasized that these were theoretic plans and not actual treatments. Currently, proton facilities are not using intensity-modulated proton therapy; proton treatments are given with conventional (eg, anteroposterior-posteroanterior, lateral) proton beams.

ALTERED FRACTIONATION WITH INTENSITY-MODULATED RADIOTHERAPY AND IMAGE-GUIDED RADIATION THERAPY

In addition to the unproved benefit of some of the technology and the possibility of long-term toxicity, such as secondary cancers, there are several other challenges with the new radiotherapy technology. One issue is the incorporation of twice-daily treatments or accelerated radiotherapy schedules. Radiotherapy delivery given more than once per day has been termed "hyperfractionation," and when the time course of radiotherapy is reduced (eg, from 6–7 weeks to 4–5 weeks) it is termed "accelerated radiotherapy." The theory behind hyperfractionated and accelerated radiotherapy is that it can decrease tumor repopulation that occurs during the radiotherapy course. There are several randomized trials[68,69] examining alternate radiotherapy schedules; although these trials did not use chemotherapy, they are considered landmark advances in nonoperative treatment of head and neck cancer. RTOG 9003[68] randomized patients to one of several radiation fractionation regimens and found that patients who received radiation twice daily had an improvement in local control and disease-free survival. The Danish Head and Neck Cancer study Group[69] randomized patients between five and six radiotherapy treatments a week and found that local control and disease-free survival were both improved in patients receiving six treatments a week. A current RTOG trial (0522) allows for six treatments per week in combination with systemic therapy.

IMRT and IGRT increase the daily treatment time, making twice-daily therapy even more difficult than usual. Although accelerated therapy has been proved to be useful with conventional therapy, it is possible that this benefit will be reduced or negated by the benefit of IMRT and IGRT. The current standard of care for patients receiving radiotherapy alone, as demonstrated in the previously mentioned trials, is with accelerated or hyperfractionated radiotherapy, and radiation oncologists may be forced to make a decision between the unproved benefits of IMRT and the more established benefits of accelerated therapy.

In response to this challenge, IMRT and the improved precision offered by IMRT and IGRT allow for another type of alternate radiotherapy delivery, termed "accelerated hypofractionation," in which radiation is delivered in higher than standard daily doses (>2.2 Gy) using IMRT safely to provide the dose escalation. This concept has been termed "simultaneous modulated accelerated radiotherapy." Using IMRT to limit the higher dose to normal structure and IGRT in better defining high-risk areas and decreasing daily set-up error make radiotherapy by simultaneous modulated accelerated radiotherapy more feasible and potentially beneficial. Clinical information on this technique is limited at this time but it is possible that the future of radiotherapy will involve differential dose targeting (dose painting) based on PET scan uptake similar to the project by Lee and coworkers[49] previously described.

INDUCTION CHEMOTHERAPY WITH INTENSITY-MODULATED RADIOTHERAPY AND IMAGE-GUIDED RADIATION THERAPY

Another uncertainty is how to incorporate planning techniques in patients who have had induction chemotherapy. There are no data to prove that induction chemotherapy is superior to immediate concurrent chemoradiotherapy. Based on recent impressive results with induction chemotherapy using TPF (docetaxel, cisplatin, and 5FU) followed by concurrent chemoradiotherapy,[70,71] however, many patients are now being treated with induction regimens. It is important to note that the induction TPF trials used conventional radiotherapy fields and techniques; they did not use either IMRT or IGRT technology. After completing induction therapy, target volumes, such as lymph nodes and the primary tumor, are not as apparent (indeed they may be completely resolved); this is almost certainly a good prognostic sign for the patient, but it complicates radiotherapy planning. It should not be assumed that induction chemotherapy, even with an apparent complete response, has sterilized the area that was originally positive. It is important that the radiation oncologist has access to detailed preinduction imaging. It is possible that in the future, the size of radiation treatment volumes or radiotherapy doses might be modified in response to induction chemotherapy, but at this time prudence requires that IMRT planning and delivery remain the same whether or not induction chemotherapy was given.

SUMMARY

Head and neck cancer remains a difficult cancer to treat; most patients have advanced disease on presentation and aggressive therapy is warranted to increase the chances of cure, but at the same time this aggressive therapy can result in significant and permanent morbidity. Thankfully, advances are being made in head and neck cancer treatments. In addition to advances from the medical oncology side, radiotherapy has made significant strides in being able to deliver more radiation that better targets the tumor and at the same time better avoids normal tissues and structures. Some of these advances include IMRT and IGRT techniques, such as incorporation of diagnostic imaging technology, repeating CT scans during therapy, and the use of daily CBCT scans. It is hoped that these advances, and other technologic advances to come, will yield improvements not only in tumor control and cure but also in quality of life for patients.

Although the theoretic and retrospective results of these advances look promising, caution should always be used when level I evidence is not available. Rigorous training, experience, and quality assurance are mandatory for the safe delivery of these complicated forms of radiotherapy. Further information regarding the risk and benefits of high-technology radiotherapy will be forthcoming in the coming decade.

REFERENCES

1. Adelstein DJ, Lavertu P, Saxton GL, et al. Mature results of a phase III randomized trial comparing concurrent chemoradiotherapy with radiation therapy alone in patients with stage III and IV squamous cell carcinoma of the head and neck. Cancer 2000;88:876–83.
2. Bonner JA, Harari PM, Giralt J, et al. Radiotherapy plus cetuximab for squamous-cell carcinoma of the head and neck. N Engl J Med 2006;354:567–78.
3. Bernier J, Domenge C, Ozahin M, et al. Postoperative irradiation with or without concomitant chemotherapy for locally advanced head and neck cancer. N Engl J Med 2004;350:1945–52.
4. Cooper JS, Pajak TF, Forastiere AA, et al. Postoperative concurrent radiotherapy and chemotherapy for high-risk squamous-cell carcinoma of the head and neck. N Engl J Med 2004;250:1937–44.
5. Chao KS. Protection of salivary gland function by intensity modulated radiation therapy in patients with head and neck cancer. Semin Radiat Oncol 2002; 12(Suppl 1):20–5.
6. Chao KS, Deasy JO, Markman J, et al. A prospective study of salivary function sparing in patients with head-and-neck cancers receiving intensity-modulated or three-dimensional radiation therapy: initial results. Int J Radiat Oncol Biol Phys 2001;49:907–16.

7. Eisbruch A, Kim HM, Terrell JE, et al. Xerostomia and its predictors following parotid-sparing irradiation of head-and-neck cancer. Int J Radiat Oncol Biol Phys 2001;50:695–704.

8. Lin A, Kim HM, Terrell JE, et al. Quality of life after parotid sparing IMRT for head-and-neck cancer: a prospective longitudinal study. Int J Radiat Oncol Biol Phys 2003;57:61–70.

9. Graff P, Lapeyre M, Desandes E, et al. Impact of intensity modulated radiotherapy on health-related quality of life for head and neck cancer patients: matched-pair comparison with conventional radiotherapy. Head Neck 2007;67:1309–17.

10. McMillan AS, Pow EH, Kwong DL, et al. Preservation of quality of life after intensity-modulated radiotherapy for early-stage nasopharyngeal carcinoma: results of a prospective longitudinal study. Head Neck 2006;28:712–22.

11. Kam MK, Leung SF, Zee B, et al. Prospective randomized study of intensity-modulated radiotherapy on salivary gland function in early stage nasopharyngeal carcinoma patients. J Clin Oncol 2007;25(31):4873–9.

12. Pow EH, Kwong DL, McMillian AS, et al. Xerostomia and quality of life after intensity modultated radiotherapy vs. conventional radiotherapy for early-stage nasopharyngeal carcinoma: initial report on a randomized controlled clinical trial. Int J Radiat Oncol Biol Phys 2006;66:981–91.

13. Wolden SL, Chen WC, Pfister DG, et al. Intensity-modulated radiation therapy (IMRT) for nasopharyngeal cancer: update of the memorial Sloan-Kettering experience. Int J Radiat Oncol Biol Phys 2006;64:57–62.

14. Kam MK, Teo PM, Chau RM, et al. Treatment of nasopharyngeal carcinoma with intensity-modulated radiotherapy: the Hong Kong experience. Int J Radiat Oncol Biol Phys 2004;60:1440–50.

15. Lee N, Xia P, Quivey JM, et al. Intensity-modulated radiotherapy in the treatment of nasopharyngeal carcinoma: an update of the UCSF experience. Int J Radiat Oncol Biol Phys 2002;53:12–22.

16. Bucci M, Xia P, Lee N, et al. Intensity modulated radiation therapy for carcinoma of the nasopharynx: an update of the UCSF experience. Int J Radiat Oncol Biol Phys 2004;60:S317–8.

17. Kwong DL, Pow EH, Sham JS, et al. Intensity-modulated radiotherapy for early-stage nasopharyngeal carcinoma: a prospective study on disease control and preservation of salivary function. Cancer 2004;101:1584–93.

18. Al-Sarraf M, LeBlanc M, Giri PG, et al. Chemoradiotherapy versus radiotherapy in patients with advanced nasopharyngeal cancer: phase III randomized intergroup study 0099. J Clin Oncol 1998;16(4):1310–7.

19. Chao KS, Low DA, Perez CA, et al. Intensity-modulated radiation therapy in head and neck cancers: the Mallinckrodt experience. Int J Cancer 2000;90:92–103.

20. Garden AS, Morrison W, Rosenthal D, et al. Intensity modulated radiation therapy (IMRT) for metastatic cervical adenopathy from oropharynx carcinoma. Int J Radiat Oncol Biol Phys 2004;60:S318.

21. Huang K, Lee N, Xia P. Intensity-modulated radiotherapy in the treatment of oropharyngeal carcinoma: a single institutional experience. Int J Radiat Oncol Biol Phys 2003;57:S302.

22. de Arruda FF, Puri DR, Zhung J, et-al. Intensity-modulated radiation therapy for the treatment of oropharyngeal carcinoma: the memorial Sloan-Kettering cancer center experience. In J Radiat Oncol Biol Phys 2006;64(2):363–73.

23. Yao M, Dornfield KJ, Buatti JM, et al. Intensity-modulated radiation treatment for head-and-neck squamous cell carcinoma: the University of Iowa experience. Int J Radiat Oncol Biol Phys 2005;63:410–21.

24. Dawson LA, Anzai Y, Marsh L, et al. Patterns of local-regional recurrence following parotid-sparing conformal and segmental intensity-modulated radiation therapy for head and neck cancer. Int J Radiat Oncol Biol Phys 2000;46:1117–26.

25. Zhen W, Lydiatt W, Lydiatt D. A preliminary analysis of patterns of failure in patients treated with intensity modulated radiotherapy (IMRT) for head and neck cancer: the University of Nebraska Medical Center experience. Int J Radiat Oncol Biol Phys 2004;60:S318.

26. Garden AS, Morrison W, Wong PF, et al. Disease-control rates following intensity-modulated radiation therapy for small primary oropharyngeal carcinoma. Int J Radiat Oncol Biol Phys 2007;67:438–44.

27. Chao KS, Ozyigit G, Tran BN, et al. Patterns of failure in patients receiving definitive and postoperative IMRT for head-and-neck cancer. Int J Radiat Oncol Biol Phys 2003;55:312–21.

28. Lee N, Xia P, Fischbein NJ, et al. Intensity-modulated radiation therapy for head-and-neck cancer: the UCSF experience focusing on target volume delineation. Int J Radiat Oncol Biol Phys 2003;57:49–60.

29. Daly ME, Lieskovsky Y, Pawlicki T, et al. Evaluation of patterns of failure and subjective salivary function in patients treated with intensity modulated radiotherapy for head and neck squamous cell carcinoma. Head Neck 2007;29:211–20.

30. Puri DR, Chou W, Lee N. Intensity-modulated radiation therapy in head-and-neck cancers: dosimetric advantages and update of clinical results. Am J Clin Oncol 2005;28:415–23.

31. Milano MT, Vokes EE, Kao J, et al. Intensity-modulated radiation therapy in advanced head and neck patients treated with intensive chemoradiotherapy: preliminary experience and future directions. Int J Radiat Oncol Biol Phys 2006;28:1141–51.

32. Daly ME, Chen AM, Bucci MK. Intensity-modulated radiation therapy for malignancies of the nasal cavity and paranasal sinuses. Int J Radiat Oncol Biol Phys 2007;67(1):151–7.

33. Biagioli MC, Harvey M, Roman E, et al. Intensity-modulated radiotherapy with concurrent chemotherapy for previously irradiated, recurrent head and neck cancer. Int J Radiat Oncol Biol Phys 2007;69(4):1067–73.

34. Sulman EP, Schwartz DI, Le TT, et al. IMRT reirradiation of head and neck cancer: disease control and morbidity outcomes. Int J Radiat Oncol Biol Phys 2008; [epub ahead of print].

35. Eisbruch A, Dawson LA, Kim HM, et al. Conformal and intensity modulated irradiation of head and neck cancer: the potential for improved target irradiation, salivary gland function and quality of life. Acta Otorhinolaryngol Belg 1999;53(3):271–5.

36. Eisbruch A, Schwartz M, Rasch C, et al. Dysphagia and aspiration after chemoradiotherapy for head-and-neck cancer: which anatomic structures are affected and can they be spared by IMRT? Int J Radiat Oncol Biol Phys 2004;60:1425–39.

37. Mock U, Georg D, Bogner J, et al. Treatment planning comparison of conventional, 3D conformal, and intensity-modulated photon (IMRT) and proton therapy for paranasal sinus carcinoma. Int J Radiat Oncol Biol Phys 2004;58:147–54.

38. Ang KA, Trotti A, Brown BW, et al. Randomized trial addressing risk features and time factors of surgery plus radiotherapy in advanced head-and-neck cancer. Int J Radiat Oncol Biol Phys 2001;51(3):571–8.

39. Cannon DM, Lee NY. Recurrence in region of spared parotid gland after definitive intensity-modulated radiotherapy for head and neck cancer. Int J Radiat Oncol Biol Phys 2008;70:660–5.

40. Rosenthal DI, Chambers MS, Fuller CD, et al. Beam path toxicities to non-target structures during intensity-modulated radiation therapy for head and neck cancer. Int J Radiat Oncol Biol Phys 2008;69(3):S1.

41. Lee N, Chuang C, Quivey JM, et al. Skin toxicity due to intensity-modulated radiotherapy for head-and-neck carcinoma. Int J Radiat Oncol Biol Phys 2002;53(3):630–7.

42. Heron DE, Andrade RS, Flickinger J, et al. Hybrid PET-CT simulation for radiation treatment planning in head-and-neck cancers: a brief technical report. Int J Radiat Oncol Biol Phys 2004;60:1419–24.

43. Scarfone C, Lavely WC, Cmelak AJ, et al. Prospective feasibility trial of radiotherapy target definition for head and neck cancer using 3-dimensional PET and CT imaging. J Nucl Med 2004;45:543–52.

44. Nishioka T, Shiga T, Shirato H, et al. Image fusion between 18 FDG-PET and MRI/CT for radiotherapy planning of oropharyngeal and nasopharyngeal carcinomas. Int J Radiat Oncol Biol Phys 2002;53:1051–7.

45. Koshy M, Paulino AC, Howell R, et al. F-18 PET-CT fusion in radiotherapy treatment planning for head and neck cancer. Head Neck 2005;27:494–502.

46. Wang D, Schultz CJ, Jursinic PA, et al. Initial experience of FDG-PET/CT guided IMRT of head-and-neck carcinoma. Int J Radiat Oncol Biol Phys 2006;65:143–51.

47. Vernon MR, Maheshwari M, Schultz CJ, et al. Clinical outcomes of patients receiving integrated PET/CT-guided radiotherapy for head and neck carcinoma. Int J Radiat Oncol Biol Phys 2006;70:678–84.

48. Nurani RD, Rajendran J, Austin-Seymour J. The predictive utility of PET-misonidazolein locally advanced head and neck cancer treated with radiotherapy. Int J Radiat Oncol Biol Phys 2007;69:S1.

49. Lee NY, Mechalakos JG, Nehmeh S, et al. Fluorine-18-labeled fluoromisonidazole positron emission and computed tomography-guided intensity-modulated radiotherapy for head and neck cancer: a feasibility study. Int J Radiat Oncol Biol Phys 2008;70:2–13.

50. Smitsmans MH, de Bois J, Sonke JJ, et al. Automatic prostate localization on cone-beam CT scans for high precision image-guided radiotherapy. Int J Radiat Oncol Biol Phys 2005;63(4):975–84.

51. Hong TS, Wolfgang AT, Chappell RJ, et al. The impact of daily setup variations on head-and-neck intensity-modulated radiation therapy. Int J Radiat Oncol Biol Phys 2005;61:779–88.

52. Li H, Zhu XR, Zhang L, et al. Comparison of 2D radiographic images and 3D cone beam computed tomography for positioning head-and-neck radiotherapy patients. Int J Radiat Oncol Biol Phys 2008;71(3):916–25.

53. Sharpe M, Brock K, Rehbinder H, et al. Adaptive planning and delivery to account for anatomical changes induced by radiation therapy of head and neck cancer. Int J Radiat Oncol Biol Phys 2005;63:S3.

54. Vakilha M, Hwang D, Breen SL. Changes in position and size of parotid glands assessed with daily cone-beam CT during image-guided IMRT for head and neck cancer: implications for dose received. Int J Radiat Oncol Biol Phys 2007;69(3):S1.

55. van Asselen B, Dehnad H, Raaijmakers CP, et al. The dose to the parotid glands with IMRT for oropharyngeal tumors: the effect of reduction of positioning margins. Radiother Oncol 2002;64(2):197–204.

56. Islam MK, Purdie TG, Norrlinger BD, et al. Patient dose from kilovoltage cone beam computed tomography imaging in radiation therapy. Med Phys 2006;33:1573–82.

Martin[2] and became the standard of care until work by Bocca and colleagues[3] and Suarez[4] in the 1960s and 1970s demonstrated that more functional or structure-preserving neck dissections could be offered to patients without compromising regional disease control.

More recently, selective procedures, in which nodal areas deemed not at risk are left undissected, have been introduced and applied widely. The selective procedures were developed to control regional metastases while reducing the morbidity associated with neck dissection. The basis for description of selective neck dissection procedures is the classification system of lymph node levels published by the American Head and Neck Society.[5] Level 1 includes the submental and submandibular nodes; levels 2–4 include the upper, middle, and lower jugular nodes, respectively; and level 5 represents the posterior triangle nodes. Levels and sublevels are depicted in **Fig. 1**. The spinal accessory nerve crosses level 2, as depicted in **Fig. 1**, dividing it into level 2a anteroinferiorly and the smaller level 2b posterosuperiorly.

The fundamental morbidity of neck dissection relates to the anatomic structures mobilized or resected with the majority of the morbidity associated with dysfunction of the accessory nerve. The accessory nerve enters the upper neck through the jugular foramen medial to the jugular vein. It then crosses the jugular vein in a medial to lateral direction (levels IIa and IIb); penetrates the medial border of the sternomastoid muscle, where it provides a motor branch to the muscle; and descends in the posterior triangle (levels 5a and 5b). After exiting the muscle the nerve usually picks up a branch of the cervical motor plexus to innervate the pars descendens and pars horizontalis of the trapezius muscle. Nerve injury or trapezius dysfunction is associated with considerable shoulder disability relating to the inability to fully abduct and internally rotate the shoulder. Permanent loss of function often results in significant pain, shoulder

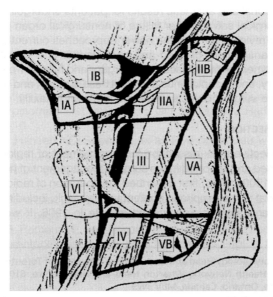

Fig. 1. Neck levels. (*From* Robbins KT, Clayman G, Levine PA, et al. Neck dissection classification update: revisions proposed by the American Head and Neck Society and the American Academy of Otolaryngology-Head and Neck Surgery. Arch Otolaryngol Head Neck Surg 2002;128(7):751–8; with permission.)

dysfunction, and deformity as a result of subluxation of the sternoclavicular joint and the associated shoulder drop.

The oncologic basis for selective neck dissection comes from analysis of histopathologic findings in comprehensive neck dissection specimens. The underlying principle is that the pattern of neck metastases from upper aerodigestive tract carcinomas occurs is predictable based on the location of the lesion. Shah and colleagues[6] provided evidence with a review of 1081 previously untreated patients who had squamous cell carcinoma (SCC) of the upper aerodigestive tract, all of whom underwent comprehensive neck dissection. Almost half of these patients had primary lesions in the oral cavity. In patients who had oral carcinoma and clinical evidence of neck disease, the rate of pathologic involvement of level 5 nodes was 4%. All these patients had metastases present in the anterior triangle, and all had tumors of the floor of mouth and lower alveolus.

Woolgar[7] used a review of histopathologic findings to define expected and aberrant patterns of neck metastases. Included were 439 patients who had oral and oropharyngeal SCC who underwent comprehensive or selective neck dissection. The expected pattern was described as an inverted cone, with maximal disease volume and maximal extracapsular extension at levels 1 and 2, with progressive diminution inferiorly. Aberrant patterns included isolated metastasis at level 1a or 2b, involvement of the contralateral neck, skipping of a level other than level 1, presence of a solitary micrometastasis, and multiple micrometastases in absence of conventional metastasis. Micrometastasis was defined as a deposit less than 2 mm in maximal dimension. Of patients who had clinically evident metastasis, 67% had a typical pattern, 14% had a solitary micrometastasis, and 10% had skip metastasis.

A similar study by Byers and colleagues[8] reviewed pathologic findings at each level after neck dissection for oral tongue carcinomas in 277 patients. In that study, the investigators reported a 16% rate of skip metastasis and advocated that selective neck dissection, when performed for prognostic purposes in oral tongue carcinoma, should include levels 1–4, an extension of the commonly used supraomohyoid dissection.

Currently, the major controversy revolves around whether or not to dissect levels 2b (requiring mobilization of the accessory nerve in the anterior triangle) and whether or not to dissect level 5 (requiring mobilization of the accessory nerve in the posterior triangle) in the clinically N0 and N+ neck.

Several studies have addressed the oncologic efficacy of leaving level 2b undissected. Kraus and coworkers,[9] in a study of 44 clinically N0 patients who had oral and oropharyngeal carcinoma, found a 2% rate of metastasis to level 2b. Lim and colleagues[10] found a 5% rate in a review of 74 patients with oral carcinoma. Elsheikh and colleagues[11] reported that 6% of 48 N0 patients who had oral carcinoma had metastasis to level 2b. In all three studies, all patients who had positive level 2b also had positive nodes at level 2a. The latter study identified oral tongue primary tumors as more likely to result in level 2b metastases than those from other oral cavity sites.

In the presence of clinical neck metastasis, the rate of level 2b involvement is higher. Silverman and colleagues[12] reported that 3 of 27 (11%) clinically positive necks demonstrated metastasis at level 2b; the presence of extracapsular extension and pathologic metastasis to level 2a were predictors of level 2b involvement—clinical N stage was not a predictor nor was it a primary site; slightly under half of the patients in this study had primary tumors in the oral cavity. Talmi and colleagues[13] reviewed results of 102 neck dissections, of which 4% were positive at level 2b. Of 22 patients who had clinical N2 or larger disease, level 2b was positive in 18%. In this study there were no patients who had proved metastasis at levels 2a and 2b.

Finally, Villaret and colleagues,[14] in a recent prospective multicenter study, found metastasis to level 2b in 10% of patients who had oral cavity primary. In patients who had clinical evidence of metastasis, the rate was 13% whereas it was 2% in patients who did not have clinical evidence of metastasis.

Many investigators have sought to determine the oncologic validity of not dissecting level V. Davidson and colleagues[15] reviewed a series of 1277 comprehensive neck dissections, of which 569 were performed for oral cavity carcinoma. Metastasis was confirmed at level 5 in 2.4% of patients who had oral carcinoma and who presented with clinical neck disease and in 0.6% of patients who had subsequent neck dissection after initial observation.

Dias and colleagues[16] also provided data on 339 patients who had oral carcinoma who underwent elective or therapeutic neck dissection. Only 2% of patients had positive nodes at level 5; all had clinical neck disease and all had involvement of multiple other node levels. De Zinis and colleagues[17] reported a series of 89 patients treated for oral carcinoma with selective or comprehensive neck dissection; level 5 was involved in 1 of 89 (1%). Four of the five neck failures in this series occurred within the previously dissected field, which likely would not have been prevented by inclusion of additional nodal levels.

Based on this evidence, for patients undergoing elective neck dissection (N0), most centers offer a highly selective neck dissection limited to levels 1, 2a, 3, and 4. Patients who have N1 disease should be offered a selective neck dissection with preservation of level 5 and for advanced disease a comprehensive clearance of all neck regions is required.

SENTINEL NODE IN ORAL CAVITY

Sentinel node biopsy has been used widely in breast and melanoma to select patients for regional lymphadenectomy and, therefore, reduce the need for elective regional dissection and the inherent morbidity. This concept has been advocated for early-stage tumors of the oral cavity based on the premise that the majority of patients who have T1 and T2 oral squamous cell carcinomas are managed with transoral procedures, which do not require entry into the neck (whereas more advanced tumors require neck exposures for reconstructive procedures).[18,19] Currently, the majority of the patients undergo elective dissections based on a risk for subclinical nodal disease that ranges from 10% to 30%. If sentinel node identification could identify subclinical nodal disease reliably then up to 70% of patients could forego a neck dissection and the associated morbidity.

The technique of sentinel node biopsy has been well described in the literature and includes the injection of radiocolloid and blue dye to identify the sentinel node or nodes for a particular primary site. Prospective studies have demonstrated a high sensitivity for the technique with most investigators reporting between 80% and 100% sensitivity. The current controversy in the widespread adoption of this technique revolves around several of questions. The most dominant of these is the question of whether or not a sentinel node biopsy is less morbid than a highly selective neck dissection. This is controversial because in the majority of prospective series, multiple sentinel nodes (as many as three or four) in multiple nodal basins have been identified, requiring multiple incisions. The other major question is whether or not sentinel node and neck dissection for node-positive patients is as effective in disease control as an elective neck dissection. A recent review[20] has suggested that the therapeutic efficacy of sentinel node is dependent on the risk for regional nodal disease. In patients at low risk for regional disease, 20% or less, there was no difference in regional recurrence or disease-free survival difference between sentinel node and elective neck dissection. For patients who had a 40% risk for subclinical disease, however, the extrapolated regional and disease-free survival advantage to elective neck dissection could be as high as 2%.

Currently, prospective trials evaluating sentinel node biopsy in early oral squamous cell carcinoma are underway and likely will answer these questions. This technique and its application in early mucosal lesions will have the potential to reduce the morbidity associated with surgical management of the neck.

TRANSORAL CO_2 LASER EXCISION OF LARYNGEAL TUMORS

The treatment of early-stage glottic (Tis, T1, and T2) and supraglottic tumors remains controversial. Options in treatment include external beam radiation (XRT), open partial laryngectomy, and transoral laser excision (TOL). The concept of transoral excision of early-stage lesions was first described by Strong and Jako[21] in 1972 and more recently has been popularized by Steiner[22] and his colleagues in Gottingen, Germany. The surgical premise of TOL is that patients can undergo an oncologically sound surgical procedure, using a minimally invasive technique performed through the mouth with the assistance of the CO_2 laser. The procedure usually can be done on an outpatient basis, is of short duration, and has limited treatment related morbidity. Advocates of the procedure argue that the local regional and overall survival associated with TOL are equivalent to those achieved with open approaches or XRT and that the voice results are similar.

In addition, there is an evolving interest in the use of this technique in more advanced tumors (integrated with neck management and adjuvant therapy). This interest is based on the belief among some of the surgical oncology community that the functional results associated with these approaches, particularly with regard to speech and swallowing, may be better than those achieved with primary chemoradiation, with equivalent survival.

The evidence in support of any treatment for early-stage laryngeal cancer is problematic. There are no well designed and executed randomized trials that address the treatment of this group of patients, with most centers reporting retrospective or prospective series of patients. Head-to-head comparison of TOL is difficult because of problems with patient selection in the existing publications. The advocates of XRT suggest that the surgical series are populated with highly selected patients (better performance status and appropriate anatomy to allow TOL) and do not represent the complete spectrum of patients reported in the XRT series.

Many publications have reported consecutive series of major approaches and the results are summarized in **Tables 1** and **2**.[23–35] In assessing the outcomes with an understanding of the inherent flaws in the data, it seems that these two techniques likely offer equivalent results in terms of locoregional control, that the voice results of TOL are somewhat inferior to XRT, and that the laryngectomy-free survival is higher in patients treated primarily with TOL. This evidence suggests that patients should be offered the options of TOL or XRT for early-stage glottic tumors.

The role of TOL in more advanced tumors awaits further study but is of interest to many surgical oncologists treating laryngeal malignancy.

ENDOSCOPIC SKULL BASE SURGERY

Surgical management of advanced tumors of the nose and paranasal sinuses has evolved dramatically over the past 2 decades.[36] The concept of craniofacial resection and en bloc resection of paranasal sinus tumors dramatically improved the local regional control for advanced sinus tumors not involving the brain or dura and has been the standard of care for surgical management of these tumors for the past

Table 1
Results of radiation series

Study	Number of Subjects	Stages	Overall Survival	Local Control
Fletcher[23]	330	T1, T2	—	80%
Harwood[24]	378	Tis, T1a, T1b	95%	87%
Horiot[25]	415	Tis, T1a, T1b	—	83%
Johansen[26]	707	T1, T2	—	77%
Le[27]	398	T1, T2	43%	80%
Mendenhall[28]	519	T1, T2	78%	86%
Wang[29]	902	T1, T2	95%	88%
Warde[30]	735	T1, T2	75%	82%

decade. In the late 1980s and early 1990s the concept of minimally invasive endoscopic sinus surgery evolved and developed to essentially replace the standard open procedures to the nose and paranasal sinuses for benign tumors and inflammatory disease. Improved understanding of the endoscopic landmarks and instrumentation has allowed these techniques to be extended to tumors involving the anterior skull base and paranasal sinuses. This new approach incorporates teams of surgeons (usually a neurosurgeon and otolaryngologist) working through both nostrils removing tumors in a piecemeal fashion without the need for facial access incisions or open craniotomy approaches. The surgical approach to tumors involves a transnasal debulking of tumors usually with powered instrumentation with endoscopic excision of the cranial base or bony margins of the tumor. Advocates of this approach[17,37,38] argue that the standard open craniofacial resection often results in a fragmented or less than en bloc resection and, therefore, is not technically different from the minimally invasive approaches. Additionally, advocates argue that the endoscopic visualization of tumor margins improves the completeness of resection. The limitation of the endoscopic approaches is that the limited surgical approach makes it technically difficult to repair the inherent dural defects, resulting in high rates of CSF leak and, therefore, risk for meningitis. There is, however, little doubt that the surgical morbidity (other than CSF leak) in experienced hands is dramatically reduced with this technique. Some institutions have developed techniques that include robotic approaches to further refine the surgical technique and potentially extend the scope of minimally invasive skull base surgery.

There is no level I evidence to support the use of endoscopic approaches for malignancies involving the paranasal sinuses and anterior skull base. The majority of reports

Table 2
Series transoral laser

Study	Number of Subjects	Stages	Overall Survival	Local Control
Gallo[32]	151	Tis, T1, T2	94%	94%
Motta[34]	482	T1a, T1b, T2	79%	75%
Eckel[33]	285	Tis, T1, T2	70%	85%
Steiner[22]	159	Tis, T1, T2	87%	93%
Steiner[31]	263	T1a, T1b, T2	76%	88%
Rudert[34]	114	Tis, T1, T2	99%	91%

are prospective data collections with small patient numbers and usually a variety of histologies. The specific indications for this technique likely are low-grade tumors (esthesioneuroblastoma) or tumors confined to the nasal cavity without intracranial or orbital involvement. Without clinical trials or multicenter prospective data collection it likely will be a least a decade before it is known if the promise of low-morbidity, minimally invasive skull base procedures will deliver equivalent local control rates to the more widely used and reported open craniofacial procedures.

MANDIBULAR AND MAXILLARY RECONSTRUCTION

It is likely that the most significant innovation in the surgical treatment of head and neck malignancy has been the introduction of free tissue transfer for reconstruction of the postablative defects. The first free flap was described in the 1972 by Taylor and Daniel[39] and was a transfer of a free groin flap to reconstruct a skin defect. The concept of transferring tissue based on its anatomic blood supply had been developed for several decades but the availability of instrumentation and, in particular, small needles that could be used to sew vessels of less than 1.5 mm was the fundamental limitation. In the decade after the first transfer a better understanding of the vascular anatomy of the skin, muscle, and bone provided a plethora of free tissue transfer options, including skin, mucosal constructs, muscle transfers, and transfers of tissue composites, including muscle skin or bone. The development of these techniques dramatically changed the landscape of surgical reconstruction as essentially any defect of the oral cavity or mandible could be reliably reconstructed. Currently, most experienced centers report flap success rates from 95% to 100%.

MANDIBULAR RECONSTRUCTION

Perhaps the most dramatic change in reconstruction in the past 2 decades has been in mandibular reconstruction. Defects in the mandible of up to 12 to 15 cm can be reconstructed with a variety of free vascularized bone transfers, including the fibula, lateral border of the scapula, iliac crest, or the radius. Each of these available transfers is associated with a certain length of available bone and each has an associated skin island or muscle transfer and associated morbidity.

The most widely used bone transfer for mandibular reconstruction is the free fibular transfer. This flap based on the peroneal branch of the tibioperoneal trunk of the popliteal artery has the advantages of a long length of available bone; up to 20 cm, a reliable skin paddle based on perforating vessels arising from the peroneal artery; and a relatively consistent anatomy. The major disadvantages of this transfer are that it is not ideal in individuals who have peripheral vascular disease or venous insufficiency and the blood supply to the skin on the lateral leg is not reliable in a small percentage of patients. The donor site is well tolerated provided the portion of the fibula that abuts the proximal tibia and supports the ankle mortice is not disrupted. The fibular transfer may be osteotomized into several segments allowing surgeons to transform a straight bone into a replica of the native mandible based on the periosteal supply provided to each segment of bone by the peroneal artery. The bone segments usually are held together with a low-profile reconstruction plate usually made of titanium (**Fig. 2**). Current limitations of the fibular donor site is that the vertical height of the mandible created with the fibula usually is shorter than the native mandible creating problems for dental rehabilitation in terms of osseointegration or fit and retention of a standard dental prosthesis. The other limitation is in temporomandibular joint reconstruction where there remains no ideal solution to reconstruction of a functional joint.

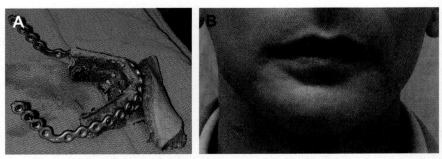

Fig. 2. (*A*) Lateral view of free fibular transfer with reconstruction plate. (*B*) AP postoperative view of same patient 2 years post surgery and radiotherapy.

In patients in whom the fibula is not an option because of peripheral vascular disease or abnormal anatomy, the scapular flap based on the circumflex scapular vessels or the iliac crest based on the deep circumflex iliac artery and venae commitantes represents an excellent alternative.

MAXILLARY RECONSTRUCTION

Traditionally, surgical defects of the maxilla and palate have been reconstructed with a prosthesis similar to a denture with a bulb or obturator projecting into the maxillary or palatal defect to close the defect and provide retention of the prosthesis. These prostheses work well for limited defects but often are associated with leakage of food or fluids into the nose or nasopharynx and when not in place dramatically change the aesthetics of the face and the resonance of the voice. In addition, in patients who have extensive defects (greater than one half the palate) or defects of the anterior maxilla, there is not adequate native tissue or muscle function to support and retain the

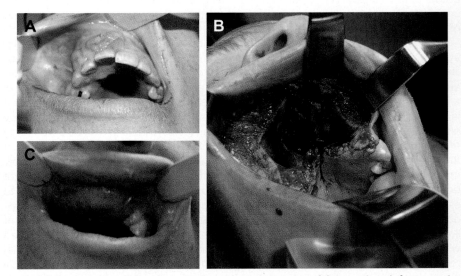

Fig. 3. (*A*) Preoperative view of maxillary osteogenic sarcoma. (*B*) Resection defect anterior maxilla. (*C*) AP postoperative view 4 months after reconstruction.

prosthesis. Recently there has been increasing interest in reconstruction of the maxilla with soft tissue or myo-osseous free tissue transfers. These reconstructions potentially offer the opportunity for anatomic restoration of midface structures with a closed palate or maxilla and the potential for dental rehabilitation through the use of osseointegrated retained or standard dentures. Controversy exists over which patients and associated defects are best suited to reconstruction, but most would agree that extremely large defects not well rehabilitated with standard prosthesis are ideally managed in this fashion. The concept of transfer of a free vascularized bone and muscle flap first was described by Brown[40] in 1995. They described the use of the free iliac crest and internal oblique muscle with the bone oriented vertically to recreate the maxillary alveolus and the muscle rotated into the maxilla defect to recreate the palate. Clark and colleagues[41] recently described the angular artery tip of scapular flap incorporating the tip of the scapula and the teres major muscle for the same purpose (**Fig. 3**). Many other free tissue transfers have been advocated and used. Reconstruction of the maxilla continues to be an area of development and innovation in head and neck surgery.

SUMMARY

The surgical management of head and neck tumors continues to evolve with a focus on reducing treatment related morbidity. The major changes in the past 2 decades have been the introduction of function-preserving and minimally invasive surgical approaches along with a dramatic change in the ability to reconstruct ablative defects and restore form and function. The future certainly will include better evidence regarding the efficacy and appropriate application of these new techniques. Reconstructive techniques will continue to evolve with introduction of tissue engineering and cell therapy to further improve the quality of life of the patients afflicted with head and neck malignancies.

REFERENCES

1. Crile G. Excision of cancer of the head and neck with special reference to the plan of dissection. JAMA 1906;47:1780–6.
2. Martin H. Surgery of the Head and Neck. New York: Harper and Row; 1957.
3. Bocca E, Pignataro O, Oldini C, Cappa C. Functional neck dissection: an evaluation and review of 843 cases. Laryngoscope 1984;94(7):942–5.
4. Suarez O. El problema de las metastasis linfaticus y alejadas del cancer laringe e hipofaringe. Rev Otorhinolaringol 1963;28:83–9.
5. Robbins KT, Clayman G, Levine PA, et al. Neck dissection classification update: revisions proposed by the American Head and Neck Society and the American Academy of Otolaryngology-Head and Neck Surgery. Arch Otolaryngol Head Neck Surg 2002;128(7):751–8.
6. Shah JP. Patterns of cervical lymph node metastasis from squamous carcinomas of the upper aerodigestive tract. Am J Surg 1990;160(4):405–9.
7. Woolgar JA. The topography of cervical lymph node metastases revisited: the histological findings in 526 sides of neck dissection from 439 previously untreated patients. Int J Oral Maxillofac Surg 2007;36(3):219–25.
8. Byers RM, Weber RS, Andrews T, McGill D, Kare R, Wolf P-. Frequency and therapeutic implications of "skip metastases" in the neck from squamous carcinoma of the oral tongue. Head Neck 1997;19(1):14–9.
9. Kraus DH, Rosenberg DB, Davidson BJ, et al. Supraspinal accessory lymph node metastases in supraomohyoid neck dissection. Am J Surg 1996;172(6):646–9.

10. Lim YC, Song MH, Kim SC, Kim KM, Choi EC. Preserving level IIb lymph nodes in elective supraomohyoid neck dissection for oral cavity squamous cell carcinoma. Arch Otolaryngol Head Neck Surg 2004;130(9):1088–91.
11. Elsheikh MN, Mahfouz ME, Elsheikh E. Level IIb lymph nodes metastasis in elective supraomohyoid neck dissection for oral cavity squamous cell carcinoma: a molecular-based study. Laryngoscope 2005;115(9):1636–40.
12. Silverman DA, El-Hajj M, Strome S, Esclamado RM. Prevalence of nodal metastases in the submuscular recess (level IIb) during selective neck dissection. Arch Otolaryngol Head Neck Surg 2003;129(7):724–8.
13. Talmi YP, Hoffman HT, Horowitz Z, et al. Patterns of metastases to the upper jugular lymph nodes (the "submuscular recess"). Head Neck 1998;20(8):682–6.
14. Villaret AB, Piazza C, Peretti G, et al. Multicentric prospective study on the prevalence of sublevel IIb metastases in head and neck cancer. Arch Otolaryngol Head Neck Surg 2007;133(9):897–903.
15. Davidson BJ, Kulkarny V, Delacure MD, Shah JP. Posterior triangle metastases of squamous cell carcinoma of the upper aerodigestive tract. Am J Surg 1993; 166(4):395–8.
16. Dias FL, Lima RA, Kligerman J, et al. Relevance of skip metastases for squamous cell carcinoma of the oral tongue and the floor of the mouth. Otolaryngol Head Neck Surg 2006;134(3):460–5.
17. De Zinis LO, Bolzoni A, Piazza C, Nicolai P. Prevalence and localization of nodal metastases in squamous cell carcinoma of the oral cavity: role and extension of neck dissection. Eur Arch Otorhinolaryngol 2006;263(12):1131–5.
18. Stoeckli SJ. Sentinel Node Biopsy for Oral and Oropharyngeal Squamous Cell Carcinoma of the Head and Neck. The Laryngoscope 2007;117(9):1539–51.
19. Civantos F, Zitsch R, Bared A. Sentinel node biopsy in oral squamous cell carcinoma. J Surg Oncol 2007;96(4):330–6.
20. Paleri V, Rees G, Arullendran P, Shoaib T, Krishman S. Sentinel node biopsy in squamous cell cancer of the oral cavity and oral pharynx: a diagnostic meta-analysis. Head Neck 2005;27(9):739–47.
21. Strong M, Jako G. Laser surgery in the larynx: early clinical experience with continuous Co2 laser. Ann Otol Rhinol Laryngol 1972;81:791–8.
22. Steiner W. Results of curative laser microsurgery of laryngeal carcinomas. Am J Otolaryngol 1993;14(2):116–21.
23. Fletcher GH, Lindberg RD, Hamberger A, Horiot JC. REASONS FOR IRRADIATION FAILURE IN SQUAMOUS CELL CARCINOMA OF THE LARYNX. The Laryngoscope 1975;85(6):987–1003.
24. Harwood AR, Hawkins NV, Keane T, et al. RADIOTHERAPY OF EARLY GLOTTIC CANCER. The Laryngoscope 1980;90(3):465–70.
25. Horiot JC, Fletcher GH, Ballantyne AI, Lindberg RD. Analysis of failures in early vocal cord cancer. Radiiology 1972;103:663–5.
26. Johansen LV, Grau C, Overgaard J. Glottic carcinoma–patterns of failure and salvage treatment after curative radiotherapy in 861 consecutive patients. Radiotherapy and Oncology 2002;63(3):257–67.
27. Le QT, Fu KK, Kroll S, et al. Influence of fraction size, total dose, and overall time on local control of T1-T2 glottic carcinoma. Int J Radiat Oncol Biol Phys 1997; 39(1):115–26.
28. Mendenhall WM, Amdur RJ, Morris CG, Hinerman RW. T1-T2N0 Squamous Cell Carcinoma of the Glottic Larynx Treated With Radiation Therapy. Journal of Clinical Oncology 2001;19(20):4029–36.

29. Wang CC. Treatment of glottic carcinoma by mega voltage radiation therapy and results 1974; 120: 157-63. Am J Roentgenol Radium Ther Nucl Med 1974;120(1): 157–63.

30. Warde P, O'Sullivan B, Bristow RG, et al. T1/T2 glottic cancer managed by external beam radiotherapy: the influence of pretreatment hemoglobin on local control. Int J Radiat Oncol Biol Phys 1998;41(2):347–53.

31. Steiner W, Ambrosch P, Rödel RMW, Kron M. Impact of Anterior Commissure Involvement on Local Control of Early Glottic Carcinoma Treated by Laser Microresection. The Laryngoscope 2004;114(8):1485–91.

32. Gallo A, Marco de Vincentiis MD, Manciocco V, Simonelli M, Fiorella ML, Shah JP. CO_2 Laser Cordectomy for Early-Stage Glottic Carcinoma: A Long-Term Follow-up of 156 Cases. The Laryngoscope 2002;112(2):370.

33. Eckel HE, Schneider C, Jungehuelsing M, Damm M, Schroeder U, Voessing M. Potential role of transoral laser surgery for larynx carcinoma. Lasers in Surgery and Medicine 1998;23(2):79–86.

34. Motta G, Esposito E, Cassiano B, Motta S. T1-T2-T3 Glottic Tumors: Fifteen Years Experience with CO_2 Laser. Acta Oto-Laryngologica 1997;117:155–9.

35. Rudert H, Werner JA. Partial endoscopic resection with the CO_2 laser in laryngeal carcinomas. II. Results. Laryngorhinootologie 1995;74(5):294–9.

36. Shah JP. Skull base surgery: the first 50 years. European Archives of Oto-Rhino-Laryngology 2007;264(7):711–2.

37. Snyderman CH, Carrau RL, Kassam AB, et al. Endoscopic skull base surgery: Principles of endonasal oncological surgery. J Surg Oncol 2008;97(8):658–64.

38. Snyderman CH, Kassam AB, Carrau R, Mintz A. Endoscopic Reconstruction of Cranial Base Defects following Endonasal Skull Base Surgery. Skull Base 2007; 17(1):73.

39. Taylor GI, Daniel RK. The Free Flap;composite tissue transfer by vascular anastomosis. Aust N Z J Surg 1973;43(1):1–3.

40. Brown JS. Deep circumflex iliac artery free flap with internal oblique muscle as a new method of immediate reconstruction of maxillectomy defect. Head Neck Sep-Oct 1996;18(5):412–21.

41. Clark JR, Vesely M, Gilbert R. Scapular angle osteomyogenous flap in postmaxillectomy reconstruction: defect, reconstruction, shoulder function, and harvest technique. HEAD AND NECK 2008;30(1):10–20.

Incorporation of Molecularly Targeted Agents in the Primary Treatment of Squamous Cell Carcinomas of the Head and Neck

Jacques Bernier, MD, PD

KEYWORDS
- Head and neck • Molecularly targeted agents • Radiotherapy
- Chemotherapy • Squamous cell carcinoma

Head and neck cancers represent approximately 5% of all cancers worldwide.[1] Most head and neck cancers are squamous cell in origin and around 60% of patients will present with advanced disease (stage III or IV).[2] The treatment of patients who have locally advanced (stages III and IVa, b) squamous cell carcinomas of the head and neck (HNSCC) is generally curative in intent and approaches are multimodal, involving either surgery and adjuvant radiotherapy/chemoradiotherapy (CRT) or definitive radiotherapy/CRT. Induction chemotherapy before definitive therapy may be beneficial in patients who have resectable disease or for whom organ preservation is desirable.[3,4] The introduction of the concurrent delivery of chemo- and radiotherapy was a significant advance in the treatment of locally advanced disease, offering overall survival benefits compared with radiotherapy alone.[5,6] Improvements in treatment have also been made with the use of altered radiation fractionation regimens.[7] Although more efficacious in terms of treatment outcome, combining radiotherapy with chemotherapy and altering the radiation schedules are associated with an increase in acute toxicities compared with conventionally fractionated radiotherapy.[5,7–9] Attempts to change the doses and schedules of chemotherapy and radiotherapy need to be

The author has received remuneration for serving on advisory boards for Amgen, GlaxoSmithKline, Merck Serono, and Sanofi-Aventis.
Department of Radio-Oncology, Genolier Swiss Medical Network, CH 1272 Genolier, Switzerland
E-mail address: jbernier@genolier.net

performed within the constraints of tolerability and it is unlikely that, with current techniques, the resulting chemotherapy dose elevations or radiation intensification will lead to clinically relevant improvements in outcome. Testing novel cytostatic agents administered concomitantly with radiotherapy should therefore be encouraged.

The considerable variation in efficacy of, and toxicity to, a particular treatment approach among patients who have the same tumor type and stage according to conventional classification systems has driven the search for clinical and biologic factors that will help in the tailoring of appropriate treatment approaches.[10] The identification of molecular markers also presents the opportunity to use targeted agents directed at disrupting signaling pathways involved in the growth, development, and progression of tumors. The specificity of such agents offers the hope of improved antitumor activity with minimal toxicity to normal tissues. This article discusses the use of predictive and prognostic molecular markers in the initial treatment of locally advanced HNSCC.

PROGNOSTIC AND PREDICTIVE MOLECULAR MARKERS IN HEAD AND NECK CANCER

Given the complexity of the signaling pathways involved in head and neck cancer,[11] a host of molecular markers with potential prognostic and predictive value has been identified.[12] Several such markers appear more promising than others, and these include the epidermal growth factor receptor (EGFR), vascular endothelial growth factors (VEGF), and p53.

EGFR-mediated signaling by way of a complex of pathways is involved in cellular proliferation and differentiation in normal tissue. The EGFR is widely recognized as playing an important role in many malignancies, including those of the head and neck, in which it shows high expression in more than 90% of tumors.[13] EGFR expression has been associated with poor prognosis and poor response to treatment with chemotherapy or radiotherapy. Radiation stimulates EGFR signaling pathways and the EGFR may assist in the repopulation of clonogenic cells during fractionated radiation.[14] The usefulness of EGFR status in predicting the outcome of radiotherapy-based treatment in patients who have head and neck cancer has been demonstrated. In a study in patients receiving radiotherapy, high levels of tumor EGFR expression were associated with a reduction in disease-free and overall survival and an increase in locoregional relapse compared with patients who had lower tumor EGFR expression.[15] A similar association between tumor EGFR expression and overall survival was reported in patients who had unresectable pharyngeal cancer and were receiving cisplatin/5-fluorouracil (FU)-based CRT.[16] In a phase III study of 803 patients, incorporating a multivariate analysis, the use of moderately accelerated radiotherapy led to better locoregional control in tumors with high EGFR expression compared with tumors with lower EGFR expression.[17] The combination of high tumor EGFR expression and good/moderate tumor differentiation was associated with improved locoregional control and disease-specific survival following accelerated radiotherapy compared with tumors with low EGFR or poor differentiation.[17] Similar findings were reported for continuous hyperfractionated accelerated radiotherapy compared with conventionally fractionated radiotherapy.[18] The EGFR may also be predictive for tumor response to chemotherapy, with significantly higher levels of EGFR expression being reported in patients who had cisplatin-resistant HNSCC compared with those who had sensitive disease ($P = .04$).[19]

In addition, patients who have advanced HNSCC have been reported to show significantly elevated serum levels of VEGF,[20] and high serum or tumor tissue levels of VEGF expression are associated with poor survival.[21] Radiation-induced release of VEGF has been observed in a range of tumor cell lines, including HNSCC, and it is thought to be involved in promoting tumor cell survival.[22] The degree of radiation resistance corresponded with the absolute level and the relative increase in the level of VEGF.[22] The EGFR and VEGF pathways have some interaction and in vitro and in vivo studies have shown the addition of EGFR inhibitors leads to a reduction in the production of VEGF.[23] Furthermore, tumors that have developed resistance to prolonged administration of EGFR inhibitors have increased VEGF expression.[23]

High levels of the cell cycle regulatory protein cyclin D1, as a result of gene amplification, can lead to unregulated tumor cell proliferation. Increases in the levels of cellular cyclin D1 are associated with a poor prognosis in HNSCC.[24] Studies have shown that high levels are associated with increased resistance to cisplatin in HNSCC xenografts[25] and that transfection of HNSCC cells with antisense cyclin D1 increases cellular cisplatin sensitivity.[26] High levels of cyclin D1 are also associated with a reduction in the antitumor activity of the EGFR tyrosine kinase inhibitor gefitinib in HNSCC cell lines.[27] The tumor suppressor protein p53 is widely regarded as an important molecular marker in head and neck cancers,[28] and alterations in p53 function, frequently caused by gene mutations, are common in these cancers. High levels of p53 expression are associated with an increase in the incidence of all-cause and cancer-specific mortality in patients who have head and neck cancers compared with lower levels.[29] High-level p53 expression is predictive of a poor response to radiotherapy[29] and tumors with high-level p53 expression or p53 gene mutations are often resistant to chemotherapy.[30,31] In patients who had locally advanced HNSCC and received surgery with curative intent, those with tumors harboring TP53 mutations survived for a significantly shorter time than those without mutations (median survival 3.2 versus 5.4 months, hazard ratio 1.4, $P = .009$).[32]

MOLECULARLY TARGETED THERAPIES

As our knowledge of the molecular determinants of HNSCC widens, it is likely that biologic markers with predictive usefulness will be increasingly instrumental in determining appropriate treatment approaches in HNSCC. Currently, however, only a proportion of the markers identified have feasibility as potential therapeutic targets. Few molecularly targeted agents have entered clinical development for locally advanced head and neck cancer; data are available in the literature mainly from early phase trials and only one published trial reports the effects of targeted therapy in a phase III setting in locally advanced disease **(Table 1)**. Many of the targeted agents being investigated in clinical trials in head and neck cancers already have regulatory approval for the treatment of other malignancies.

Epidermal Growth Factor Receptor Inhibition

The largest bank of clinical data with molecularly targeted agents in the treatment of locally advanced head and neck cancer comes from the use of the EGFR inhibitors.

Cetuximab

To date, the only targeted therapy that has demonstrated significant improvements in the outcome of patients who have locally advanced HNSCC compared with standard therapy alone in a controlled, phase III trial, is the EGFR-targeting immunoglobulin (Ig) G1 monoclonal antibody (MAb) cetuximab (Erbitux). In this trial, reported by Bonner and colleagues,[33] 424 patients received a 6- to 7-week course of radiotherapy (once daily, twice daily or concomitant boost) either alone or in combination with cetuximab (400 mg/m[2] initial dose followed by subsequent doses of 250 mg/m[2]/week). The addition of cetuximab to radiotherapy significantly prolonged the duration of locoregional control compared with radiotherapy alone (hazard ratio for locoregional

Table 1
Targeted agents under clinical investigation in locally advanced squamous cell carcinoma of the head and neck

Type of Agent	Agent	Latest Phase of Development[a]			Selected ongoing Randomized Trials (Phase III unless Otherwise Specified)
		Phase I	Phase II	Phase III	
EGFR inhibitors	Cetuximab (Erbitux)		+ Platinum-based CRT [41] (71% 3-year LRC rate, 76% 3-year OS rate among 22 patients) + Platinum-based chemotherapy (induction) (65% pCR rate among 40 patients[42]) (95% response rate among 16 patients[43])	RT versus cetuximab/RT[33] (see **Table 2**)	Platinum-based CRT ± cetuximab Cetuximab + RT versus cetuximab + platinum-based CRT
	Panitumumab (Vectibix)	+ Platinum-based CRT[45] (4 CR among 4 patients)			
	Zalutumumab (HuMax-EGFr)		Single-agent in advanced HNSCC[46]		(C)RT ± zalutumumab
	Nimotuzumab (CIMAher, TheraCIM h-R3, Theraloc)	+ RT[47] (88% response rate among 16 patients)			
	Gefitinib (Iressa)		+ Platinum-based CRT[50] (52% CR rate among 46 patients) Docetaxel + carboplatin + gefitinib (induction)[51] (47% response rate among 60 patients)		Platinum-based CRT ± gefitinib

	Erlotinib (Tarceva)	+ Cisplatin-based CRT[53] (84% pCR rate among 25 patients)	CRT ± erlotinib (phase II) Erlotinib post-CRT in resected patients
VEGF inhibitor	Bevacizumab (Avastin)	+ Docetaxel-based CRT[63] (75% CR rate among 12 patients)	
Multitargeted agents	Lapatinib (Tyverb)	+ Cisplatin-based CRT[66]	Cisplatin-based CRT ± lapatinib (phase II)
	Vandetanib (Zactima)		Docetaxel ± vandetanib (phase II)
Proteasome inhibitor	Bortezomib (Velcade)	Early phase studies ongoing	

Abbreviations: CR, complete response; LRC, locoregional control; OS, overall survival; pCR, complete pathologic response; RT, radiotherapy.
[a] Based on findings from the literature (from PubMed database and ASCO abstracts).

progression 0.68, P = .005). The median duration of locoregional control was 24.4 months with radiotherapy plus cetuximab and 14.9 months with radiotherapy alone. Patients in the cetuximab arm also had a statistically significant 26% reduction in the risk for death compared with those receiving radiotherapy (hazard ratio 0.74, P = .03). The median duration of overall survival was 49 months in the cetuximab arm and 29.3 months in the radiotherapy alone arm. The investigators noted that the clinical benefits of cetuximab appeared to be independent of tumor stage, primary tumor site, and type of radiation. In addition, the improvements in outcome were not associated with any statistically significant increase in the incidence of toxicities greater than or equal to grade 3, commonly associated with radiotherapy, including radiation-induced dermatitis. The only adverse events greater than or equal to grade 3 that differed in incidence between the treatment arms were acneiform rash and infusion reactions, both of which were reported significantly more frequently in the cetuximab arm (acneiform rash 17% versus 1%, P < .001, and infusion reactions 3% versus 0%, P = .01). Both events are associated with EGFR inhibitors or monoclonal antibodies. Several studies in patients receiving cetuximab plus chemotherapy for recurrent or metastatic HNSCC have reported a positive relationship between the development or grade of skin reactions and outcome (in terms of progression-free survival, overall survival, or time to progression).[34–36] Whether such a relationship exists in patients receiving cetuximab in combination with radiotherapy remains to be seen.

A separate analysis of the data from Bonner and colleagues[37] reported that adding cetuximab to radiotherapy did not adversely affect quality of life. The tolerability of the cetuximab/radiotherapy combination reported in the Bonner trial was reflected in the good treatment compliance recorded. Most (90%) of the patients receiving cetuximab received all planned doses and cetuximab did not interfere with the delivery of radiotherapy as scheduled.

The results achieved with cetuximab plus radiotherapy in the Bonner trial led to the regulatory approval of this combination as an alternative to CRT. The option to treat a patient with either cetuximab plus radiotherapy or with CRT is currently at the discretion of the treating physician.

To define further the relative roles of radiotherapy plus cetuximab and CRT in locally advanced disease, a comparison of the efficacy and tolerability of the two approaches is necessary. To date, no phase III trial has directly compared radiotherapy plus cetuximab with CRT. However, between-study comparison of phase III trials shows that the survival advantage over radiotherapy alone of adding cetuximab to radiotherapy is similar to that achieved with CRT (20 months and up to 18 months, respectively).[5,6,33,38,39] Bonner and colleagues[33] sought to put the clinical benefit achieved with cetuximab into context with CRT. They conducted a retrospective analysis of data comparing the outcome of 29 patients who had locally advanced HNSCC and were receiving radiotherapy plus cetuximab with that of 103 patients who were receiving cisplatin-based CRT at a single center.[40] No significant difference was shown between radiotherapy plus cetuximab and CRT in terms of 3-year rates of locoregional control (71% versus 75%), distant metastasis-free survival (92% versus 87%), and disease-specific survival (79% versus 77%). Three-year overall survival was significantly higher in the radiotherapy plus cetuximab group compared with the CRT group (76% versus 61%, P = .02) (**Table 2**). However, the treatment groups showed no significant difference in overall survival when controlling for T stage, an important factor, considering that the proportion of patients who had T4 tumors was higher in the CRT group and T stage was an independent predictor of survival. The investigators highlighted the fact that patients who received either radiotherapy plus cetuximab or CRT within a clinical trial (protocol patients) had significantly better survival than

Table 2
Comparison of the effects of radiotherapy, radiotherapy plus cetuximab, and chemoradiotherapy on 3-year locoregional control rates and overall survival of patients who had locally advanced squamous cell carcinoma of the head and neck: results from a multicenter, prospective, randomized trial and a single-center retrospective analysis

| End Point | Multicenter, Multinational Prospective, Randomized Trial[33] | | | Single-Center, Retrospective Analysis[40] | | | | | |
	RT (n = 213)	RT + Cetuximab (n = 211)	P	RT + Cetuximab (n = 29)	All CRT (n = 103)	P	CRT Protocol (n = 43)	CRT Nonprotocol (n = 60)	P
3-y LRC, %	34	47	<0.01	71	75	0.98	72	77	0.850
3-y OS, %	45	55	0.05	76	61	0.02	68	57	0.002

Abbreviations: LRC, locoregional control; RT, radiotherapy; OS, overall survival.

nonprotocol CRT patients ($P = .001$ and $P = .01$, respectively). However, overall survival was no different between the protocol patients receiving radiotherapy plus cetuximab or CRT. The investigators also acknowledged the increase in the locoregional control and overall survival observed in this analysis of a single center in the United States compared with the international phase III trial, which they said reflects findings in the literature comparing United States and international trials. In the absence of a phase III trial, the analysis provides convincing support for the efficacy benefits of cetuximab plus radiotherapy compared with CRT. These findings, combined with the favorable tolerability profile of radiotherapy plus cetuximab, support the use of this combination as an alternative to CRT in locally advanced HNSCC.

In light of the additive effects reported for combinations of cetuximab and chemotherapy or radiotherapy, both in vitro and in vivo, and from clinical studies in head and neck cancer, it was a logical step to investigate the combination of cetuximab and CRT in locally advanced disease. In a pilot phase II study in 22 patients, the use of weekly cetuximab with cisplatin and concomitant boost radiotherapy led to 3-year locoregional control and overall survival rates of 71% and 76%, respectively.[41] The study was terminated early when adverse events raised safety concerns, although this was a cautionary measure because the investigators were unable to establish a causal link between cetuximab and the adverse events. As highlighted by Bonner and colleagues,[33] the 3-year locoregional control rate of 71% reported in this phase II study was the same as that observed with radiotherapy plus cetuximab in their single-center analysis, and similar to that achieved with CRT alone in the same analysis. Two phase III trials are investigating the combination of cetuximab and CRT in locally advanced HNSCC. The first trial is being conducted by the Radiation Therapy Oncology Group and compares the use of the cisplatin-based CRT regimen described in the phase II trial,[41] with and without cetuximab. The second trial was initiated early in 2008 by the Groupe Oncologie Radiotherapie Tete et Cou and aims to compare the effects, primarily on progression-free survival, of radiotherapy plus cetuximab with those of cetuximab combined with carboplatin/5-FU-based CRT.

Cetuximab has also shown good antitumor activity when used as neoadjuvant therapy in locally advanced HNSCC. The combination of cetuximab with paclitaxel and carboplatin in operable, locally advanced disease was associated with a complete pathologic response rate of 65% among 40 patients.[42] The subsequent addition of cetuximab to the definitive CRT regimen of paclitaxel, carboplatin, and radiotherapy led to a complete pathologic response rate of 100% among the patients sampled. In another study, induction therapy comprising cetuximab, docetaxel, and cisplatin led to an overall response rate of 94% among 16 evaluable patients who had stage II to IV disease.[43] Recently reported randomized trials have demonstrated that a triple combination of taxane, platinum, and 5-FU (TPF) is more active as induction therapy than platinum and S-Fu alone.[3,4] A retrospective analysis of patients receiving cetuximab in combination with induction TPF reported a tumor response rate of 71%, with a complete response rate of 14%.[44] In all studies, the incorporation of cetuximab into induction therapy did not compromise the subsequent administration of definitive therapy.

Other epidermal growth factor receptor–targeted monoclonal antibodies

Initial results from part 1 of a two-part phase I study, involving eight patients, suggested that the fully human EGFR-targeted IgG2 MAb, panitumumab (Vectibix), can be added to paclitaxel/carboplatin-based CRT in locally advanced HNSCC.[45] The incidence of grade 3/4 mucositis and radiation dermatitis was 75% each. Four patients evaluated for response had a complete response in the primary tumor. Zalutumumab (HuMax-EGFr), another fully human EGFR-targeted MAb, has shown activity as a single agent in a phase I/II study in advanced HNSCC.[46] The Danish Head and Neck Cancer Group is performing a phase III study comparing the effects on locoregional control of radiotherapy (or CRT) with radiotherapy (or CRT) plus zalutumumab. Combination of the humanized EGFR-targeted MAb, nimotuzumab (CIMAher, Thera-CIM h-R3, Theraloc), with radiotherapy in patients who have unresectable head and neck cancer has also been shown to have activity in this setting.[47] Nimotuzumab appears to differ from other EGFR inhibitors in that it does not appear to cause the acnelike rash that is so common with EGFR-targeted MAbs and tyrosine kinase inhibitors.[47]

Epidermal growth factor receptor tyrosine kinase inhibitors

The use of gefitinib (Iressa) in combination with CRT in locally advanced disease has been reported in two phase I studies[48,49] and one phase II study.[50] In the phase II study, the combination of gefitinib (250 mg/day) with cisplatin and accelerated radiotherapy was active, with a complete response rate of 52% among 46 patients.[50] The incidence of grade 3/4 toxicity was in line with that expected from the individual agents. A randomized phase II trial comparing cisplatin-based CRT with or without gefitinib (at doses of 250 mg/day and 500 mg/day) in the treatment of locally advanced HNSCC was due to be completed in May 2008. A phase I/II trial has also reported the inclusion of gefitinib into induction therapy with docetaxel and carboplatin to be feasible.[51] Of 60 patients, 47% achieved a response to induction therapy. Gefitinib was also added to the subsequent CRT regimen of conventionally fractionated radiotherapy and docetaxel, and at the end of treatment, the response rate was 67% among 51 patients. The combination of erlotinib (Tarceva) and CRT has also been shown to be active and feasible. In a phase I study of erlotinib plus docetaxel-based conventionally fractionated CRT, 15 of 18 patients achieved a complete response.[52] Results from a phase II study demonstrated encouraging activity with a combination of erlotinib and cisplatin-based conventionally fractionated CRT.[53] Twenty-one of 25 patients (84%) achieved a complete pathologic response. The rates of grade 3/4 in field dermatitis, nausea, and mucositis were 56%, 52%, and 36%, respectively. The effects of adding erlotinib to cisplatin-based CRT are now being investigated in a randomized phase II trial. In addition, a phase III trial is investigating the effects of administering erlotinib post-CRT in patients who have resected HNSCC.

Tailoring the Use of Epidermal Growth Factor Receptor Inhibitors

Molecular tumor markers will have an important role to play in tailoring treatment with targeted agents. For the EGFR inhibitors, the most promising candidate markers identified in studies in other solid tumor types are EGFR and Kirsten ras (KRAS) mutations. In non–small cell lung cancer (NSCLC), somatic mutations in the tyrosine kinase domain of the EGFR were shown to be predictive of response to treatment with EGFR tyrosine kinase inhibitors in pretreated patients[54] and in the first-line setting.[55] Studies in NSCLC and colorectal cancer have demonstrated that tumors carrying mutations in the KRAS gene respond poorly to treatment with EGFR inhibitors.[55–57] In one study in NSCLC, the addition of erlotinib to platinum-based therapy led to a significant reduction in overall survival compared with chemotherapy alone (*P*<.019) among patients who had tumors with KRAS mutations.[55] In a Southwestern Oncology Group study in patients who had NSCLC and were receiving docetaxel-based CRT, patients randomized to receive gefitinib as post-CRT maintenance therapy had a significantly shorter survival than those receiving placebo.[58] No reasons were obvious for this effect, but the influence of KRAS mutations and an interaction between the effects of radiation and EGFR signaling were raised by the investigators as areas worth exploring. It is not clear how applicable the findings from other tumors are to the HNSCC setting. Certainly, studies suggest the absence of tumor EGFR tyrosine kinase mutations[59] and KRAS mutations,[60,61] as previously described for NSCLC and CRC, in head and neck cancers, and so they could be expected to have little influence on treatment efficacy. The negative effect on survival of gefitinib post-CRT in NSCLC raises the possibility that treatment scheduling may play an important role in the efficacy of EGFR inhibitors in combination with other treatment modalities. It will be interesting to observe the results of the phase III trial in which erlotinib is being administered after CRT in patients who have resected HNSCC. Some evidence suggests an interaction between the scheduling of radiation and cetuximab in studies on A431 tumor xenografts, which demonstrated that the administration of cetuximab during and after radiation led to greater antitumor activity than the administration of cetuximab before and during radiation.[62] Whether the scheduling of EGFR inhibitors with respect to CRT affects outcome in the head and neck setting remains to be seen.

VASCULAR ENDOTHELIAL GROWTH FACTOR INHIBITION

A phase II study in 12 patients showed the VEGF inhibitor bevacizumab (Avastin) in combination with docetaxel and standard once-daily radiotherapy to be a feasible approach, with 9/12 complete responses.[63] In a phase I study in patients who had poor prognosis head and neck cancer (recurrent and treatment naïve), the addition of bevacizumab to 5-FU plus hydroxyurea-based CRT demonstrated activity.[64] However, the association of bevacizumab with side effects including fistula formation (11%) and ulceration/tissue necrosis (9%) was uncertain. The activity of bevacizumab in locally advanced HNSCC is being investigated in several phase II studies.

In vitro studies have shown the activity of a triple combination of a novel VEGF inhibitor, AZD2171 (Recentin), gefitinib, and radiation in a VEGF-secreting, EGFR-expressing head and neck tumor xenograft.[65] The triple combination reduced cell proliferation markedly, and beyond that achieved with radiotherapy alone or AZD2171 plus gefitinib.

AGENTS DIRECTED AT MULTIPLE MOLECULAR TARGETS

Lapatinib (Tyverb), a dual inhibitor of EGFR and human EGFR 2 tyrosine kinase activity, has been investigated in combination with cisplatin-based CRT in a phase I study in patients who had locally advanced disease.[66] A randomized, phase II trial comparing cisplatin-based CRT with or without lapatinib is ongoing.

Vandetanib (Zactima) is a dual VEGF receptor/EGFR tyrosine kinase inhibitor that has shown antitumor efficacy in HNSCC xenografts.[67] The antitumor activity of single-agent vandetanib appears to be confined to EGFR-expressing tumor xenografts.[68] Although the combination of vandetanib and radiation was active in both EGFR-expressing and nonexpressing tumors, activity was schedule dependent in EGFR nonexpressing tumors, such that concomitant application was more active than vandetanib given before or after radiation. Vandetanib is currently being investigated in combination with docetaxel in a randomized phase II study in patients who have locally advanced HNSCC (with or without metastases) not amenable to treatment with surgery or radiotherapy.

OTHER MOLECULARLY TARGETED AGENTS

Proteasomes are critical to the regulation of a wide variety of proteins involved in cell cycle regulation (including cyclin-dependent kinases), apoptosis (including nuclear factor κB), and angiogenesis. Bortezomib (Velcade) is a proteasome inhibitor that is currently licensed for the treatment of hematologic malignancies. Data from a phase I study investigating the combination of bortezomib and radiotherapy in patients receiving reirradiation for recurrent HNSCC[69] suggest that, although the dosing regimens investigated were not clinically useful in this study, with the use of alternative schedules, this approach may be suitable for investigation in the context of primary radiotherapy.[69] Several studies are investigating the combination of bortezomib and cetuximab in the treatment of solid tumors, including locally advanced HNSCC.

SUMMARY

Increasing numbers of clinical studies are identifying molecular markers that indicate patient prognosis and the likelihood of a tumor responding to particular treatments or that provide an opportunity for direct, potentially therapeutic targeting. To date, although the data are persuasive, the use of prognostic and predictive markers that can direct treatment with radiotherapy or CRT in patients who have HNSCC remains investigational. However, the use of biologic agents directed at potentially therapeutic molecular targets now forms an integral part of treatment of several malignancies. The first, and currently only, biologic agent to be given regulatory approval in Europe or the United States for the treatment of locally advanced HNSCC in combination with radiotherapy is the EGFR antagonist, cetuximab. The combination of cetuximab and radiotherapy led to statistically and clinically significant benefits over radiotherapy alone and was well tolerated. Radiotherapy plus cetuximab provides us with a valuable treatment option in this setting, although its place opposite CRT in the treatment algorithm has not been defined. It is up to the treating physician to decide which is the most appropriate approach. Because the two treatment approaches are not being compared in a definitive trial, we must turn to retrospective comparisons for interpretation, and such comparisons indicate that the efficacy of radiotherapy plus cetuximab, and CRT, are similar. Radiotherapy plus cetuximab has in its favor a better tolerability profile than CRT, although skin reactions may be a problem for some patients. As a matter of fact, the efficacy results and safety profile observed so far strongly suggest that adding cetuximab to radiotherapy significantly increases the therapeutic index of this latter modality. The cost of treatment will also be a consideration. Results from ongoing trials will tell us if the addition of cetuximab improves the efficacy of CRT, without exacerbating toxicities. The clinical investigation of other molecularly targeted agents in locally advanced HNSCC has lagged behind that of cetuximab. Several phase III or randomized phase II trials are ongoing with several of these agents, but it is likely to be some time before we have the results showing how they perform in a randomized setting.

REFERENCES

1. Parkin DM, Bray F, Ferlay J, et al. Global cancer statistics, 2002. CA Cancer J Clin 2005;55(2):74–108.
2. Vernham GA, Crowther JA. Head and neck carcinoma–stage at presentation. Clin Otolaryngol Allied Sci 1994;19(2):120–4.
3. Posner MR, Hershock DM, Blajman CR, et al. Cisplatin and fluorouracil alone or with docetaxel in head and neck cancer. N Engl J Med 2007;357(17):1705–15.
4. Vermorken JB, Remenar E, van Herpen C, et al. Cisplatin, fluorouracil, and docetaxel in unresectable head and neck cancer. N Engl J Med 2007;357(17): 1695–704.

5. Calais G, Alfonsi M, Bardet E, et al. Randomized trial of radiation therapy versus concomitant chemotherapy and radiation therapy for advanced-stage oropharynx carcinoma. J Natl Cancer Inst 1999;91(24):2081–6.

6. Huguenin P, Beer KT, Allal A, et al. Concomitant cisplatin significantly improves locoregional control in advanced head and neck cancers treated with hyperfractionated radiotherapy. J Clin Oncol 2004;22(23):4665–73.

7. Fu KK, Pajak TF, Trotti A, et al. A Radiation Therapy Oncology Group (RTOG) phase III randomized study to compare hyperfractionation and two variants of accelerated fractionation to standard fractionation radiotherapy for head and neck squamous cell carcinomas: first report of RTOG 9003. Int J Radiat Oncol Biol Phys 2000;48(1):7–16.

8. Bernier J, Domenge C, Ozsahin M, et al. Postoperative irradiation with or without concomitant chemotherapy for locally advanced head and neck cancer. N Engl J Med 2004;350(19):1945–52.

9. Cooper JS, Pajak TF, Forastiere AA, et al. Postoperative concurrent radiotherapy and chemotherapy for high-risk squamous-cell carcinoma of the head and neck. N Engl J Med 2004;350(19):1937–44.

10. Almadori G, Bussu F, Paludetti G. Should there be more molecular staging of head and neck cancer to improve the choice of treatments and thereby improve survival? Curr Opin Otolaryngol Head Neck Surg 2008;16(2):117–26.

11. Perez-Ordonez B, Beauchemin M, Jordan RC. Molecular biology of squamous cell carcinoma of the head and neck. J Clin Pathol 2006;59(5):445–53.

12. Lothaire P, de Azambuja E, Dequanter D, et al. Molecular markers of head and neck squamous cell carcinoma: promising signs in need of prospective evaluation. Head Neck 2006;28(3):256–69.

13. Waksal HW. Role of an anti-epidermal growth factor receptor in treating cancer. Cancer Metastasis Rev 1999;18(4):427–36.

14. Petersen C, Eicheler W, Frommel A, et al. Proliferation and micromilieu during fractionated irradiation of human FaDu squamous cell carcinoma in nude mice. Int J Radiat Biol 2003;79(7):469–77.

15. Ang KK, Berkey BA, Tu X, et al. Impact of epidermal growth factor receptor expression on survival and pattern of relapse in patients with advanced head and neck carcinoma. Cancer Res 2002;62(24):7350–6.

16. Magne N, Pivot X, Bensadoun RJ, et al. The relationship of epidermal growth factor receptor levels to the prognosis of unresectable pharyngeal cancer patients treated by chemo-radiotherapy. Eur J Cancer 2001;37(17):2169–77.

17. Eriksen JG, Steiniche T, Overgaard J. The influence of epidermal growth factor receptor and tumor differentiation on the response to accelerated radiotherapy of squamous cell carcinomas of the head and neck in the randomized DAHANCA 6 and 7 study. Radiother Oncol 2005;74(2):93–100.

18. Bentzen SM, Atasoy BM, Daley FM, et al. Epidermal growth factor receptor expression in pretreatment biopsies from head and neck squamous cell carcinoma as a predictive factor for a benefit from accelerated radiation therapy in a randomized controlled trial. J Clin Oncol 2005;23(24):5560–7.

19. Hasegawa Y, Goto M, Hanai N, et al. Prediction of chemosensitivity using multigene analysis in head and neck squamous cell carcinoma. Oncology 2007;73(1–2):104–11.

20. Teknos TN, Cox C, Yoo S, et al. Elevated serum vascular endothelial growth factor and decreased survival in advanced laryngeal carcinoma. Head Neck 2002; 24(11):1004–11.

21. Tse GM, Chan AW, Yu KH, et al. Strong immunohistochemical expression of vascular endothelial growth factor predicts overall survival in head and neck squamous cell carcinoma. Ann Surg Oncol 2007;14(12):3558–65.

22. Brieger J, Kattwinkel J, Berres M, et al. Impact of vascular endothelial growth factor release on radiation resistance. Oncol Rep 2007;18(6):1597–601.

23. Ciardiello F, Troiani T, Bianco R, et al. Interaction between the epidermal growth factor receptor (EGFR) and the vascular endothelial growth factor (VEGF) pathways: a rational approach for multi-target anticancer therapy. Ann Oncol 2006; 17(Suppl 7):vii109–14.

24. Michalides RJ, van Veelen NM, Kristel PM, et al. Overexpression of cyclin D1 indicates a poor prognosis in squamous cell carcinoma of the head and neck. Arch Otolaryngol Head Neck Surg 1997;123(5):497–502.

25. Henriksson E, Baldetorp B, Borg A, et al. p53 mutation and cyclin D1 amplification correlate with cisplatin sensitivity in xenografted human squamous cell carcinomas from head and neck. Acta Oncol 2006;45(3):300–5.

26. Wang MB, Yip HT, Srivatsan ES. Antisense cyclin D1 enhances sensitivity of head and neck cancer cells to cisplatin. Laryngoscope 2001;111(6):982–8.

27. Kalish LH, Kwong RA, Cole IE, et al. Deregulated cyclin D1 expression is associated with decreased efficacy of the selective epidermal growth factor receptor tyrosine kinase inhibitor gefitinib in head and neck squamous cell carcinoma cell lines. Clin Cancer Res 2004;10(22):7764–74.

28. Partridge M, Costea DE, Huang X. The changing face of p53 in head and neck cancer. Int J Oral Maxillofac Surg 2007;36(12):1123–38.

29. Geisler SA, Olshan AF, Weissler MC, et al. p16 and p53 protein expression as prognostic indicators of survival and disease recurrence from head and neck cancer. Clin Cancer Res 2002;8(11):3445–53.

30. Lassaletta L, Brandariz JA, Benito A, et al. p53 expression in locally advanced pharyngeal squamous cell carcinoma. Arch Otolaryngol Head Neck Surg 1999; 125(12):1356–9.

31. Cabelguenne A, Blons H, de Waziers I, et al. p53 alterations predict tumor response to neoadjuvant chemotherapy in head and neck squamous cell carcinoma: a prospective series. J Clin Oncol 2000;18(7):1465–73.

32. Poeta ML, Manola J, Goldwasser MA, et al. TP53 mutations and survival in squamous-cell carcinoma of the head and neck. N Engl J Med 2007;357(25):2552–61.

33. Bonner JA, Harari PM, Giralt J, et al. Radiotherapy plus cetuximab for squamous-cell carcinoma of the head and neck. N Engl J Med 2006;354(6):567–78.

34. Baselga J, Trigo JM, Bourhis J, et al. Phase II multicenter study of the anti-epidermal growth factor receptor (EGFR) monoclonal antibody cetuximab in combination with platinum-based chemotherapy in patients with platinum-refractory metastatic and/or recurrent squamous cell carcinoma of the head and neck (SCCHN). J Clin Oncol 2005;23:5568–77.

35. Burtness B, Goldwasser MA, Flood W, et al. Phase III randomized trial of cisplatin plus placebo compared with cisplatin plus cetuximab in metastatic/recurrent head and neck cancer: an Eastern Cooperative Oncology Group study. J Clin Oncol 2005;23(34):8646–54.

36. Herbst RS, Arquette M, Shin DM, et al. Phase II multicenter study of the epidermal growth factor receptor antibody cetuximab and cisplatin for recurrent and refractory squamous cell carcinoma of the head and neck. J Clin Oncol 2005;23(24): 5578–87.

37. Curran D, Giralt J, Harari PM, et al. Quality of life in head and neck cancer patients after treatment with high-dose radiotherapy alone or in combination with cetuximab. J Clin Oncol 2007;25(16):2191–7.
38. Budach VG, Stuschke M, Budach W, et al. Accelerated hyperfractionated chemoradiation (C-HART) plus 5-FU/MMC is superior to HART for inoperable locally advanced head and neck cancer. Final results of the German ARO 95-06 multicentre trial. J Clin Oncol 2004;22(14S) [Abstract 5503].
39. Semrau R, Mueller RP, Stuetzer H, et al. Efficacy of intensified hyperfractionated and accelerated radiotherapy and concurrent chemotherapy with carboplatin and 5-fluorouracil: updated results of a randomized multicentric trial in advanced head-and-neck cancer. Int J Radiat Oncol Biol Phys 2006;64(5):1308–16.
40. Caudell JJ, Sawrie SM, Spencer SA, et al. Locoregionally advanced head and neck cancer treated with primary radiotherapy: a comparison of the addition of cetuximab or chemotherapy and the impact of protocol treatment. Int J Radiat Oncol Biol Phys 2008 [E-pub].
41. Pfister DG, Su YB, Kraus DH, et al. Concurrent cetuximab, cisplatin, and concomitant boost radiotherapy for locoregionally advanced, squamous cell head and neck cancer: a pilot phase II study of a new combined-modality paradigm. J Clin Oncol 2006;24(7):1072–8.
42. Wanebo HJ, Ghebremichael M, Burtness B, et al. Phase II evaluation of cetuximab (C225) combined with induction paclitaxel and carboplatin followed by C225, paclitaxel, carboplatin, and radiation for stage III/IV operable squamous cancer of the head and neck (ECOG, E2303). J Clin Oncol 2007;25(18S) [Abstract 6015].
43. Argiris A, Karamouzis MV, Heron DE, et al. Phase II trial of docetaxel (T), cisplatin (P), and cetuximab (E) followed by concurrent radiation (RT), P, and E in locally advanced head and neck squamous cell carcinoma (HNSCC). J Clin Oncol 2007;25(18S) [Abstract 6051].
44. Kuperman DI, Nussenbaum B, Thorstad W, et al. Retrospective analysis of the addition of cetuximab to induction chemotherapy (IC) with docetaxel, cisplatin and 5-fluorouracil (TPF-C) for locally advanced squamous cell carcinoma of the head and neck (LA-HNSCC). J Clin Oncol 2007;25(18S) [Abstract 6072 and virtual presentation]. Available at: http://www.asco.org/ASCO/Abstracts+%26+Virtual+Meeting/Abstracts?&vmview=abst_detail_view&confID=47&abstractID=35471#.
45. Wirth LJ, Posner MR, Tishler RB, et al. Phase I study of panitumumab, chemotherapy and intensity-modulated radiotherapy (IMRT) for head and neck cancer (HNC): early results. J Clin Oncol 2007;25(18S) [Abstract 6083].
46. Bastholt L, Specht L, Jensen K, et al. Phase I/II clinical and pharmacokinetic study evaluating a fully human monoclonal antibody against EGFr (HuMax-EGFr) in patients with advanced squamous cell carcinoma of the head and neck. Radiother Oncol 2007;85(1):24–8.
47. Crombet T, Osorio M, Cruz T, et al. Use of the humanized anti-epidermal growth factor receptor monoclonal antibody h-R3 in combination with radiotherapy in the treatment of locally advanced head and neck cancer patients. J Clin Oncol 2004;22(9):1646–54.
48. Chen C, Kane M, Song J, et al. Phase I trial of gefitinib in combination with radiation or chemoradiation for patients with locally advanced squamous cell head and neck cancer. J Clin Oncol 2007;25(31):4880–6.
49. Morris JC, Allen CT, Citrin D, et al. Pilot phase I study of gefitinib (GEF) in combination with paclitaxel (PAC) and radiation therapy (RT) in patients with locally advanced head and neck squamous cell carcinoma (HNSCC) and effects on

epidermal growth factor receptor (EGFR) signaling pathway. J Clin Oncol 2007; 25(18S) [Abstract 16526].

50. Rueda A, Medina JA, Mesia R, et al. Gefitinib plus concomitant boost accelerated radiation (AFX-CB) and concurrent weekly cisplatin for locally advanced unresectable squamous cell head and neck carcinomas (SCCHN): a phase II study. J Clin Oncol 2007;25(18S) [Abstract 6031].

51. Doss HH, Greco FA, Meluch AA, et al. Induction chemotherapy + gefitinib followed by concurrent chemotherapy/radiation therapy/gefitinib for patients (pts) with locally advanced squamous carcinoma of the head and neck: a phase I/II trial of the Minnie Pearl Cancer Research Network. J Clin Oncol 2006;24(18S) [Abstract 5543].

52. Savvides P, Agarwala SS, Greskovich J, et al. Phase I study of the EGFR tyrosine kinase inhibitor erlotinib in combination with docetaxel and radiation in locally advanced squamous cell cancer of the head and neck (SCCHN). J Clin Oncol 2006;25(18S) [Abstract 5545].

53. Herchenhorn D, Dias FL, Pineda RM, et al. Phase II study of erlotinib combined with cisplatin and radiotherapy for locally advanced squamous cell carcinoma of the head and neck (SCCHN). J Clin Oncol 2007;25(18S) [Abstract 6033].

54. Lynch TJ, Bell DW, Sordella R, et al. Activating mutations in the epidermal growth factor receptor underlying responsiveness of non-small-cell lung cancer to gefitinib. N Engl J Med 2004;350(21):2129–39.

55. Eberhard DA, Johnson BE, Amler LC, et al. Mutations in the epidermal growth factor receptor and in KRAS are predictive and prognostic indicators in patients with non-small-cell lung cancer treated with chemotherapy alone and in combination with erlotinib. J Clin Oncol 2005;23(25):5900–9.

56. De Roock W, Piessevaux H, De Schutter J, et al. KRAS wild-type state predicts survival and is associated to early radiological response in metastatic colorectal cancer treated with cetuximab. Ann Oncol 2008;19(3):508–15.

57. Amado RG, Wolf M, Peeters M, et al. Wild-type KRAS is required for panitumumab efficacy in patients with metastatic colorectal cancer. J Clin Oncol 2008; 26(10):1626–34.

58. Kelly K, Chansky K, Gaspar LE, et al. Phase III trial of maintenance gefitinib or placebo after concurrent chemoradiotherapy and docetaxel consolidation in inoperable stage III non-small-cell lung cancer: SWOG S0023. J Clin Oncol 2008 [E-pub].

59. Cohen EE, Lingen MW, Martin LE, et al. Response of some head and neck cancers to epidermal growth factor receptor tyrosine kinase inhibitors may be linked to mutation of ERBB2 rather than EGFR. Clin Cancer Res 2005;11(22): 8105–8.

60. Anderson JA, Irish JC, Ngan BY. Prevalence of RAS oncogene mutation in head and neck carcinomas. J Otolaryngol 1992;21(5):321–6.

61. Yarbrough WG, Shores C, Witsell DL, et al. Ras mutations and expression in head and neck squamous cell carcinomas. Laryngoscope 1994;104(11 Pt 1):1337–47.

62. Milas L, Fang FM, Mason KA, et al. Importance of maintenance therapy in C225-induced enhancement of tumor control by fractionated radiation. Int J Radiat Oncol Biol Phys 2007;67(2):568–72.

63. Savvides P, Greskovich J, Bokar J, et al. Phase II study of bevacizumab in combination with docetaxel and radiation in locally advanced squamous cell cancer of the head and neck (SCCHN). J Clin Oncol 2007;25(18S) [Abstract 6068].

64. Seiwert TY, Haraf DJ, Cohen EE, et al. A phase I study of bevacizumab (B) with fluorouracil (F) and hydroxyurea (H) with concomitant radiotherapy (X) (B-FHX)

for poor prognosis head and neck cancer (HNC). J Clin Oncol 2007;24(18S) [Abstract 5530].

65. Bozec A, Formento P, Lassalle S, et al. Dual inhibition of EGFR and VEGFR pathways in combination with irradiation: antitumour supra-additive effects on human head and neck cancer xenografts. Br J Cancer 2007;97(1):65–72.

66. Harrington KJ, Bourhis J, Nutting CM, et al. A phase I, open-label study of lapatinib plus chemoradiation in patients with locally advanced squamous cell carcinoma of the head and neck (SCCHN). J Clin Oncol 2006;24(18S) [Abstract 5553].

67. Sano D, Kawakami M, Fujita K, et al. Antitumor effects of ZD6474 on head and neck squamous cell carcinoma. Oncol Rep 2007;17(2):289–95.

68. Gustafson DL, Frederick B, Merz AL, et al. Dose scheduling of the dual VEGFR and EGFR tyrosine kinase inhibitor vandetanib (ZD6474, Zactima) in combination with radiotherapy in EGFR-positive and EGFR-null human head and neck tumor xenografts. Cancer Chemother Pharmacol 2008;61(2):179–88.

69. Van Waes C, Chang AA, Lebowitz PF, et al. Inhibition of nuclear factor-kappaB and target genes during combined therapy with proteasome inhibitor bortezomib and reirradiation in patients with recurrent head-and-neck squamous cell carcinoma. Int J Radiat Oncol Biol Phys 2005;63(5):1400–12.

Molecularly Targeted Agents in the Treatment of Recurrent or Metastatic Squamous Cell Carcinomas of the Head and Neck

Christophe Le Tourneau, MD, PhD, Eric X. Chen, MD, PhD*

KEYWORDS

- Head and neck cancer • Targeted agents
- Clinical development • EGFR • VEGFR
- Molecular targets

Despite decades of research, therapeutic options are limited for patients who have recurrent or metastatic squamous cell carcinoma of the head and neck (SCCHN). Currently, the most active regimens combining either cisplatin or carboplatin with fluorouracil (FU) or a taxane have been associated with a 30% response rate, a 3- to 4-month median progression-free survival, and a median overall survival of 6 to 8 months.[1] However, cytotoxic treatment is associated with frequent and severe toxicities and treatment-related mortality in this patient population. For patients who experience treatment failure with first-line therapy for recurrent or metastatic disease, retrospective analysis has demonstrated a median overall survival of 3 to 4 months even with treatment, underscoring the aggressiveness of this malignancy and the need for more effective therapies.

Interest has been substantial in developing novel agents that specifically modulate growth factor and signaling pathways that are dysregulated in tumor cells. Cetuximab, a monoclonal antibody that targets the epidermal growth factor receptor (EGFR), was the first molecularly targeted agent to be approved for clinical use in combination with radiation therapy for patients who have locally advanced SCCHN, based on a phase III trial that demonstrated an overall survival benefit compared with radiation alone.[2] It has also been approved as monotherapy for patients who have recurrent or metastatic

Christophe Le Tourneau is supported in part by a grant from the Fondation de France.

Drug Development Program, Department of Medical Oncology and Hematology, Princess Margaret Hospital, University of Toronto, Room 5-719, 610 University Avenue, Toronto, Ontario M5G2M9, Canada

* Corresponding author.

E-mail address: eric.chen@uhn.on.ca (E. Chen).

Hematol Oncol Clin N Am 22 (2008) 1209–1220
doi:10.1016/j.hoc.2008.08.002
0889-8588/08/$ – see front matter © 2008 Elsevier Inc. All rights reserved.

SCCHN and have progressed on platinum-based therapy, based on an open-label, multicenter phase II trial.[3]

In this article, the authors summarize the current status of clinical evaluation of molecularly targeted agents, including anti-EGFR and antiangiogenic agents, in SCCHN, focusing on the recurrent or metastatic setting. They then discuss potential strategies to develop novel agents in this setting.

TARGETING THE EPIDERMAL GROWTH FACTOR RECEPTOR

The EGFR expression occurs in up to 90% of patients who have advanced SCCHN, and has been shown to be associated with poor prognosis and resistance to therapy.[4] Activation of EGFR promotes processes responsible for tumor growth and progression, including proliferation and maturation, angiogenesis, invasion, metastasis, and evasion of apoptosis.[5] Thus, anti-EGFR agents have been extensively evaluated in SCCHN, including monoclonal antibodies that target the extracellular domain of EGFR, such as cetuximab and panitumumab, and receptor tyrosine kinase inhibitors that target the intracellular domain, such as gefitinib and erlotinib. Agents that target both EGFR and human epidermal growth factor receptor 2 (HER-2), such as lapatinib, have also been studied in SCCHN because HER-2 is the preferred dimerization partner of EGFR and EGFR/HER-2 heterodimers may potentiate receptor signaling and resistance to EGFR inhibitors.

Epidermal Growth Factor Receptor Inhibitors as Single Agents

EGFR inhibitors as single agents are moderately active in recurrent or metastatic SCCHN (**Table 1**).[3,6–12] Most of these studies are uncontrolled, single-arm phase II trials. The inclusion criteria vary substantially among these studies, especially with respect to prior therapy allowed, hence precluding direct comparisons across studies. In general, monoclonal antibodies appear to have a slight advantage in terms of higher overall response rate (about 10%–13%) than small molecule tyrosine kinase inhibitors (about 2.0%–10.6%). In a large randomized trial (IMEX), 486 patients who had recurrent SCCHN were randomized to gefitinib 250 mg daily, gefitinib 500 mg daily, or weekly methotrexate. Neither gefitinib 250 mg/day nor gefitinib 500 mg/day demonstrated an improvement in overall survival over methotrexate (5.6 months, 6.0 months, and 6.7 months, respectively).[10] The dual inhibition of EGFR and HER-2 with lapatinib does not appear to be more effective than the inhibition of EGFR alone.[12]

Epidermal Growth Factor Receptor Inhibitors in Combination with Chemotherapy

Data from preclinical models suggested at least additive effects of EGFR inhibitors when administered with cisplatin,[13] thus providing the rationale for combination therapy, particularly for patients who have sufficient organ functions and performance status to receive aggressive palliative chemotherapy. Adding platinum to EGFR inhibitors appears to confer no additional benefit over platinum alone, either in response rate or overall survival (see **Table 1**).[14–17] Cetuximab has also been evaluated in combination with paclitaxel or docetaxel (see **Table 1**).[18,19] The results are difficult to interpret given the lack of a control arm but appear to be in line with those reported using cisplatin and EGFR inhibitors.

After it had been shown that the triple combination of cetuximab, cisplatin, and FU was feasible,[20] the EXTREME study randomized patients who had previously untreated recurrent or metastatic SCCHN to the classic platinum plus 5-fluorouracil (5FU) combination with or without cetuximab (see **Table 1**).[21] The overall survival was significantly improved for patients receiving chemotherapy and cetuximab (10.1

months versus 7.4 months, P = .036). Panitumumab, a fully humanized monoclonal antibody against EGFR, is currently being evaluated in a phase III study with a similar design. EGFR inhibitors have also been evaluated in combination with a platinum and a taxane as a triplet combination (see **Table 1**).[22–24] Results of these trials are encouraging; disease control rates as high as 90% have been reported. However, toxicities of triple combination are high, with rates of febrile neutropenia reaching 25%. Hence, such combinations remain investigational until randomized data are available.

Biomarkers for Epidermal Growth Factor Receptor Inhibitors' Efficacy

When EGFR inhibitors first entered the clinic, their effectiveness was anticipated only in patients who had tumors that expressed EGFR, and tumor response was expected to be proportional to the level of EGFR expression. However, studies so far have failed to demonstrate a consistent relationship between pretreatment tumor EGFR expression, typically measured by immunohistochemistry from archival specimens, and response to EGFR inhibition.[3,16] No validated markers of sensitivity or resistance to EGFR inhibitors currently exist in SCCHN, although potential markers of therapeutic benefit have been identified, including EGFR gene copy numbers on archival specimen and phosphorylated EGFR on paired tumor biopsies.[25,26] However, these biomarkers have been identified from single-arm phase II studies and therefore await validation in randomized phase III studies.

In patients who have advanced colorectal cancer, multiple studies have shown that the benefits of EGFR inhibition with monoclonal antibodies are confined to patients who have wild-type Kirsten ras (KRAS). In fact, patients harboring KRAS mutations may suffer potential harm with anti-EGFR therapy.[27] Even though KRAS mutations are rare in SCCHN, being less than 5%,[28] an urgent need exists to determine whether such an observation holds true in advanced SCCHN as well.

TARGETS BEYOND EPIDERMAL GROWTH FACTOR RECEPTOR

New targets beyond EGFR have been identified in SCCHN as playing key roles in tumor proliferation and metastases.[29] Among these targets, tumoral angiogenesis is the most active area of research because vascular endothelial growth factor (VEGF) expression has been demonstrated to be highly correlated with prognosis in patients who have SCCHN.[30] Two classes of antiangiogenic agents, monoclonal antibodies that target the VEGF, such as bevacizumab, and multitargeted receptor tyrosine kinase inhibitors that target the VEGF receptor (VEGFR), such as sorafenib or sunitinib, have been evaluated in advanced SCCHN. Agents targeting other targets, such as Src, the insulin-like growth factor 1 receptor (IGF-1R), and the proteasome are also in clinical evaluation.

Vascular Endothelial Growth Factor

It has been demonstrated that EGFR activation can up-regulate VEGF, and this phenomenon correlated with resistance to anti-EGFR agents.[31] Therefore, studies of bevacizumab in combination with cetuximab or erlotinib without any chemotherapeutic agent have been performed in patients who had recurrent or metastatic SCCHN (see **Table 1**).[32,33] In these two studies, patients were allowed up to one prior regimen for their recurrent or metastatic disease. Among 51 patients treated with bevacizumab and erlotinib, three severe adverse events related to bleeding, one of which was fatal, were reported. No hemorrhagic events were reported among 18 patients treated with bevacizumab and cetuximab. Response rates of 27% and 14% were reported with the bevacizumab/cetuximab and bevacizumab/erlotinib doublets, respectively.

Table 1
Clinical trials of molecularly targeted therapies in recurrent or metastatic squamous cell carcinoma of the head and neck

Compound	Phase	Tumor Type and Treatment Setting	Treatment	n	CR (%)	PR (%)	SD (%)	TTP (m)	PFS (m)	OS (m)
Anti-EGFR molecularly targeted therapies (single agent)										
Cetuximab (Erbitux)	II	2nd line R/M SCCHN[3]	Cetuximab 400 mg/m² followed by weekly 250 mg/m²	103	0	13	7	2.3	—	6
Gefitinib (Iressa)	II	1st or 2nd line R/M SCCHN[6]	Gefitinib 500 mg/d	52	2.1	8.5	42.6	3.4	—	8.1
	II	1st or 2nd line R/M SCCHN[7]	Gefitinib 500 mg/d	32	0	9	28	3	—	6
	II	2nd or 3rd line R/M SCCHN[8]	Gefitinib 250 mg/d	70	0	1.4	31.6	—	1.8	5.5
	II	2nd or 3rd line R/M SCCHN[9]	Gefitinib 500 mg/d	47	0	2	26	2.6	—	4.3
	III	2nd or 3rd line R/M SCCHN[10]	Gefitinib 250 mg/d	158	—	2.7	—	—	—	5.6
			Gefitinib 500 mg/d	167	—	7.6	—	—	—	6
			Methotrexate	161	—	3.9	—	—	—	6.7
Erlotinib (Tarceva)	II	1st or 2nd line R/M SCCHN[11]	Erlotinib 150 mg/d	115	0	4.3	33.9	—	2.3	6
Lapatinib (Tykerb)	II	R/M SCCHN with (A) or without (B) prior EGFR inhibitor[12]	Lapatinib 1500 mg/d (A)	27	0	0	37	1.6	—	—
			Lapatinib 1500 mg/d (B)	15	0	0	20	1.7	—	—
Anti-EGFR molecularly targeted therapies (doublet combination)										
Cetuximab (Erbitux)	II	2nd line R/M SCCHN[14]	Platinum + cetuximab	96	0	10	43	2.4	—	5
	II	2nd line R/M SCCHN[15]	Cisplatin + cetuximab (SD)	51	4	14	59	—	4.9	11.7
			Cisplatin + cetuximab (PD/1)	25	0	20	44	—	3	6.1
			Cisplatin + cetuximab (PD/2)	54	0	6	46	—	2	4.3
	III	1st line R/M SCCHN[16]	Cisplatin + cetuximab	57	—	26[a]	—	—	4.2	9.2
			Cisplatin + placebo	60	—	10	—	—	2.7	8
	II	2nd line R/M SCCHN[18]	Docetaxel + cetuximab	47	0	20	27	—	—	—
	II	1st line R/M SCCHN[19]	Paclitaxel + cetuximab	46	24	36	28	—	5	NR
Erlotinib (Tarceva)	II	1st line R/M SCCHN[17]	Cisplatin + erlotinib 100 mg/d	44	3	19	49	—	3.3	7.9
Anti-EGFR molecularly targeted therapies (triplet combination)										

Drug	Phase	Regimen	Setting	N	CR	PR	SD	PFS	TTP	OS
Cetuximab (Erbitux)	II	Platinum + 5FU + cetuximab	1st line R/M SCCHN[20]	53	4	32	38	5.1	—	9.8
	III	Cisplatin + 5FU + cetuximab	1st line R/M SCCHN[21]	220	—	36[a]	45	5.6[a]	—	10.1[a]
		Cisplatin + 5FU		222	—	20	40	3.3	—	7.4
	II	Carboplatin + paclitaxel + cetuximab	2nd line R/M SCCHN[22]	23	4	30	22	5	—	8
Gefitinib (Iressa)	II	Cisplatin + docetaxel + gefitinib 250 mg/d	1st line R/M SCCHN[23]	17	37.5	25	12.5	—	5.1	NR
Erlotinib (Tarceva)	II	Cisplatin + docetaxel + erlotinib 150 mg/d	1st line R/M SCCHN[24]	47	8	58	28	—	6	11
Antiangiogenic molecularly targeted therapies										
Bevacizumab (Avastin)	II	Bevacizumab 15 mg/kg q3w + cetuximab	1st or 2nd line R/M SCCHN[32]	18	0	27	53	—	—	—
	II	Bevacizumab 15 mg/kg q3w + erlotinib 150 mg/d	1st or 2nd line R/M SCCHN[33]	51	4	10	56	—	4	7
	II	Bevacizumab 15 mg/kg q3w + pemetrexed	1st line R/M SCCHN[34]	25	14	23	59	—	7	—
Sorafenib (Nexavar)	II	Sorafenib 800 mg/d	1st line R/M SCCHN[35]	44	0	3	45	4.2	—	8
	II	Sorafenib 800 mg/d	2nd line R/M SCCHN or NPC[36]	28	0	4	37	1.8	—	4
Sunitinib (Sutent)	II	Sunitinib 50 mg/d 4 wk on, 2 wk off	1st to 3rd line R/M SCCHN[37]	22	0	6	28	2.3	—	4.7

Abbreviations: CR, complete response; NR, not reached; OS, overall survival; PD/1, patients who have progressive disease within 3 months after platinum-based therapy; PD/2, patients who have progressive disease after platinum-based therapy; PFS, progression-free survival; PR, partial response; R/M, recurrent or metastatic; SD, stable disease; TTP, time to progression; 5FU, 5-fluorouracil.
[a] Statistically significant.

Feinstein and colleagues[34] performed a phase II trial of pemetrexed and bevacizumab in previously untreated recurrent or metastatic disease (see **Table 1**). Among 25 patients evaluable for toxicity, three hemorrhagic events were reported, one gastric and two at the tumor site. In addition, two toxic deaths were reported, one from febrile neutropenia and the other from tracheal bleeding. Among 22 patients evaluable for response, 3 (14%) had a complete response, 5 (23%) had a partial response, and 13 (59%) had stable disease. Median progression-free survival was 7 months.

Vascular Endothelial Growth Factor Receptor

Small molecule tyrosine kinase inhibitors so far included sorafenib and sunitinib. Williamson and colleagues[35] performed a phase II trial of sorafenib 400 mg twice daily in 44 patients who were chemotherapy naïve for their recurrent or metastatic SCCHN (see **Table 1**). Median time to progression and overall survival were 4 months and 8 months, respectively. Sorafenib has also been studied by Elser and colleagues[36] in 28 patients who had refractory recurrent or metastatic SCCHN or nasopharyngeal carcinoma (see **Table 1**). Results of this study were disappointing, with a time to progression of 1.8 months.

Similarly, a phase II trial was performed with sunitinib given at the dose of 50 mg daily for 4 weeks followed by a 2-week rest period in first- to third-line treatment of patients who had recurrent or metastatic SCCHN (see **Table 1**).[37] Among 22 patients evaluable for toxicity, 5 experienced hemorrhagic events. Efficacy results were comparable to those observed with sorafenib given in pretreated patients. Based on these findings, sorafenib or sunitinib given as a single agent in pretreated patients who have recurrent or metastatic SCCHN does not demonstrate sufficient antitumor activity.

In summary, antiangiogenic therapies as single agents have shown limited antitumor activity in recurrent or metastatic SCCHN. In addition, potential vascular complications will further hinder development of this class of agents in this patient population.

Src

Because EGFR can be activated by multiple ligands and can, in turn, mediate several downstream signaling pathways, in vitro studies have evaluated the possibility of blocking ligands or downstream effectors of EGFR. Src kinase is a nonreceptor cytoplasmic tyrosine kinase that plays a key role in modulating multiple cellular functions including invasion, adhesion, motility, migration proliferation, and survival. Preclinical evaluations demonstrated a strong rationale for targeting Src in SCCHN. Src inhibition using dasatinib, an ATP-binding competitive tyrosine kinase inhibitor, in SCCHN cell lines in vitro has led to cell cycle arrest and apoptosis.[38] Inhibitors of Src kinase, such as dasatinib and AZD0530, are currently undergoing phase II evaluations in recurrent or metastatic SCCHN.[39,40]

Insulin-Like Growth Factor 1 Receptor

EGFR activation can also be achieved through cross-talk with other receptors, such as G-protein-coupled receptors, platelet-derived growth factor receptor, and IGF-1R. Barnes and colleagues[41] demonstrated in a panel of SCCHN cell lines that IGF-1R expression is increased and that IGF-1R and EGFR functionally heterodimerize. Antiproliferative effects were observed with an IGF-1R inhibitor in these cell lines and tumor xenografts. In addition, combined treatment with anti–IGF-1R antibody and cetuximab yielded a more effective reduction in cellular proliferation than with either agent alone.[41] IMC-A12, which is a monoclonal antibody targeting IGF-R1, is currently being studied with or without cetuximab in a phase II trial in patients who have recurrent or metastatic SCCHN.[42]

Proteasome

The 26S proteasome is central for the ubiquitin-proteasome degradation pathway. Bortezomib is a selective inhibitor of the 26S proteasome that has been approved for the treatment of hematologic malignancies. Preclinical studies have shown that bortezomib has antitumor activity in SCCHN models.[43] Bortezomib is currently being studied in phase II trials in combination with irinotecan or docetaxel in recurrent or metastatic SCCHN.[44,45]

DEVELOPMENTAL STRATEGIES
Phase II Trial Designs

The overall response rate has often been used as a primary end point in phase II trials in advanced SCCHN. Novel agents, such as those targeting the VEGF pathway, may be cystostatic, rather than cytotoxic, in nature. These agents may induce tumor necrosis without any tumor shrinkage. Thus, relying on the response rate as the sole indicator of antitumor activity may be misleading and could potentially result in abandoning agents prematurely. Possible solutions include incorporation of the rate of prolonged stable disease (eg, >4–6 months) or progression-based end points in future trials. These end points may provide more realistic assessments of antitumor activity than those based primarily on tumor shrinkage. In addition, innovative pharmacodynamic end points, such as intratumoral blood flow perfusion parameters based on dynamic contrast-enhanced CT/MRI, may be more relevant than conventional response criteria for these agents.

The most commonly used study design for phase II studies is the Simon two-stage design. The published literature indicates that significant tumor shrinkage is only observed in a small proportion of patients who have advanced SCCHN, such that response rates of 15% to 20% typically stated in the alternative hypothesis of a two-stage design are unlikely to be attainable even with the most active compounds. For instance, based on the published data with EGFR inhibitors, the objective response rate of these agents in advanced SCCHN is fairly consistent, at less than 10% for gefitinib and erlotinib, and at 13% for cetuximab. Therefore, the development of cetuximab in advanced SCCHN would have been terminated if it was tested in a phase II study with a two-stage design using an unattainably high response rate in the alternative hypothesis (eg, ≥20%). In designing future phase II studies in advanced SCCHN, the null hypothesis should be that the objective response rate is less than or equal to 5% versus the alternative hypothesis that the objective response rate is greater than or equal to 15%. Unfortunately, such a design would necessitate a large sample size. Therefore, more innovative study designs, such as an adaptive trial design that enables continual assessment, should be actively explored in future studies in advanced SCCHN.

Randomized phase II trials may be an alternative to assess the efficacy of a novel agent in advanced SCCHN. These trials should be designed as phase II/III studies so that they can transition into phase III studies if the primary end point of the phase II portion is met. This type of design has the advantages of providing a realistic estimation of treatment benefits and a shorter time interval between the phase II and phase III portions. However, the number of patients required for the phase II portion is larger than that for single-arm studies.

Phase III Trial Designs

If the activity of a novel agent (drug X) appears to be comparable to, or better than, that of cetuximab in phase II trials, two strategies can be applied for further development in SCCHN (**Fig. 1**). The first strategy is to test drug X in the only Food and Drug Administration (FDA)-approved indication for cetuximab in the recurrent or metastatic setting, namely as a single agent for the treatment of patients for whom prior platinum-based therapy has failed. A possible trial design could be drug X versus cetuximab alone in these patients. The primary end point should be overall survival, and secondary end points should include quality of life. In the situation in which no significant difference in overall survival can be detected, a difference in quality of life would prove that drug X compares favorably to cetuximab. This strategy to benchmark directly against cetuximab may enable drug X to obtain accelerated approval in the platinum-refractory SCCHN population, but the success of such a strategy would require impressive antitumor activity of such an agent given as monotherapy. The second strategy for testing drug X is outside of FDA-approved indications for cetuximab. In this scenario, a possible trial design could be drug X versus chemotherapy alone in patients for whom cetuximab-based treatment has failed. The primary end point for such a trial should be overall survival. Secondary end points should include quality of life. Assuming that cetuximab will get FDA approval in combination with platinum and 5FU in first-line treatment based on the EXTREME study, another trial design could be drug X in combination with platinum and 5FU versus cetuximab in combination with platinum and 5FU in a first-line recurrent or metastatic setting. The primary end point should also be overall survival and secondary end points should also include quality of life.

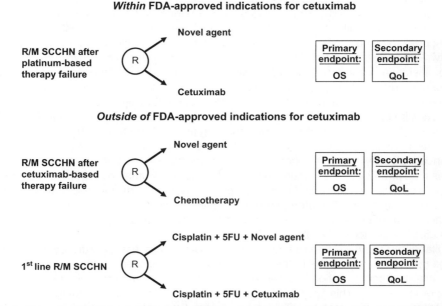

Fig. 1. Phase III clinical trial designs to develop molecularly targeted agents in recurrent or metastatic SCCHN. FDA, Food and Drug Administration; OS, overall survival; QoL, quality of life; R/M, recurrent or metastatic.

Stratification Based on Human Papilloma Virus

Recent data indicate that human papilloma virus (HPV)-related SCCHN is a distinct disease with a better prognosis.[46] The prognostic impact of HPV-related SCCHN is less clear in the recurrent or metastatic setting; hence, it may not be relevant to distinguish HPV-related from non–HPV-related SCCHN for its prognostic difference.[47] However, it seems that HPV-induced HNSCC displays distinct molecular features that may rationally lead to test-specific molecularly targeted agents. Preclinical studies recently presented show that repression of E6/E7 gene expression leads to activation of the Notch and nuclear factor–kappa B pathways only in HPV16-positive oropharyngeal cancer cell lines.[48] On the contrary, PTEN seems to be inactivated independently of AKT.[49] Future trial designs should consider distinguishing between HPV-related and non–HPV-related SCCHN as a patient selection or stratification strategy.

SUMMARY

Molecularly targeted agents already belong to the treatment strategy for patients who have SCCHN. Novel molecular targets and corresponding therapies continue to emerge. Identification of predictive biomarkers of resistance or sensitivity to these therapies remains one of the main challenges in the optimal selection of patients most likely to benefit from them. However, clinical trials with these novel agents need to be designed rationally to improve the overall outcome of patients. Given the emerging evidence that HPV-related SCCHN appears to represent a distinct entity, compared with non–HPV-related disease, these two subgroups should be evaluated prospectively in specific trials.

REFERENCES

1. Gibson MK, Li Y, Murphy B, et al. Randomized phase III evaluation of cisplatin plus fluorouracil versus cisplatin plus paclitaxel in advanced head and neck cancer (E1395): an intergroup trial of the Eastern Cooperative Oncology Group. J Clin Oncol 2005;23:3562–7.
2. Bonner JA, Harari PM, Giralt J, et al. Radiotherapy plus cetuximab for squamous-cell carcinoma of the head and neck. N Engl J Med 2006;354:567–78.
3. Vermorken JB, Trigo J, Hitt R, et al. Open-label, uncontrolled, multicenter phase II study to evaluate the efficacy and toxicity of cetuximab as a single agent in patients with recurrent and/or metastatic squamous cell carcinoma of the head and neck who failed to respond to platinum-based therapy. J Clin Oncol 2007; 25:2171–7.
4. Ang KK, Berkey BA, Tu X, et al. Impact of epidermal growth factor receptor expression on survival and pattern of relapse in patients with advanced head and neck carcinoma. Cancer Res 2002;62:7350–6.
5. Rocha-Lima CM, Soares HP, Raez LE, et al. EGFR targeting of solid tumors. Cancer Control 2007;14:295–304.
6. Cohen EE, Rosen F, Stadler WM, et al. Phase II trial of ZD1839 in recurrent or metastatic squamous cell carcinoma of the head and neck. J Clin Oncol 2003;21: 1980–7.
7. Wheeler RH, Jones D, Sharma P, et al. Clinical and molecular phase II study of gefitinib in patients (pts) with recurrent squamous cell cancer of the head and neck (H&N Ca) [abstract 5531]. In: Programs and abstracts of the American Society of Clinical Oncology meeting. Orlando: 2005.

8. Cohen EE, Kane MA, List MA, et al. Phase II trial of gefitinib 250 mg daily in patients with recurrent and/or metastatic squamous cell carcinoma of the head and neck. Clin Cancer Res 2005;11:8418–24.

9. Kirby AM, A'Hern RP, D'Ambrosio C, et al. Gefitinib (ZD1839, Iressa) as palliative treatment in recurrent or metastatic head and neck cancer. Br J Cancer 2006;94: 631–6.

10. Stewart S, Cohen E, Licitra L, et al. A phase III randomized parallel-group study of gefitinib (Iressa) versus methotrexate (IMEX) in patients with recurrent squamous cell carcinoma of the head and neck [abstract 3522]. In: Programs and abstracts of the American Association of Cancer Research meeting. Los Angeles: 2007.

11. Soulieres D, Senzer NN, Vokes EE, et al. Multicenter phase II study of erlotinib, an oral epidermal growth factor receptor tyrosine kinase inhibitor, in patients with recurrent or metastatic squamous cell cancer of the head and neck. J Clin Oncol 2004;22:77–85.

12. Abidoye OO, Cohen EE, Wong SJ, et al. A phase II study of lapatinib (GW572016) in recurrent/metastatic (R/M) squamous cell carcinoma of the head and neck (SCCHN) [abstract 5568]. In: Programs and abstracts of the American Society of Clinical Oncology meeting. Atlanta: 2006.

13. Mendelsohn J, Fan Z. Epidermal growth factor receptor family and chemosensitization. J Natl Cancer Inst 1997;89:341–3.

14. Baselga J, Trigo JM, Bourhis J, et al. Phase II multicenter study of the antiepidermal growth factor receptor monoclonal antibody cetuximab in combination with platinum-based chemotherapy in patients with platinum-refractory metastatic and/or recurrent squamous cell carcinoma of the head and neck. J Clin Oncol 2005;23:5568–77.

15. Herbst RS, Arquette M, Shin DM, et al. Phase II multicenter study of the epidermal growth factor receptor antibody cetuximab and cisplatin for recurrent and refractory squamous cell carcinoma of the head and neck. J Clin Oncol 2005;23: 5578–87.

16. Burtness B, Goldwasser MA, Flood W, et al. Phase III randomized trial of cisplatin plus placebo compared with cisplatin plus cetuximab in metastatic/recurrent head and neck cancer: an Eastern Cooperative Oncology Group study. J Clin Oncol 2005;23:8646–54.

17. Siu LL, Soulieres D, Chen EX, et al. Phase I/II trial of erlotinib and cisplatin in patients with recurrent or metastatic squamous cell carcinoma of the head and neck: a Princess Margaret Hospital phase II consortium and National Cancer Institute of Canada Clinical Trials Group study. J Clin Oncol 2007;25:2178–83.

18. Knoedler M, Gauler TC, Matzdorff A et al. Phase II trial to evaluate efficacy and toxicity of cetuximab plus docetaxel in platinum pretreated patients with recurrent and/or metastatic head and neck cancer [abstract 6066]. In: Programs and abstracts of the American Society of Clinical Oncology meeting. Chicago: 2008.

19. Hitt R, Irigoyen A, Nuñez J, et al. Phase II study of combination cetuximab and weekly paclitaxel in patients with metastatic/recurrent squamous cell carcinoma of head and neck (SCCHN): Spanish Head and Neck Cancer Group (TTCC) [abstract 6012]. In: Programs and abstracts of the American Society of Clinical Oncology meeting. Chicago: 2007.

20. Bourhis J, Rivera F, Mesia R, et al. Phase I/II study of cetuximab in combination with cisplatin or carboplatin and fluorouracil in patients with recurrent or metastatic squamous cell carcinoma of the head and neck. J Clin Oncol 2006;24: 2866–72.

21. Vermorken JB, Rivera F. Platinum-based chemotherapy plus cetuximab in head and neck cancer. N Engl J Med 2008;359:1116–27.

22. Buentzel J, de Vries A, Micke O. Experience with cetuximab plus paclitaxel/carboplatinum in primary platinum-resistant recurrent head and neck cancer [abstract 6077]. In: Programs and abstracts of the American Society of Clinical Oncology meeting. Chicago: 2007.

23. Belón J, Irigoyen A, Rodríguez I, et al. Preliminary results of a Phase II study to evaluate gefitinib combined with docetaxel and cisplatin in patients with recurrent and/or metastatic squamous-cell carcinoma of the head and neck [abstract 5563]. In: Programs and abstracts of the American Society of Clinical Oncology meeting. Orlando: 2005.

24. Kim ES, Kies MS, Glisson BS, et al. Final results of a phase II study of erlotinib, docetaxel and cisplatin in patients with recurrent/metastatic head and neck cancer [abstract 6013]. In: Programs and abstracts of the American Society of Clinical Oncology meeting. Chicago: 2007.

25. Agulnik M, da Cunha Santos G, Hedley D, et al. Predictive and pharmacodynamic biomarker studies in tumor and skin tissue samples of patients with recurrent or metastatic squamous cell carcinoma of the head and neck treated with erlotinib. J Clin Oncol 2007;25:2184–90.

26. Calvo E, Malik SN, Siu LL, et al. Assessment of erlotinib pharmacodynamics in tumors and skin of patients with head and neck cancer. Ann Oncol 2007;18:761–7.

27. Le Tourneau C, Vidal L, Siu LL. Progress and challenges in the identification of biomarkers for EGFR and VEGFR targeting anticancer agents. Drug Resist Updat 2008;11:99–109.

28. Bissada E, Abou-Chacra Z, Weng X, et al. Prevalence of K-RAS codon 12 mutations in locally advanced head and neck squamous cell carcinoma and influence with regards to response to chemoradiation therapy [abstract 17005]. In: Programs and abstracts of the American Society of Clinical Oncology meeting. Chicago: 2008.

29. Le Tourneau C, Faivre S, Siu LL. Molecular targeted therapy of head and neck cancer: review and clinical development challenges. Eur J Cancer 2007;43:2457–66.

30. Lothaire P, de Azambuja E, Dequanter D, et al. Molecular markers of head and neck squamous cell carcinoma: promising signs in need of prospective evaluation. Head Neck 2006;28:256–69.

31. O-charoenrat P, Rhys-Evans P, Modjtahedi H, et al. Vascular endothelial growth factor family members are differentially regulated by c-erbB signaling in head and neck squamous carcinoma cells. Clin Exp Metastasis 2000;18:155–61.

32. Kies MS, Gibson MK, Kim SW, et al. Cetuximab (C) and bevacizumab (B) in patients with recurrent or metastatic head and neck squamous cell carcinoma (SCCHN): An interim analysis [abstract 6072]. In: Programs and abstracts of the American Society of Clinical Oncology meeting. Chicago: 2008.

33. Vokes EE, Cohen EE, Mauer AM, et al. A phase I study of erlotinib and bevacizumab for recurrent or metastatic squamous cell carcinoma of the head and neck (HNC) [abstract 5504]. In: Programs and abstracts of the American Society of Clinical Oncology meeting. Orlando: 2005.

34. Feinstein TM, Raez LE, Rajasenan KK, et al. Pemetrexed (P) and bevacizumab (B) in patients (pts) with recurrent or metastatic head and neck squamous cell carcinoma (HNSCC): updated results of a phase II trial [abstract 6069]. In: Programs and abstracts of the American Society of Clinical Oncology meeting. Chicago: 2008.

35. Williamson SK, Moon J, Huang CH, et al. A phase II trial of BAY 43-9006 in patients with recurrent and/or metastatic head and neck squamous cell carcinoma (HNSCC): A Southwest Oncology Group (SWOG) trial [abstract 6044]. In: Programs and abstracts of the American Society of Clinical Oncology meeting. Chicago: 2007.

36. Elser C, Siu LL, Winquist E, et al. Phase II trial of sorafenib in patients with recurrent or metastatic squamous cell carcinoma of the head and neck or nasopharyngeal carcinoma. J Clin Oncol 2007;25:3766–73.

37. Choong NW, Cohen EE, Kozloff MF, et al. Phase II trial of sunitinib in patients with recurrent and/or metastatic squamous cell carcinoma of the head and neck (SCCHN) [abstract 6064]. In: Programs and abstracts of the American Society of Clinical Oncology meeting. Chicago: 2008.

38. Johnson FM, Saigal B, Talpaz M, et al. Dasatinib (BMS-354825) tyrosine kinase inhibitor suppresses invasion and induces cell cycle arrest and apoptosis of head and neck squamous cell carcinoma and non-small cell lung cancer cells. Clin Cancer Res 2005;11:6924–32.

39. Available at: http://www.cancer.gov/search/ViewClinicalTrials.aspx?cdrid=559148& version=HealthProfessional&protocolsearchid=4724336.

40. Available at: http://www.cancer.gov/search/ViewClinicalTrials.aspx?cdrid=559632& version=HealthProfessional&protocolsearchid=4724344.

41. Barnes CJ, Ohshiro K, Rayala SK, et al. Insulin-like growth factor receptor as a therapeutic target in head and neck cancer. Clin Cancer Res 2007;13:4291–9.

42. Available at: http://www.cancer.gov/search/ViewClinicalTrials.aspx?cdrid=588712& version=HealthProfessional&protocolsearchid=4724347.

43. Sunwoo JB, Chen Z, Dong G, et al. Novel proteasome inhibitor PS-341 inhibits activation of nuclear factor-kappa B, cell survival, tumor growth, and angiogenesis in squamous cell carcinoma. Clin Cancer Res 2001;7:1419–28.

44. Available at: http://www.nci.nih.gov/search/ViewClinicalTrials.aspx?cdrid=525999& version=HealthProfessional&Protocolsearchid=3056999.

45. Available at: http://www.nci.nih.gov/search/ViewClinicalTrials.aspx?cdrid=409577& version=HealthProfessional&Protocolsearchid=3056999.

46. Ragin CC, Taioli E. Survival of squamous cell carcinoma of the head and neck in relation to human papillomavirus infection: review and meta-analysis. Int J Cancer 2007;121:1813–20.

47. Worden FP, Kumar B, Lee JS, et al. Chemoselection as a strategy for organ preservation in advanced oropharynx cancer: response and survival positively associated with HPV16 copy number. J Clin Oncol 2008;26:138–46.

48. Rampias T, Sasaki C, Burtness BA et al. Gene expression differences associated with silencing of E6 and E7 viral oncogenes in HPV16+ oropharyngeal cancer cell lines [abstract 6009]. In: Programs and abstracts of the American Society of Clinical Oncology meeting. Chicago: 2008.

49. Psyrri A, Sasaki C, Burtness BA, et al. Regulation of cytoplasmic and nuclear PTEN levels by human papillomavirus (HPV) type 16 E6 and E7 oncogenes in HPV16+ oropharyngeal cancer cell lines [abstract 6034]. In: Programs and abstracts of the American Society of Clinical Oncology meeting. Chicago: 2008.

Role of Functional Imaging in Head and Neck Squamous Cell Carcinoma: Fluorodeoxyglucose Positron Emission Tomography and Beyond

Sandro V. Porceddu, BSc, MBBS, FRANZCR[a,b,]*,
Bryan H. Burmeister, MB ChB, FF Rad(T) SA, FRANZCR, MD[a,b],
Rodney J. Hicks, MBBS, MD, FRACP[c,d,e]

KEYWORDS
- PET • Head and neck • Squamous cell carcinoma
- Radiotherapy • Chemotherapy

Accurate staging and restaging of head and neck cancers is paramount to clinical practice because of its prognostic implications, role in tailoring treatment, and assisting with avoidance of futile aggressive therapies in the case of incurable disease.[1–6]

With the move toward organ preservation treatment of locally advanced head and neck squamous cell carcinoma (HNSCC) accurate restaging allows avoidance of unnecessary posttherapy surgery in the absence of residual disease.[2]

Conventional work-up, which includes physical examination, panendoscopy, biopsy, and CT or MRI, provides much of the information required for clinical staging and restaging.

[a] Division of Cancer Services, Princess Alexandra Hospital, Ipswich Road, Woolloongabba, Brisbane, Queensland, Australia 4102
[b] University of Queensland, School of Medicine, Brisbane, Queensland, Australia, 4102
[c] Centre for Molecular Imaging, Peter MacCallum Cancer Centre, St Andrews Place, Locked Bag 1, A'Beckett Street, East Melbourne, Victoria 8006, Australia
[d] Department of Medicine, University of Melbourne, Parkville, Victoria 3052, Australia
[e] Department of Radiology, University of Melbourne, Parkville, Victoria 3052, Australia
* Corresponding author. Division of Cancer Services, Princess Alexandra Hospital, Ipswich Road, Woolloongabba, Brisbane, Queensland 4102, Australia.
E-mail address: sandro_porceddu@health.qld.gov.au (S.V. Porceddu).

Hematol Oncol Clin N Am 22 (2008) 1221–1238
doi:10.1016/j.hoc.2008.08.009   hemonc.theclinics.com
0889-8588/08/$ – see front matter © 2008 Elsevier Inc. All rights reserved.

There are inherent limitations with conventional work-up, however, which include

Poor sensitivity for the detection of disease smaller than 1 cm
Limited ability to distinguish between residual or recurrent tumor from scar
Inability to biologically characterize disease
Inability to provide early prognostic information regarding treatment outcome

Positron emission tomography (PET) has emerged as a diagnostic tool that is superior to conventional work-up in these areas. It therefore provides additional information and complements conventional work-up in the management of HNSCC. In addition, it now plays a role in the planning of radiotherapy (RT), and may potentially play a role in the long-term surveillance of these patients.[7,8]

PET provides an assessment of biochemical processes by way of uptake and retention of radiopharmaceuticals by tissues. Although structural imaging, such as CT and MRI, allows identification of enlarged or distorted internal structures, PET provides information about whether these derangements are likely tumor, scarring from previous treatment, or other biologic processes. Although its diagnostic value has been limited in the past by its spatial resolution, its role has been enhanced with the development of PET/CT.[9,10]

PET scans are commonly performed with fluorine-18 fluorodeoxyglucose (18-F FDG), an analog of glucose. Malignant cells, particularly squamous cell carcinoma (SCC), have increased glucose metabolism and ability to incorporate more glucose analog compared with surrounding normal tissues. Because of the high FDG avidity of tumors compared with normal tissues FDG-PET provides an improved level of diagnostic contrast.

Novel tracers, such as fluorine-18 fluoromisonidazole (FMISO) and fluorine-18 fluoro-deoxy-L-thymidine (FLT), are being evaluated in their ability to biologically characterize disease and provide prognostic information. Tumor characterization may lead to more targeted therapy, such as the use of hypoxic cytotoxins in patients demonstrating tumor hypoxia on PET imaging.[11]

This article addresses the usefulness of FDG-PET and FDG-PET/CT, ongoing dilemmas, cost effectiveness, and the potential role of emerging novel markers in the management of mucosal HNSCC, excluding paranasal and salivary gland tumors.

STAGING
Primary Tumor Staging (T Stage)

The extent of local disease in patients amenable for curative treatment affects the decision to treat with definitive surgery with or without postoperative RT or radical RT with or without chemotherapy. Conventional work-up often provides sufficient information to determine the extent of primary disease.

PET has been shown to be highly sensitive and specific in detecting clinically evident primary disease in more than 90% to 95% of patients; however, it has a limited role in providing additional information with regard to the extent of primary disease following conventional work-up.[12–14]

Although PET scanning has minimal impact on T staging following conventional assessment, it does provide valuable additional information in relation to nodal and distant disease staging, as discussed later.

Occult Primary Staging

PET has superior resolution for disease smaller than 1 cm compared with conventional imaging.[1,12] Consequently there has been an expectation that PET and PET/CT would be useful in the detection of occult primary disease in patients presenting with malignant cervical lymphadenopathy.[15,16]

There have been conflicting reports with respect to the usefulness of PET in this setting. In a review of the published series by Rusthoven and colleagues[17] the overall ability of PET to detect the occult primary was 25%, with a sensitivity, specificity, and accuracy of 88%, 75%, and 79%, respectively. This finding has not been universal, however, with some studies not reporting a high level of detection following workup by members of an established head and neck unit.[12,15]

The rate of detection of the occult primary with PET may possibly reflect the level of experience by the examining team. PET is still worth performing in this context because it may direct potential regions for biopsy. A proportion of these sites turn out to be false positive, however.[12,15,18,19] It is possible that reporting PET specialists read for sensitivity rather than specificity in the knowledge that no definite primary had been identified.

Nodal Staging (N Stage)

Management differs depending on whether the neck is involved, if there are single or multiple positive nodes, and if the involvement is unilateral or bilateral.

Accurate N staging provides important prognostic information and affects how aggressively the neck is treated. The prognostic significance of nodal involvement is well established, with 5-year survival of 30% in node-positive compared with greater than 50% in node-negative patients.[20]

PET has a high positive predictive value, greater than 90% to 95%, and is superior to CT and MRI with respect to sensitivity and specificity in the detection of nodal disease.[1,6,7,12] As a result, it has now become integral in the routine management of these patients in many centers.

Table 1 summarizes studies that have compared the accuracy of the preoperative PET or PET/CT with CT or MRI in the detection of nodal metastatic disease.

The likelihood of nodal metastases is partly related to the primary site, size, and differentiation of the tumor. Physical examination may miss up to 30% to 40% of cases with nodal involvement. Whereas 20% to 30% of nodes less than 1 cm may harbor occult disease following conventional imaging.[21] The sensitivity and specificity of CT and MRI are essentially reliant on nodal size for the detection of disease. For nodes greater than 1 to 1.5 cm the specificity of CT and MRI is 90%, but this value decreases for nodes smaller than 1 cm.

Although the sensitivity of PET increases in the presence of enlarged nodes it is less reliant on nodal size compared with conventional imaging, and has the ability to detect disease in nodes smaller than 1 cm, although its resolution for disease less than 5 mm remains limited.[1,12]

Fig. 1 illustrates the role of PET in detecting unsuspecting disease in the radiologically negative neck.

Distant Metastases Staging (M0) and Detection of Synchronous Primary Tumors

Based on Bayesian principles the likelihood of distant metastases increases in concert with increasing locoregional disease burden. Patients who have locally advanced HNSCC are at risk for having distant metastases or a synchronous second malignancy in 15% and 5% of cases, respectively.[22]

PET is useful in identifying distant metastases and synchronous second malignancies that may not have been detected on routine conventional imaging. Some series have reported a detection rate of previously unrecognized distant metastases of 27%.[17,23]

Table 1
Sensitivity and specificity of positron emission tomography (PET/CT) compared with CT or MRI in the detection of nodal disease in the neck confirmed on pathologic findings

Author	No. of patients	PET[a] or PET/CT[b] Sens/Spec (%)	CT Sens/Spec (%)	MRI Sens/Spec	Significance
Adams et al (1998)[6,a]	60	90/94	82/85	80/79	S
Benchaou et al (1997)[58,a]	48	72/99	67/97	NP	NS
Braams et al (1995)[59,a]	12	91/88	NP	36/94	NP
Di Martino et al (2000)[60,a]	50	82/87	82/94	NP	NS
Hannah et al (2002)[61,a]	40	82/100	81/81	NP	NP
Jeong et al (2007)[5,b]	47	92/99	90/94	NP	S
Laubenbacher et al (1995)[13,a]	22	90/96	NP	78/71	S
Mattei et al (1998)[62,a]	24	87/99	53/87 (CT/MRI)	—	S
Myers et al (1998)[63,a]	14	78/100	57/90	NP	NS
McGuirt et al (1998)[12,a]	45[c]	83/82	95/86	NP	NP
Ng et al (2005)[64,a]	134	74/95	74/93 (CT/MRI)	—	S
Nowak et al (1999)[65,a]	71	80/92	80/84 (CT/MRI)	—	NS
Paulus et al (1998)[66,a]	25	50/100	40/100	NP	NP
Schwartz et al (2005)[67,b]	63	100/96	96/99	NP	NS
Stuckensen et al (2000)[68,a]	106	70/82	66/74	64/69	NP
Wong et al (1997)[14,a]	16	67/100	—	67/25 (CT/MRI)	NP

Abbreviations: NP, not performed; NS, not statistically significant; S, statistically significant; Sens/Spec (%), sensitivity/specificity percentage.
[a] PET performed.
[b] PET/CT performed.
[c] Neck dissections.

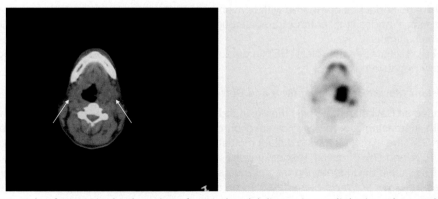

Fig. 1. Role of PET/CT in the detection of cervical nodal disease in a radiologic node negative neck.

The reasons for this include detection of disease beyond regions that are routinely scanned as part of the conventional work-up, and the superior ability of PET to detect smaller volume disease.

In addition, PET is useful in determining the relevance of equivocal (1–1.5 cm) lung nodules on conventional imaging, which are not infrequent in head and neck patients. A recent meta-analysis has demonstrated the superiority of PET/CT compared with conventional imaging for the characterization of solitary lung nodules.[24] The resolution for pulmonary nodules less than 5 mm remains limited. Because of its high positive predictive value, if a pulmonary nodule is FDG avid then it is likely to be a malignant lesion.

Assessment of an FDG-avid pulmonary lesion needs to be made in the context of the clinical scenario. In the presence of a head and neck cancer with bulky nodal disease or low neck involvement the lesion is more suspicious of metastatic disease, whereas if there is either no nodal disease or small-volume nodal disease high in the neck then it is more likely to be a primary pulmonary lesion, particularly in an older patient who has a smoking history.

In patients who have HNSCC with non–FDG-avid pulmonary nodules smaller than 1 to 1.5 cm it is not unreasonable to assume the lesions are nonmalignant. When compared with conventional imaging, PET staging may also detect additional benign lesions, such as inflammatory lung conditions and bowel polyps, potentially necessitating further investigations.[12]

Given its ability to detect unsuspected metastatic disease or synchronous primaries, PET can have a significant impact in altering treatment plans or preventing futile aggressive therapy.

INITIAL MANAGEMENT
Treatment

The ability of PET to alter the TNM staging following conventional imaging, mainly N and M staging, is well recognized and can result in alteration in the overall surgical or RT management.[7,21,25,26]

Connell and colleagues[7] found PET/CT altered the TNM staging in 34% of patients, with 10/35 patients up-staged and 2/35 down-staged. In most cases the alteration was attributable to a change in N staging. Twenty-nine percent had the RT technique or dose altered and in 1 patient the treatment intent was altered from curative to palliative because of the detection of distant disease.

Clinically Node-Negative Neck (N0)

The decision to omit elective neck management in the clinical/radiologic N0 neck is generally based on the perceived risk for less than 15% to 20% occult neck disease.[27–29]

Although the overall positive predictive value of PET for the presence of nodal disease is in the order of 90% to 95%, the negative predictive value ranges between 50% and 85%.[9,30,31]

Ng and colleagues[32] assessed the usefulness of PET, CT, and MRI in patients who had oral cavity SCC and a palpably N0 neck. Of the 134 patients, 26% were found to have neck metastases. PET was superior to CT/MRI in detecting palpably occult neck disease. The sensitivity of PET on a patient-by-patient basis was 51% and this increased after visual correlation with CT/MRI to 57%. The probability of occult neck disease following a negative PET for T1–3 tumors was less than 15%, and 25% for T4 tumors. These results make a compelling case for observation of the neck in patients who have a palpable, radiologic, and PET-negative neck for T1–3 oral cavity SCC.

At this point in time, interpretation of the PET findings must still be made in the context of the clinical scenario. For example, in the case of a well-lateralized oropharyngeal lesion with a clinical and radiologic N0 neck, the absence of PET avidity in the contralateral neck strengthens the case for observation of that neck.

Elective treatment should still be considered in the clinical/radiologic/PET N0 neck when the perceived risk for occult nodal disease remains greater than 15% to 20%. In this setting, because of the superior sensitivity of PET for the detection of smaller-volume disease, the absence of PET avidity supports the notion that if disease is present it is of low volume and therefore elective doses of RT or a limited neck dissection is justified.

Clinically Node-Positive Neck (N+)

PET can either confirm the initial surgical or RT management or lead to treatment alterations in the event further disease is detected, such as the addition of a contralateral neck dissection or tailoring the RT dose to address previously unrecognized nodal disease.

Equivocal Findings

In some cases there may be equivocal findings detected on structural imaging, such as a 1.5-cm node in the neck. PET can be useful in determining the likelihood of whether the node is benign or malignant, given a benign or scarred node is likely to be non–FDG avid.

In other instances the PET may be equivocal (eg, a reactive/inflammatory node that may be FDG avid). This finding is discussed in further detail in the section about dilemmas in PET/CT imaging.

Radiotherapy Planning

Accurate definition of the gross tumor volume (GTV) underpins the ability to deliver highly conformal RT with either three-dimensional conformal RT or intensity-modulated RT. The fusing of diagnostic MRI and PET/CT images with planning CT scans has gained popularity. Fusion is particularly useful when it is difficult to distinguish between involved nodes and surrounding blood vessels with noncontrast planning scans or certain primary tumors, such as infiltrative base of tongue tumors, where it can be difficult to distinguish tumor from surrounding normal tissues.

Several series have assessed the usefulness of PET and PET/CT in RT planning.[7,25,33] Ha and colleagues[33] found PET/CT confirmed the RT plan in 25/36 (69%) patients. Eleven (31%) patients had their plan altered because of either up-staging, resulting in the addition of concomitant chemotherapy, or inclusion or exclusion of the contralateral neck in the RT field and alteration of RT dose.

Daisne and colleagues[34] found the GTV for locally advanced oropharyngeal HNSCC was on average 37% larger when MRI and PET were co-registered with the planning CT compared with CT alone.

Although several studies have examined the impact of fusing the PET/CT with planning scans it is difficult to assess what significance this has had on overall treatment outcome.[35] Nonetheless, the fusion of PET/CT with planning scans along with the physical examination, endoscopic findings, and conventional imaging all complement each other in defining the GTV and improving RT design.

Fig. 2 demonstrates PET/RT planning scan fusion to assist with definition of a tongue base GTV.

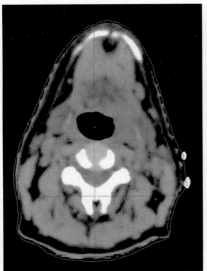 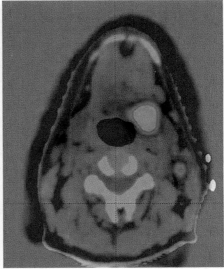

Fig. 2. PET fusion with RT planning CT scans to assist with definition of tongue base tumor.

Post-Radiotherapy Restaging

One of the greatest impacts of PET/CT has been its role in the restaging of patients who have HNSCC following RT with or without chemotherapy.

Controversy remains regarding the need for a planned neck dissection in patients who have bulky (N2–3) disease following RT. Improvement in radiologic techniques and the introduction of PET and PET/CT have strengthened the argument for observation following a complete response in the neck with RT.

The isolated failure rate in the neck following a complete response of the primary and neck based on clinical and radiologic findings is less than 5%.[2] Corry and colleagues[36] reported on the isolated neck failure of patients who have N2–3 neck disease treated with chemotherapy and RT on the Trans Tasman Radiation Oncology Group (TROG 98–02) trial. Of the 102 patients who achieved a complete clinical and CT or MRI response at the primary site and neck there were no isolated neck failures, with a median follow up of 4.3 years.

Assessment of the neck to determine whether there has been a complete response following chemotherapy and RT can be difficult because of residual clinical or radiologic abnormalities. Following RT, PET/CT has the ability to distinguish whether there is ongoing metabolic activity within residual structural abnormalities and has a high negative predictive value, in excess of 95%.[37–39] Yao and colleagues[40] assessed the role of PET at a median of 15 weeks following definitive RT and found the negative predictive value was 100%.

The optimal time for a restaging PET seems to be 12 to 15 weeks following treatment. Studies have consistently shown a lower positive predictive value, between 43% and 89%, when the scan is performed too early following treatment. The probability of false-positive results diminishes with time following treatment because of resolution of the inflammatory response and opportunity for residual tumor to resolve.[7,37–42]

In addition, if scans are performed too early, this may be during a period when tumor response is maximal but not reflective of whether cure has been achieved, leading to false-negative results. Greven and colleagues[42] found a higher false-negative rate when the posttherapy PET was performed within 1 month compared with 4, 12, and 24 months following treatment. Seven of 25 (28%) patients had a recurrence following a negative PET at 1 month compared with none of 18 when the PET was negative at 4 months. Yao and colleagues reported on 3- to 5-month posttherapy PET and found only 1 of 45 were false negative at the primary site and none of 49 in the neck. Our series also found a high negative predictive value if the restaging PET was performed at 12 weeks.[37,40]

The timing of the PET around this period also means that if a neck dissection is required it can be performed before the establishment of late radiation fibrosis.

The value of restaging PET to assess primary tumor response seems as effective as for the neck. Chen and colleagues[39] found a PET accuracy of 86% for the detection of residual primary disease after treatment of oropharyngeal cancer. Connell and colleagues found that PET, performed around 12 weeks following RT, altered primary tumor response in 8/30 (27%) compared with conventional imaging alone. Six of the 8 patients who had residual abnormality on CT were negative on PET and were all true negative. Two of the 8 patients had a partial response on PET and were both found to be biopsy-proven false positive.

As a result of the high negative predictive value of a restaging PET performed more than 12 weeks following treatment it would seem safe to omit a planned neck dissection in patients who have achieved a complete response at the primary site and neck.[37] Some still advocate a neck dissection if a residual node greater than 2 to 3 cm persists beyond 12 to 15 weeks, even if the PET is negative.[41] Patients who have persisting avidity at the primary site or neck beyond 12 weeks require further evaluation, which may include a biopsy and possibly salvage surgery.

PET/CT-guided management of the neck protocol is described in **Fig. 3**.

THERAPEUTIC MONITORING AND PROGNOSTICATION

PET response following RT seems to have some role in predicting long-term outcome. Brun and colleagues[8] evaluated the metabolic response (MR) and standardized uptake value (SUV) in 47 patients who had HNSCC. Patients underwent a preatment PET followed by another PET after 1 to 3 weeks of radical RT. Low and high MR FDG PET, with median value as cutoff, was associated with complete response in 96% and 62% ($P = .007$), respectively. A significant difference was also seen with local control, 96% versus 55% ($P = .002$), and 5-year survival, 72% versus 35% ($P = .0042$), respectively.

Connell and colleagues[7] found a significant difference in disease-free survival and overall survival favoring those who had a complete response on PET/CT at 12 weeks.

At this stage the value of FDG PET as a prognostication tool seems promising. How this information will be used requires further evaluation.

RESTAGING AT RELAPSE AND SURVEILLANCE

There are potential benefits to the individual if a recurrence or new secondary primary is detected early. In patients treated with HNSCC the 5-year rate of locoregional recurrence, second malignancy, and development of distant metastases are 40% to 50%, 10% to 30%, and 15% to 20%, respectively.

Although treatment options are limited for those who have asymptomatic metastases, expedient detection of an early small recurrence is important because successful salvage is more likely, compared with more advanced recurrences.[7,8] One study demonstrated patients who had early recurrent disease who underwent salvage surgery

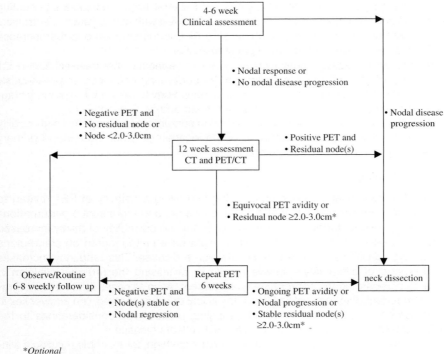

Fig. 3. PET/CT guided management of the neck following radiation therapy and complete response at the primary site.

had a 70% 2-year relapse-free survival compared with 22% in patients who had advanced recurrence.[4]

Confirming suspected relapse following RT can be difficult because of the resulting scar tissue, which hinders interpation of the physical examination and radiologic findings. Biopsy is helpful if positive but uncertainty remains if negative. Several studies have shown superiority of PET compared with conventional imaging in detecting recurrent locoregional disease.[4] Serial CT scans may help support the diagnosis of recurrence, if progression is seen. Serial scans performed over time can delay the diagnosis and miss the opportunity for curative salvage therapy.

PET/CT is not readily available in all centers and is a costly imaging modality. Optimal frequency and cost effectiveness of PET/CT surveillance following treatment of HNSCC remains unresolved.

DILEMMAS IN POSITRON EMISSION TOMOGRAPHY/CT IMAGING

It is possible to make a case for going directly to the staging modality that has the highest sensitivity for locoregional and distant metastatic disease. FDG PET/CT is currently the modality fulfilling this requirement. Since the first commercial release of PET/CT scanners in 2001, when the most advanced device had only a 4-slice multidetector CT (MDCT) and most had either single- or dual-slice configurations, the sophistication of the MDCT component has increased markedly. Entry-level scanners are now typically equipped with a 16-slice MDCT and 64-slice scanners are becoming commonplace. The PET component has also improved with new crystals, electronics, and processing algorithms, including iterative reconstruction methods that increase lesion-to-background contrast and spatial resolution.

There is an increasing motivation to perform diagnostic, contrast-enhanced CT (ceCT) as part of the PET/CT examination. By performing ceCT contemporaneously with FDG PET/CT it would be feasible for this technology to become the primary staging tool in many high-risk cancers, including head and neck cancer.[43]

Acquisition of a study in RT treatment position contemporaneous with a high-quality ceCT would provide precise definition of the location of lymph nodes and primary tumor in relation to normal structures.

Equivocal Findings

One of the theoretical disadvantages of the improving sensitivity of PET related to technological advancement is that it can detect more and more subtle perturbations of tissue glucose metabolism. A corollary of this is the possibility of mildly increased uptake in a lymph node, which previously might have been ignored on stand-alone PET, being considered as possible small-volume disease. This tendency increases the likelihood of either false-positive results or of leaving the referring clinician in a quandary regarding the appropriate management. As in all cases relating to integration of imperfect diagnostic standards into clinical decision making, the answer lies in rating competing clinical priorities and applying probabilistic considerations to the likelihood that a faint abnormality on FDG PET reflects disease.

If the clinical consequences of missing disease are high, for example missing a window of opportunity for cure, a high sensitivity is appropriate, whereas if the likelihood of disease is low and the morbidity is high, it is may be more appropriate to interpret the scan for high specificity—that is, to seek to achieve a high positive predictive value. With respect to the PET interpretation alone, it is important to apply oncologic and physical principles to scan reading.

Because nodal spread of head and neck cancers is generally a hierarchal process, knowledge of patterns of spread is important to image interpretation. A faint node just inferior to a chain of positive nodes is likely to harbor disease on oncologic grounds alone. Furthermore, partial volume effects could reasonably explain the low uptake observed. Partial volume effects result in lesions that are smaller than the resolution of the imaging device having less perceived activity than they actually contain. This effect leads to reduced contrast between the lesion itself and surrounding tissue, which, necessarily, is also sampled within the imaging element (voxel).

For PET scanners the diameter of lesion at which partial volume effects diminish apparent compared with actual counts in a lesion varies from about 15 mm for older generation stand-alone PET scanners to about 8 mm or less for modern high-resolution PET/CT systems. For both generations of scanners this reflects a spectrum of nodal size that also carries significant uncertainty for CT interpretation. The availability of ceCT can help to increase diagnostic confidence regarding the nature of equivocal abnormalities on FDG PET.

If the node is enlarged but faint, when the uptake in other large disease sites is intense, a benign basis is likely because partial volume effects cannot be invoked to explain the low signal intensity. The exception to this is when there are CT features suggesting nodal necrosis, in which case the small volume of viable tumor cells at the periphery of the node may contribute to partial volume effects.

Conversely, if the node can be measured to be small but has higher uptake than similar-sized nodes elsewhere in the imaging field of view, the faint uptake should be considered more likely to be attributable to partial volume effects. Although somewhat counterintuitive, the rule is that faint and small is much more worrying than faint and big.

The Use of Standardized Uptake Value Measurements

As a digital technology, PET can be used as a quantitative technique. Radioactive decay leads to release of energy in a predictable way, characterized by the physical half-life of a given radioisotope. After correction for the effects of decay, tissue attenuation, and the intrinsic sensitivity of the scanner, it is possible to measure the concentration of a radiotracer in any given tissue at any given time. By applying a calibration factor, obtained by measuring a sample of known activity, it is possible to express tissue radioactivity in counts/tissue mass/time. This capability has led to various quantitative and semiquantitative measures being applied to analysis of FDG uptake in lesions identified on PET.

The most widely used technique is SUV. The SUV basically assumes that if the entire administered activity of a radiotracer were evenly distributed within the body, the SUV would be equal to 1.0 at all time points. Because of excretion and differential tracer uptake by some tissues relative to others, however, the relative uptake and retention is higher in some tissues than others. Cancers typically have maximum SUV (SUVmax) of 2.5 or more. Accordingly, there are those who have advocated various SUVmax thresholds for differentiating benign lesions from malignancy.

Such thresholds fail to correctly characterize those lesions that have low apparent uptake because of partial volume effects, unless partial volume correction algorithms are applied. In the case of lymph nodes and, to a lesser extent, primary lesions, the structural volume of a lesion does not necessarily reflect its functional volume. A thin rim of viable cells in a necrotic lymph node can be subject to partial volume effects but cannot necessarily be demarcated and measured volumetrically by CT independent of the necrotic cellular elements.

Furthermore, many inflammatory conditions can have SUV recordings that are higher than the somewhat arbitrary thresholds selected. Technical factors and altered metabolic conditions may also influence the measured SUV. These factors include the method of attenuation correction, blood glucose level, body fat content, and time after injection of the tracer that the measurement is made.[44] Although useful for confirming the visual impression of high or low uptake, the routine use of SUV to characterize the nature of lesions is discouraged.

Measurement of the SUV may, however, be useful in further characterizing therapeutic response in patients not achieving a complete metabolic response.

Cost Effectiveness

Since soon after the introduction of FDG PET whole-body imaging it has been recognized that more sensitive and specific detection of metastatic disease than achieved by conventional cancer staging techniques has the potential to avoid futile or unnecessary interventions.[45]

Although FDG PET/CT has been more expensive than conventional imaging, enhanced throughput allows greater amortization of equipment costs and efficient use of isotope and staff. Accordingly, the cost of performing PET scans can be reduced, provided sufficient patient numbers are available. Added to improved cost efficiency, the ability to prevent expensive additional tests or therapeutic interventions significantly increases the potential cost effectiveness. There are, however, relatively few formal studies that have addressed the cost effectiveness of this modality in head and neck cancer. Those that have, suggest benefits.[46] Some of the benefits in avoiding futile treatments because of PET may be offset because of its increased sensitivity leading to the detection of benign lesions and further investigations, such as colonoscopy for benign polyps.

NOVEL TRACERS AND CLINICAL IMPLICATIONS
Hypoxic Imaging

Hypoxia has long been recognized as an adverse determinant of RT treatment outcome in head and neck cancer.[47] The theoretical gold standard for evaluating tumor hypoxia is the direct measurement of oxygen saturation using polarographic probes. There are several drawbacks with this invasive procedure, however, which include limited access to this technology, the requirement for meticulous calibration, and the inability to access some tumor sites.

Functional imaging to detect hypoxia is currently being evaluated and offers the advantage of being less invasive and more practical than probes. In addition, several new approaches to overcoming hypoxia are currently being investigated, including the use of hypoxic cytotoxins, such as tirapazamine.[11]

Functional imaging with radiolabeled nitroimidazoles has considerable promise as a means of detecting and monitoring hypoxia in human tumors.[48] The most widely reported method of hypoxia imaging has been 18F-labelled FMISO PET. This agent has increased uptake and retention in hypoxic tumors.[11,49,50]

The Peter MacCallum Cancer Center group reported on a phase I trial of tirapazamine in advanced head and neck cancer and imaging with FMISO PET at baseline and during treatment. This trial demonstrated a high prevalence of positive scans for hypoxia and its resolution with treatment. This outcome was associated with an excellent locoregional control rate in a group of patients who would ordinarily be expected to have a poor response to RT.[50]

A subsequent randomized phase II trial, reported that "imageable" hypoxia on FMISO PET predicted for a markedly higher locoregional failure to RT without tirapazamine but very low local failure in such patients if they received hypoxia-targeting therapy.[11]

The images obtained with this agent suffer from high nonspecific background activity leading to generally low contrast between normal tissues and sites of presumed hypoxia. Accordingly there have been efforts to develop hypoxia tracers with superior imaging characteristics. One such agent is fluorine-18 fluoroazomycin arabinoside (FAZA). Recent reports suggest that this agent has more rapid soft tissue clearance leading to higher lesion contrast.[51,52] In addition, this would facilitate the ability to define hypoxic subvolumes for RT dose painting.[53]

Fig. 4 demonstrates uptake at the tongue base and level II node on FDG PET, with FAZA PET demonstrating hypoxia in the node only.

There is increasing interest in the use of therapies directed against vascular targets, such as vascular-endothelial growth factor receptors and epithelial growth factor receptors. These include monoclonal antibodies, such as bevacizumab and cetuximab. These therapies could increase tumor hypoxia by reducing vascularity or reduce it by improving the efficiency of oxygen delivery to the tumor by way of "vascular normalization."[54] The ability of hypoxia imaging with PET to demonstrate changes in hypoxia during treatment with small tyrosine kinase inhibitors has been demonstrated in preclinical models of SCC and offers promise for evaluating these agents in clinical practice.[55]

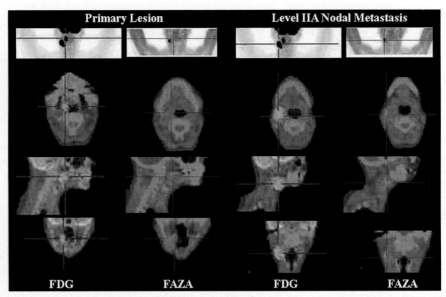

Fig. 4. FDG PET demonstrating uptake at the tongue base and level II node with the FAZA PET demonstrating hypoxia in the node only.

Proliferation Imaging

Increased proliferation is one of the hallmarks of cancer cells. Recent development of PET tracers to evaluate this biologic process has opened the way for in vivo evaluation of tumor aggressiveness and assessment of drugs that may induce growth arrest as opposed to cell death. FLT has been the most extensively evaluated tracer. Preclinical and early clinical studies suggest promise; however, further evaluation is needed at this stage to assess how this knowledge can be integrated into clinical practice.[56,57]

SUMMARY
Staging with Positron Emission Tomography and Positron Emission Tomography/CT

PET and PET/CT are highly sensitive and specific in confirming clinical and radiologic findings, and useful in detection of additional disease not seen on routine staging and in altering TNM staging and management in approximately 34% of HNSCC.

The detection rate of an occult primary with PET following conventional imaging can be as high as 25%. Its role following assessment in a head and neck unit may be limited. It may play a role in identifying potential biopsy sites and aids in completing the staging work-up.

PET is less reliant on size for the detection of nodal disease but at this stage elective neck treatment in the clinical/radiologic N0 neck following a negative PET cannot be safely omitted if the perceived risk for occult involvement is greater than 15% to 20%.

PET can detect distant metastases and synchronous secondary primary malignancies not seen on routine work-up and therefore assists in avoiding inappropriate or futile aggressive treatments.

Therapeutic Planning

Fusion of PET and PET/CT to RT planning scans facilitates the delineation of the tumor volumes and enhances the ability to deliver conformal radiation therapy.

Posttherapy Restaging

The optimal timing of the restaging PET seems to be 12 to 15 weeks post-RT and has a high negative predictive value. It is therefore safe to observe the neck if the PET is negative and residual nodes are less than 2 to 3 cm.

PET has a lower positive predictive value attributable to the occurrence of false positives associated with ongoing inflammatory/tumor response; however, positive PET findings should not be ignored.

PET is useful in distinguishing between scar and residual tumor.

Therapeutic Monitoring and Outcome, Restaging at Relapse, and Surveillance

PET response to RT seems predictive of long term outcome.

PET is useful in the early detection of recurrence, particularly in the presence of scar.

Dilemmas in Positron Emission Tomography/CT Imaging

The management of an equivocal PET or CT/PET finding should be based on the clinical scenario and knowledge of the tumor behavior.

Cost effectiveness remains unresolved.

SUV is useful in confirming the visual impression of uptake; however, its routine use to characterize the nature of lesions is discouraged.

Hypoxia imaging is likely to play a key role in future molecular targeted therapies of head and neck cancer, particularly in association with RT.

Imaging of cellular proliferation may provide novel insights into tumor biology.

PET is rapidly becoming an integral diagnostic tool in the management of head and neck cancer. It is highly sensitive and specific in the detection of disease and is invaluable in restaging following chemoradiotherapy or RT. It is now entering new frontiers with its role in facilitating RT planning and tumor characterization.

ACKNOWLEDGMENT

The authors thank Germain Thompson for her administrative support.

REFERENCES

1. Ahn PH, Garg MK. Positron emission tomography/computed tomography for target delineation in head and neck cancers. Semin Nucl Med 2008;38(2):141–8.
2. Pellitteri PK, Ferlito A, Rinaldo A, et al. Planned neck dissection following chemoradiotherapy for advanced head and neck cancer: is it necessary for all? Head Neck 2006;28(2):166–75.
3. Vernon MR, Maheshwari M, Schultz CJ, et al. Clinical outcomes of patients receiving integrated PET/CT-guided radiotherapy for head and neck carcinoma. Int J Radiat Oncol Biol Phys 2008;70(3):678–84.
4. Vermeersch H, Loose D, Ham H, et al. Nuclear medicine imaging for the assessment of primary and recurrent head and neck carcinoma using routinely available tracers. Eur J Nucl Med Mol Imaging 2003;30(12):1689–700.

5. Jeong H, Baek C, Son Y, et al. Use of integrated 18F-FDG PET/CT to improve the accuracy of initial cervical nodal evaluation in patients with head and neck squamous cell carcinoma. Head Neck 2007;29(3):203–10.

6. Adams S, Baum RP, Stuckensen T, et al. Prospective comparison of 18F-FDG PET with conventional imaging modalities (CT, MRI, US) in lymph node staging of head and neck cancer. Eur J Nucl Med 1998;25(9):1255–60.

7. Connell CA, Corry J, Milner AD, et al. Clinical impact of, and prognostic stratification by, F-18 FDG PET/CT in head and neck mucosal squamous cell carcinoma. Head Neck 2007;29(11):986–95.

8. Brun E, Kjellén E, Tennvall J, et al. FDG PET studies during treatment: prediction of therapy outcome in head and neck squamous cell carcinoma. Head Neck 2002;24(2):127–35.

9. Schoder H, Carlson DL, Kraus DH, et al. 18F-FDG PET/CT for detecting nodal metastases in patients with oral cancer staged N0 by clinical examination and CT/MRI. J Nucl Med 2006;47:755–62.

10. Schöder H, Yeung HW, Gonen M, et al. Head and neck cancer: clinical usefulness and accuracy of PET/CT image fusion. Radiology 2004;231:65–72.

11. Rischin D, Hick RJ, Fisher R, et al. Prognostic significance of [18f]-misonidazole positron emission tomography-detected tumor hypoxia in patients with advanced head and neck cancer randomly assigned to chemoradiation with or without tirapazamine: a substudy of Trans-Tasman Radiation Oncology Group study 98.02. J Clin Oncol 2006;24:2098–104.

12. McGuirt WF, Greven K, Williams D III, et al. PET scanning in head and neck oncology: a review. Head Neck 1998;20(3):208–15.

13. Laubenbacher C, Saumweber D, Wagner-Manslau C, et al. Comparison of fluorine-18-fluorodeoxyglucose PET, MRI and endoscopy for staging head and neck squamous-cell carcinomas. J Nucl Med 1995;36(10):1747–57.

14. Wong WL, Chevton E, McGurk M, et al. A prospective study of PET-FDG imaging for the assessment of head and neck squamous cell carcinoma. Clin Otolaryngol 1997;22(3):209–14.

15. Fogarty GB, Peters LJ, Stewart J, et al. The usefulness of fluorine 18-labelled deoxyglucose positron emission tomography in the investigation of patients with cervical lymphadenopathy from an unknown primary tumor. Head Neck 2003;25(2):138–45.

16. Miller FR, Hussey D, Beeram M, et al. Positron emission tomography in the management of unknown primary head and neck carcinoma. Arch Otolaryngol Head Neck Surg 2005;131(7):626–9.

17. Rusthoven KE, Koshy M, Paulino AC, et al. The role of fluorodeoxyglucose positron emission tomography in cervical lymph node metastases from an unknown primary tumor. Cancer 2004;101(11):2641–9.

18. Hanasono MM, Kunda LD, Segall GM, et al. Uses and limitations of FDG positron emission tomography in patients with head and neck cancer. Laryngoscope 1999;109:880–5.

19. Kole AC, Nieweg OE, Pruim J, et al. Detection of unknown occult primary tumours using positron emission tomography. Cancer 1998;82:1160–6.

20. Whitehurst JO, Droulias CA. Surgical treatment of squamous cell carcinoma of the oral tongue: factors influencing survival. Arch Otolaryngol 1977;103(4):212–5.

21. Heron DE, Andrade RS, Flickinger J, et al. Hybrid PET-CT simulation for radiation treatment planning in head-and-neck cancers: a brief technical report. Int J Radiat Oncol Biol Phys 2004;60:1419–24.

22. Erkal HS, Mendenhall WM, Amdur RJ, et al. Synchronous and metachronous squamous cell carcinomas of the head and neck mucosal sites. J Clin Oncol 2001;19:1358–62.

23. Goerres GW, Schmid DT, Grätz KW, et al. Impact of whole body positron emission tomography on initial staging and therapy in patients with squamous cell carcinoma of the oral cavity. Oral Oncol 2003;39(6):547–51.

24. Cronin P, Dwamena B, Kelly A, et al. Solitary pulmonary nodules: meta-analytic comparison of cross-sectional imaging modalities for diagnosis of malignancy. Radiology 2008;246(3):772–82.

25. Koshy M, Paulino AC, Howell R, et al. F-18FDGPET-CT fusion in radiotherapy treatment planning for head and neck cancer. Head Neck 2005;27(6):494–502.

26. Agarwal V, Branstetter BF IV, Johnson JT. Indications for PET/CT in the head and neck. Otolaryngol Clin North Am 2008;41(1):23–49.

27. Narayan K, Crane CH, Kleid S, et al. Planned neck dissection as an adjunct to the management of patients with advanced neck disease treated with definitive radiotherapy: for some or for all? Head Neck 1999;21(7):606–13.

28. Vandenbrouck C, Sancho-Garnier H, Chassagne D, et al. Elective versus therapeutic radical neck dissection in epidermoid carcinoma of the oral cavity: results of a randomized clinical trial. Cancer 1980;46(2):386–90.

29. Kligerman J, Lima RA, Soares JR, et al. Supraomohyoid neck dissection in the treatment of T1/T2 squamous cell carcinoma of oral cavity. Am J Surg 1994; 168(5):391–4.

30. Layland MK, Sessions DG, Lenox J, et al. The influence of lymph node metastasis in the treatment of squamous cell carcinoma of the oral cavity, oropharynx, larynx and hypopharynx: N0 versus N+. Laryngoscope 2005;115(4):629–39.

31. Stoekli SJ, Steinert H, Pfaltz M, et al. Is there a role for positron emission tomography with 18F-fluorodeoxyglucose in the initial staging of nodal negative oral and oropharyngeal squamous cell carcinoma. Head Neck 2002;24:345–9.

32. Ng SH, Yen TC, Chang JT, et al. Prospective study of [18F]fluorodeoxyglucose positron emission tomography and computed tomography and magnetic resonance imaging in oral cavity squamous cell carcinoma with palpably negative neck. J Clin Oncol 2006;24(27):4371–6.

33. Ha PK, Hdeib A, Goldenberg D, et al. The role of positron emission tomography and computed tomography fusion in the management of early-stage and advanced-stage primary head and neck squamous cell carcinoma. Arch Otolaryngol Head Neck Surg 2006;132(1):12–6.

34. Daisne J, Duprez T, Weynant B, et al. Impact of image coregistration with computed tomography (CT), magnetic resonance (MR) and positron emission tomography with fluorodeoxyglucose (FDG-PET) on delineation of GTV's in oropharyngeal, laryngeal and hypopharyngeal tumors. Int J Radiat Oncol Biol Phys 2002;54(S):15–6.

35. Wang D, Schultz CJ, Jursinic PA, et al. Initial experience of FDG-PET/CT guided IMRT of head and neck carcinoma. Int J Radiat Oncol Biol Phys 2006;65(1): 143–51.

36. Corry J, Peters L, Fisher R, et al. N2–N3 neck nodal control without planned neck dissection for clinical/radiologic complete responders—Results of Trans Tasman Radiation Oncology Group Study 98.02. Head Neck 2008 Feb [Epub ahead of print].

37. Porceddu SV, Jarmolowski E, Hicks RJ, et al. Utility of positron emission tomography for the detection of disease in residual neck nodes after (chemo)radiotherapy in head and neck cancer. Head Neck 2005;27(3):175–81.

38. Ware RE, Matthews JP, Hicks RJ, et al. Usefulness of fluorine-18 fluorodeoxyglucose positron emission tomography in patients with a residual structural abnormality following definitive treatment for squamous cell carcinoma of the head and neck. Head Neck 2004;26:1008–17.

39. Chen AY, Vilaseca I, Hudgins PA, et al. PET-CT vs contrast-enhanced CT: what is the role for each after chemoradiation for advanced oropharyngeal cancer? Head Neck 2006;28(6):487–95.

40. Yao M, Smith RB, Graham MM, et al. The role of FDG PET in management of neck metastasis from head-and-neck cancer after definitive radiation treatment. Int J Radiat Oncol Biol Phys 2005;63(4):991–9.

41. Yao M, Graham MM, Smith RB, et al. Value of FDG PET in assessment of treatment response and surveillance in head-and-neck cancer patients after intensity modulated radiation treatment: a preliminary report. Int J Radiat Oncol Biol Phys 2004;60:1410–8.

42. Greven KM, Williams DW III, McGuirt WF Sr, et al. Serial positron emission tomography scans following radiation therapy of patients with head and neck cancer. Head Neck 2001;23:942–6.

43. Hicks RJ, Ware RE, Lau EW. PET/CT: will it change the way that we use CT in cancer imaging? Cancer Imaging 2006;6:S52–62.

44. Visvikis D, Costa DC, Croasdale I, et al. CT-based attenuation correction in the calculation of semi-quantitative indices of [18F]FDG uptake in PET. Eur J Nucl Med Mol Imaging 2003;30:344–53.

45. Valk PE, Pounds TR, Tesar RD, et al. Cost-effectiveness of PET imaging in clinical oncology. Nucl Med Biol 1996;23:737–43.

46. Hollenbeak CS, Lowe VJ, Stack BC Jr. The cost-effectiveness of fluorodeoxyglucose 18-F positron emission tomography in the N0 neck. Cancer 2001;92(9): 2341–8.

47. Brizel DM, Sibley GS, Prosnitz LR, et al. Tumor hypoxia adversely affects the prognosis of carcinoma of the head and neck. Int J Radiat Oncol Biol Phys 1997;38:285–9.

48. Lee ST, Scott AM. Hypoxia positron emission tomography imaging with 18f-fluoromisonidazole. Semin Nucl Med 2007;37:451–61.

49. Hicks RJ, Rischin D, Fisher R, et al. Utility of FMISO PET in advanced head and neck cancer treated with chemoradiation incorporating a hypoxia-targeting chemotherapy agent. Eur J Nucl Med Mol Imaging 2005;32:1384–91.

50. Thorwarth D, Eschmann SM, Scheiderbauer J, et al. Kinetic analysis of dynamic 18F-fluoromisonidazole PET correlates with radiation treatment outcome in head-and-neck cancer. BMC Cancer 2005;5:152.

51. Sorger D, Patt M, Kumar P, et al. [18F]Fluoroazomycinarabinofuranoside (18FAZA) and [18F]Fluoromisonidazole (18FMISO): a comparative study of their selective uptake in hypoxic cells and PET imaging in experimental rat tumors. Nucl Med Biol 2003;30:317–26.

52. Piert M, Machulla HJ, Picchio M, et al. Hypoxia-specific tumor imaging with 18F-fluoroazomycin arabinoside. J Nucl Med 2005;46:106–13.

53. Grosu AL, Souvatzoglou M, Roper B, et al. Hypoxia imaging with FAZA-PET and theoical considerations with regard to dose painting for individualization of radiotherapy in patients with head and neck cancer. Int J Radiat Oncol Biol Phys 2007;69:541–51.

54. Jain RK. Normalization of tumor vasculature: an emerging concept in antiangiogenic therapy. Science 2005;307:58–62.

55. Solomon B, Binns D, Roselt P, et al. Modulation of intratumoral hypoxia by the epidermal growth factor receptor inhibitor gefitinib detected using small animal PET imaging. Mol Cancer Ther 2005;4:1417–22.

56. Vesselle H, Grierson J, Muzi M, et al. In vivo validation of 3′deoxy-3′-[(18)F]fluorothymidine ([(18)F]FLT) as a proliferation imaging tracer in humans: correlation of [(18)F]FLT uptake by positron emission tomography with Ki-67 immunohistochemistry and flow cytometry in human lung tumors. Clin Cancer Res 2002;8: 3315–23.

57. Buck AK, Halter G, Schirrmeister H, et al. Imaging proliferation in lung tumors with PET: 18F-FLT versus 18F-FDG. J Nucl Med 2003;44:1426–31.

58. Benchaou M, Lehmann W, Slosman DO, et al. The role of FDG-PET in the preoperative assessment of N-staging in head and neck cancer. Acta Otolaryngol 1996;116:332–5.

59. Braams JW, Pruim J, Freling NJM, et al. Detection of lymph node metastases of squamous-cell cancer of the head and neck with FDG-PET and MRI. J Nucl Med 1995;36:211–6.

60. Di Martino E, Nowak B, Hassan HA, et al. Diagnosis and staging of head and neck cancer: a comparison of modern imaging modalities (positron emission tomography, computed tomography, colour-coded duplex sonography) with pan-endoscopic and histopathologic findings. Arch Otolarnygol Head Neck Surg 2000;126:1457–61.

61. Hannah A, Scott AM, Tochon-Danguy H, et al. Evaluation of 18 F-fluorodeoxyglucose positron emission tomography and computed tomography with histopathologic correlation in the initial staging of head and neck cancer. Ann Surg 2002; 236(2):208–17.

62. Mattei R, Rubello D, Ferlin G, et al. Positron emission tomography (PET) with 18-fluorodeoxyglucose (FDG) in the diagnosis and preoperative staging of head and neck tumors: a prospective study. Acta Otorhinolarynhol Ital 1998;18:387–91.

63. Myers LL, Wax MK, Nabi H, et al. Positron emission tomography in the evaluation of the N0 neck. Laryngoscope 1998;108(2):232–6.

64. Ng SH, Yen TC, Liao CY, et al. 18F-FDG PET and CT/MRI in oral cavity squamous cell carcinoma: A prospective study of 124 patients with histologic correlation. J Nucl Med 2005;46:1136–43.

65. Nowak B, Di Martino E, Janicke S, et al. Diagnostic evaluation of malignant head and neck cancer by F-18-FDG PET compared to CT/MRI. Nuklearmedizin 1999; 38:312–8.

66. Paulus P, Sambon A, Vivegnis D, et al. [F-18]FDG-PET for the assessment of primary head and neck tumors. Clinical, computed tomography, and histopathological correlation in 38 patients. Laryngoscope 1998;108:1578–83.

67. Schwartz DL, Ford E, Rajendran J, et al. FDG-PET/CT imaging for preradiotherapy staging of head and-neck squamous cell carcinoma. Int J Radiat Oncol Biol Phys 2005;61:129–36.

68. Stuckensen T, Kovacs AF, Adams S, et al. Staging of the neck in patients with oral cavity squamous cell carcinomas: a prospective comparison of PET, ultrasound, CT and MRI. J Craniomaxillofac Surg 2000;28:319–24.

Evaluation of Quality of Life and Organ Function in Head and Neck Squamous Cell Carcinoma

Rosemary Martino, MA, MSc, PhD[a,b,*], Jolie Ringash, BSc, MD, MSc[c,d]

KEYWORDS

- Speech • Swallowing • Quality of life
- Measurement outcomes • Xerostomia
- Head and neck cancer

Despite contributing only 3% of incident cancer cases and cancer deaths, affecting approximately 4,000 Canadians each year, head and neck squamous cell cancer (HNC) has a significant impact on function and quality of life (QOL).[1] Treatment is becoming increasingly complex, long, and toxic;[2] currently, as an extreme example, a selected patient may undergo 6 months of therapy, including 3 months of induction chemotherapy, followed by 7 weeks of concurrent chemoradiotherapy (CRT), a 4-week break, and a surgical neck dissection. Other strategies combine accelerated fractionation radiotherapy (RT) with chemotherapy, again followed by neck surgery in selected patients.[3] How biologic agents will be optimally integrated with other therapies is an open question, but some current clinical trials are using such agents as the anti-epidermal growth-factor receptor (EGFR) antibody cetuximab as a further addition to standard therapies, such as CRT (eg, Radiation Therapy Oncology Group 0522).[4] Each intensification has shown small benefits in survival or local control: for example, 6% to 8% improvement in 5-year overall survival with CRT versus standard RT; 3% with altered fractionation versus standard RT;[5] 10% improvement in 3-year overall survival with RT-cetuximab versus standard RT.[6] However, the cost in terms

[a] Department of Speech Language Pathology, University of Toronto, 160-500 University Avenue, Toronto, Ontario, Canada M5G 1V7
[b] Health Care and Outcomes Research, Toronto Western Research Institute, 399 Bathurst Street, MP 11-331, Toronto, Ontario, Canada M5T 2S8
[c] Department of Radiation Oncology, The Princess Margaret Hospital, 610 University Avenue, Toronto, Ontario, Canada M5G 2M9
[d] The University of Toronto, 27 King's College Circle, Toronto, Ontario, Canada M5S 1A1
* Corresponding author. Department of Speech Language Pathology, University of Toronto, 160-500 University Avenue, Toronto, Ontario, Canada M5G 1V7.
E-mail address: rosemary.martino@utoronto.ca (R. Martino).

Hematol Oncol Clin N Am 22 (2008) 1239–1256
doi:10.1016/j.hoc.2008.08.011
hemonc.theclinics.com

of toxicity has been ill-defined. Trotti and colleagues[7] have shown that traditional toxicity reporting may systematically underestimate the toxicity of aggressive regimens. Using their proposed TAME system, they suggest that the relative risk for acute toxicity of concurrent CRT, as compared with standard RT, may be 320, and accelerated RT (concomitant boost) with chemotherapy may result in a relative risk of 590, with risk class value ranges of low (100–140), moderate (150–390), high (400–490), and extreme ($\geq$500).

In recent years, recognition of the multidimensional impact on patients of HNC tumors and their treatment has led to an explosion of interest in concepts such as toxicity, function, and patient-reported outcomes (PROs).[8] Both an excellent overall review of PROs and guidelines on their use in clinical trials have been recently published.[9,10] **Fig. 1** shows a classification of selected PROs applicable to cancer patients. A variety of disease, condition, function, and treatment-specific PRO instruments designed for this patient population have been published, mainly within the past 10 years.[11] Functional outcomes related to speech, swallowing, and salivary flow may also be measured by clinician-rated or biologic instruments.

Common concerns of HNC patients include concerns about illness and their future, general physical and emotional well being, speech, body image, and financial issues; patients receiving RT report high levels of problems with swallowing, eating, and dry mouth.[12,13] This article focuses on several of the most common and severe lasting issues for HNC patients: impairments of overall QOL, xerostomia, speech, and swallowing. While the authors focus on the tools and techniques for measuring such effects, more practical clinical advice on supportive care has been provided in a recent review.[14]

CLASSIFICATION OF OUTCOMES

Over the years there has been an evolving recognition of differences in practice behaviors among clinicians treating the same clinical problem.[15–17] As a result, there has emerged a growing need for clinicians to know more about these practice variations and what they mean in relation to the patient's recovery.[18] With this awareness, clinicians would then be able to select the most appropriate and effective intervention based on evidence rather than assumption.[19] This has lead to an explosion of patient-based outcome measures targeting either specific diseases or general health. In a recent survey there were more than 75 instruments developed to measure QOL in cancer patients alone.[20]

Despite the plethora of available indices for cancer in general, there is a paucity of measurement tools available specific to HNC. Of those HNC-specific tools available, most measure QOL and few measure the common comorbidities of speech and swallowing. As a result, there is a gap of outcome measures specific to speech and

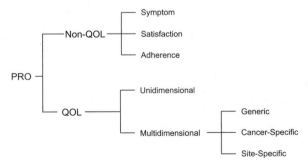

Fig. 1. Classification of patient reported outcomes.

swallowing that requires addressing. The presence of speech abnormalities and dysphagia are not only common but also associated with poorer rehabilitation outcomes and, in the case of dysphagia, even death. There is a need for a standardized method by which to compare and contrast the influence of HNC on, not only QOL, but also speech and swallowing. Instruments such as these will delineate the interventions most effective to reduce these poor comorbidities of HNC, thereby fostering evidenced-based practice and clinician accountability.

A necessary step in the development of any tool is to establish a framework within which three dimensions are detailed: (1) a conceptual definition of the topic being measured with reference to how it links to a broader theory; (2) the purpose of what it measures and how the results should be interpreted; and (3) the specifics of the population for whom it will be designed.[21–23] For the purpose of this article, the target population will be the HNC patient.

The conceptual foundation sets the stage for the comprehensive selection of items.[24] The relevant constructs and domains of the new tool, along with the necessary linkages to other outcome components, should be detailed.[25] These details will not only ensure its proper development, but once developed they will also allow other clinicians to assess it more critically for inclusion in their own practice or clinical trials.[23] A sound theoretic model will permit hypotheses to test multiple relationships between patient characteristics, interventions, and the outcome. These hypotheses will serve to assess both benefiting and confounding influences to the intervention.[24] By controlling multiple comparisons in this way, considerations about sample size and statistical analyses could be incorporated when planning new trials using the given tool.[26] Despite these known benefits, the majority of published functional disability[27] and QOL tools failed to declare a conceptual basis.[28] Hence, the broader interrelationships among physiologic impairment, disability, and QOL outcomes are ignored.[25]

The impetus toward a broader definition for outcomes came from the Institute of Medicine.[29] In 1980, the World Health Organization (WHO) developed a three-way classification system for the different types of patient outcomes: impairment, function, and handicap.[30] This WHO model was formulated to create a taxonomic classification that was compatible with the International Classification of Disease. According to the WHO, "impairment" represents the traditional marker of abnormal physiology, "disability" represents the functional consequence of the impairment, and "handicap" represents the perceived disadvantage experienced as a result of the impairment or disability that limits or prevents personal fulfillment. This original WHO taxonomy has since been criticized and recently replaced with a new classification, also developed by the WHO, called the International Classification of Functioning, Disability and Health (ICF).[31] The ICF evolved over several years and is a revision of several earlier versions. The latest ICF classifies disability and handicap along the same three dimensions of the original WHO version, with only a few exceptions: a new taxonomy that is neutral rather then pejorative, incorporates the influences of environmental and personal factors, and that details interactions among the three dimensions rather than making them distinct.[32]

PRINCIPLES OF MEASUREMENT

The purpose of an instrument refers to the type of question it best answers.[33] Proper construction and validation of a new tool are guided by its purpose, and for this reason it is critical that this purpose is declared.[34] Several frameworks have been proposed to capture the various purposes that tools can serve.[35–37] Among these frameworks, three common fundamental purposes are (1) measurement at a single point in time,

(2) prediction of a future event, and (3) assessment of change in status either in response to treatment or simply in time.

Measures may be used with large groups or individuals irrespective of purpose. It is important to specify whether comparisons will be made between groups or at the individual level, because this choice has implications on the maximum acceptable level of random error.[38,39] Reliability refers to the degree to which scores are free from errors in measurement.[40] Errors in measures may add to the total variance in scores, which reduces the study's power to detect statistically significant differences. Comparisons between large groups are more forgiving to error and can be done with less reliable measures than comparisons between individuals. Individual tools require high internal-consistency reliability (ie, Cronbach's alpha coefficients) and high inter-rater reliability (ie, intraclass correlation coefficients), ranging from 0.90 to preferably greater than 0.95.[40]

Measurement tools can be of three types: generic, disease-specific, or patient-specific. Generic measures target a broad spectrum of health issues and are especially useful for comparisons across different disorders, severities of disease, and interventions.[23,27,41] Disease-specific measures are applicable to specific patient populations, typically defined by disease.[23,27] Patient-specific tools are an extension of disease-specific measures in that these tools target not only the disease but also the particular preferences of the individual patient.[23,41] Although there are advantages and disadvantages for each, treating clinicians tend to favor disease-specific tools because of greater perceived value in clinical decision-making and influencing patient outcomes.[26] Unlike patient-specific tools, disease-specific tools use the same items to assess patients with the same disease rather than different items for each patient. Their common item inventories allow for comparisons between patients and within patients over time.[42] Unlike generic tools, disease-specific tools capture only a few dimensions but each dimension is captured comprehensively for the patient group being measured.[42]

Regardless of purpose or type, outcome measures can be developed according to one of two apposing principles: psychometric or clinimetric.[43,44] Although both methods include item generation, item reduction, and a standardization process ensuring reliability and validity, these processes will depend on whether they were developed according to clinimetric, psychometric, or blended methods. Clinimetric methods generate items primarily from judgments of both clinicians and patients and have been used mainly for the development of clinically related tools assessing benefit from treatment interventions.[45,46] Their items are selected based on perceived relevance, rather than any statistical properties.[43] In contrast, psychometric methods rely on conceptual frameworks and previous literature to generate items and then statistical strategies, such as internal consistency and factor analysis, to select items.[43]

A measure is not valid for all people and in all institutions; hence, it is critical that the population for which the measure has been validated be clearly stated.[47] Validation studies essentially assess two hypotheses: how well the measure discriminates the target population from another (ie, discriminatory validity), and how well the measure relates to other measures that are similar (ie, criterion and convergent validity) or predictably different (ie, divergent validity).[48] Within these broad categories are many different types of validity tests and which of these is necessary depend on the purpose of the measure. For example, a measure that captures an outcome at a single point in time needs at a minimum to establish discriminatory validity. Unlike item generation and selection, the validation of any measure can be an ongoing process. Over time, measures can be validated for additional purposes or patient groups not originally targeted.

QUALITY OF LIFE

Health-related QOL is a subjective, multi-attribute construct defined by the WHO as follows: "an individual's perception of their position in life in the context of the culture and value systems in which they live and in relation to their goals, standards and concerns. It is a broad ranging concept affected in a complex way by the person's physical health, psychosocial state, level of independence, social relationships, and their relationships to salient features of their environment."[49] All QOL instruments are PROs, but not all PROs measure QOL (examples of non-QOL PROs would include patient-reported adherence to medication or satisfaction with care).

The steps in developing a QOL instrument have been summarized elsewhere.[50] Similarly, standardized criteria to evaluate QOL questionnaires are available.[51] The general measurement principles of reliability, validity, responsiveness, and interpretability apply, but an ideal measurement instrument must also suit the patient population, setting and practical needs of a given application. Research has shown that generic QOL instruments (with general population norms) are insufficiently sensitive on their own to the special concerns of HNC patients; frequently, both a general or cancer-specific instrument will be administered concurrently with a HNC-specific questionnaire.[52] Choosing which instrument to use thus poses a challenge for investigators of QOL in HNC; frequently, other PROs may be of interest in the same study or cohort, and excess patient burden must be avoided.

A recent literature review using the Medical Outcomes Trust (MOT) criteria[51] for instrument development identified three PRO instruments specific for surgically-treated HNC for which all criteria were met.[53] All three were QOL instruments: EORTC HN35 (The European Organization for Research into the Treatment of Cancer QOL Questionnaire for HNC),[54] HNQOLQ (University of Michigan Head and Neck Quality-of-Life Questionnaire),[55] and the HNCI (University of Iowa HNC Inventory).[56] An older structured review predating the development of the MOT criteria,[57] but not limited to surgical issues, additionally found acceptable measurement properties for the FACT-H&N (Functional Assessment of Cancer Therapy–Head and Neck),[58,59] the UW QOL (University of Washington QOL Questionnaire),[60] and two instruments aimed specifically at patients receiving RT or CRT: the QOL-RTI/H&N (University of South Florida QOL–Radiation Therapy Instrument Head & Neck Module)[61,62] and the HNRQ (McMaster Head and Neck Radiotherapy Questionnaire).[63] In today's environment of international multicenter trials and multicultural patient populations, the availability of language translations and cross-cultural validations of PRO instruments can often be an important factor in instrument selection; it is perhaps in part for this reason that the most commonly used instruments are the EORTC QLQ-C30 and HN35.[8]

It is important to recognize that a statistically significant difference on a QOL instrument or subscale does not always reflect a clinically important difference. Much recent work has centered on defining the "minimally important difference" for QOL tools, although a reasonable rough guide may be provided by 5% to 10% of the instrument range.[56,64]

More recent work has shown the value of QOL instruments in predicting survival or locoregional control, both for cancer patients in general and specifically for HNC patients.[13,65–68] As treatment options proliferate, in time it may be feasible to select treatment strategies with a favorable risk: benefit profile based in part on prognostic indicators, including baseline QOL.

In the past few years, more publications of HN QOL results from prospective clinical trials have become available. To date there has been no systematic overview; however, in general such studies show impairment in overall QOL during treatment and in early follow-up (eg, 3 months), either for radiotherapy or surgically based treatment. Subsequently, most patients recover to baseline on overall QOL by 1 year.[13,67] However, symptoms and concerns specific to HNC and its treatment modalities can remain impaired in the long-term, with specific impairments varying according to tumor site and treatment modality.[11] Voice impairment is mainly problematic with laryngeal cancer, and is most severe with laryngectomy. While patients treated in all ways may experience general emotional and functional impairment, those receiving RT or CRT tend to have more issues with xerostomia and dysphagia, whereas surgical patients are more likely to experience pain and concerns about facial disfigurement.[69,70]

Few publications have assessed long-term QOL. One article has suggested a late decline in survivors' QOL scores at 10 years after treatment as compared with 1- and 2-year follow-up.[71] Another interesting study used a general health survey, SF-36, with the EORTC QLQ-C30 and HN35 instruments in 3-year HNC survivors from a clinical trial, comparing them with age- and sex-matched controls from the general Swedish population.[72] While overall QOL did not differ significantly from the normal population, disease-specific problems, including swallowing, local pain, and dry mouth were much more common in the HNC patients.

XEROSTOMIA

Xerostomia is a complex problem. Both acute and late phases of xerostomia exist and differ in both their pathophysiology and in their response to preventive strategies.[73] Salivary fraction from the parotid glands, submandibular/submental glands, and minor salivary glands may play different roles in baseline dryness and in eating-related difficulties. Similarly, xerostomia is not an isolated symptom. Both swallowing and speech performance have been shown to be impaired in xerostomic patients.[74,75] Consequently, prevention of the subjective sensation of dry mouth, in contrast to reduction in salivary flow, may require different strategies; evidence to link xerostomia-prevention strategies to reduction in late complications, such as dental caries, osteoradionecrosis, and chronic malnutrition, is lacking.

The relationship between reduced salivary flow, patient-reported dry mouth, and overall QOL is complex. Reduction in salivary flow to less than or equal to 25% of baseline has been arbitrarily classified as xerostomia, with measurement using either parotid-specific methods (eg, Lashley cup) or whole salivary production; both stimulated and unstimulated flow may be measured.[76] Physician-rated outcomes include the Radiation Therapy Oncology Group (RTOG)/EORTC grading scale, although more recently the Late Effects Normal Tissue–Subjective, Objective, Management, Analytic (LENT-SOMA) and National Cancer Institute Common Toxicity Criteria (CTC version 3) systems have also been proposed.[77-79] These measures have rarely been validated against salivary flow or PRO data. All common HNC-specific QOL instruments include at least one item related to xerostomia; however, non-QOL PROs specific to xerostomia have also been developed. Two popular instruments have been a six-item linear analog scale (LAS)[80] and the eight-item University of Michigan XQ.[81] Though less rigorously developed and validated as most HNC QOL questionnaires, these instruments have performed as expected in research use.

Prospective data on 130 patients with HNC treated with conventional RT showed that PROs (xerostomia LAS and a single question on the HNRQ) by 1-month after RT showed a statistically and clinically significant worsening; at 6 months, no recovery was seen, although overall QOL scores on HNRQ did show recovery.[82] In addition to providing validation of the LAS outcome, this result raises the issue of "response shift," a known phenomenon whereby QOL may recover in time despite ongoing objective toxicity because of a readjustment of patient expectations.[83]

Two small randomized, controlled trials have compared conventional RT with intensity-modulated RT (IMRT) for prevention of xerostomia in patients with early stage nasopharyngeal cancer (NPC).[84,85] Because of a high risk of bilateral nodal failure, NPC represents the most technically challenging subgroup of HNC for parotid sparing. Nevertheless, both studies showed improved outcomes in the IMRT group, with better parotid and whole salivary flow at 12 months after treatment. Kam and colleagues'[84] study failed to show any PRO difference between groups on the LAS, whereas Pow and colleagues,[85] using the SF-36 generic QOL instrument and the EORTC-QLQ-C30/HN35, showed better scores for the IMRT group on SF-36 role-physical and bodily pain scores and EORTC role-function, speech, and swallowing at 12 months. Neither article reported on xerostomia-associated complications or on outcomes beyond 12 months.

For non-NPC HNC, no randomized trials of IMRT are available. Prospective cohort data are available for parotid sparing using non-IMRT techniques. One study showed recovery of patient-reported xerostomia at 24 months on the EORTC QLQ-C30/HN35 in 55 subjects treated with homolateral RT, whereas 95 subjects treated with bilateral RT showed persistently worse xerostomia at 6 to 24 months after treatment.[86] The best available evidence for IMRT, outside of the NPC population, comes from a retrospective review of patients included in a prospective QOL database in whom data were collected at baseline, 3, 6 and 12 months on the HNCI.[87] Although the 26 IMRT patients were slightly older, had more advanced disease, and were more likely to have received CRT than the 27 treated with standard fractionation RT, at 12-months' follow-up their QOL scores were better in the eating domain, with favorable trends on speech and aesthetics; xerostomia was not reported directly. Importantly, not all patients are suitable for parotid-sparing RT, even with IMRT techniques. Patients with bilateral lymph node involvement and those with nonlateralized tumors may require treatment to the upper level two lymph nodes on both sides of the neck, limiting the ability to reduce mean dose to either parotid gland to the recommended level of less than or equal to 25 Gy.[88] One report linked parotid sparing to recurrence in three cases, illustrating the importance of patient selection.[89]

Administration of radioprotectant chemicals during radiotherapy has also been attempted. Amifostine has shown benefit in a randomized open-label trial of 303 subjects undergoing standard fractionation RT.[90] Subjects who received an intravenous infusion of the drug daily had a reduced incidence of physician-rated xerostomia ($\geq$ grade 2 RTOG), both acute (51% versus 78%) and late (34% versus 57%), with up to 1 year of follow-up. Whole salivary flow at 1 year was greater than or equal to 0.1 mL in 72% of amifostine subjects as compared with 49% of controls, and the mean score on the LAS xerostomia PRO was modestly higher in treated subjects. At 2 years, amifostine patients had better scores on "mouth dryness," and a greater proportion had meaningful unstimulated saliva production.[91] However, the inconvenience of daily injections and the potential for side effects, including a risk of severe hypotension, has limited the popularity of this strategy in North America.

A third interesting strategy is surgical salivary gland transfer. Jha and colleagues[92,93] have pioneered this approach for selected patients requiring postoperative RT. During the primary surgical resection, the contralateral submandibular gland is repositioned in the submental space, allowing it to be shielded during subsequent RT. With this approach, 83% of patients had normal salivary flow 2 years after RT. However, in their largest study, 17 of 60 subjects underwent the procedure unnecessarily (RT was subsequently not given, or the submental space was not shielded).[94]

Table 1
Tools identified to measure speech and swallowing specific outcomes in head and neck cancer patients

Tools	Outcome	Perspective	Domains (Themes)	Validation Population	Test-Retest Reliability	Validity
Performance Status Scale for Head and neck Cancer (PSS-HN)[113]	Speech and swallowing function	Items generated by clinicians; Tool completed by clinicians	Eating (eating in public, normalcy of diet) Speech (understandability of speech)	181 adult cancer patients of the oral cavity (28%), pharynx (36%), larynx (29%), and other head and neck areas (7%)	Public subscale: Kappa = 0.78 (SE = 0.11) Normalcy subscale: Kappa = 0.88 (SE = 0.08) Understandability subscale: Kappa = 0.64 (SE = 0.08)	Differentiated patients with head and neck cancer from breast cancer on all three subscales (P<.001) Severity of all subscales aligned with extent of surgery (P<.02)
Swedish Self-Evaluation of Communication Experiences after Laryngeal Cancer (S-SECEL)[107]	Voice, QOL	Items generated by patients; Tool completed by patients	Coping ability (general, environmental, attitude)	102 adult patient after laryngectomy	Agreement for total score = 87%	Severity subscales aligned with global rating of adjustment (P<.001)
Voice Handicap Index (VHI)[108]	Voice, function, and QOL	Items generated from patients; Tool completed by patients	Functional Emotional Physical	65 adult patients with mixed etiologies including mass lesions (32%), neurologic (26%), laryngectomy (26%), musculoskeletal tension (8%), inflammation (5%), and other (3%)	Functional subscale: r = 0.84 Emotional subscale: r = 0.92 Physical subscale: r = 0.86 Total score: r = 0.92	Severity subscales aligned with global severity rating (r = 0.60)

Instrument	Purpose	Item source	Domain	Population	Subscale results	Findings
MD Anderson Dysphagia Inventory (MDADI)[109]	Swallowing, function, and QOL	Items generated by clinicians and patients; Tool completed by patients	Psychosocial (global, emotional, functional, physical)	100 adult cancer patients of the oral cavity (12%), oropharynx (8%), hypopharynx (6%), larynx (64%), and other head and neck areas (10%)	Global subscale:[a] 0.69 Emotional subscale: 0.88 Functional subscale: 0.88 Physical subscale: 0.86	Moderately correlated with all PSS-HN subscales (r_s = 0.47–0.61) Moderately correlated with all SF-36 subscales (r_s = 0.21–0.54) Severity of all subscales aligned with extent of surgery (P<.001)
Swallowing Quality of Life (SWAL-QOL)[110–112]	Swallowing, QOL	Items generated by patients and caregivers; Tool completed by patients	Psychosocial (food selection, burden, mental health, social functioning, fear, eating duration, eating desire, communication, sleep, fatigue)	386 adult outpatients with mixed etiologies including cancer (28%), vascular (16%), degenerative neurologic (13%), other neurologic (9%), respiratory (6%), trauma (4%), chronic medical (4%), dementia (1%), other (7%), and unknown (12%)	Food selection subscale: r = 0.83 Burden subscale: r = 0.60 Mental health subscale: r = 0.80 Social functioning subscale: r = 0.88 Fear subscale: r = 0.74 Eating duration subscale: r = 0.64 Eating desire subscale: r = 0.91 Communication subscale: r = 0.76 Sleep subscale: r = 0.80 Fatigue subscale: r = 0.85	Differentiated patients with dysphagia and no dysphagia on all subscales (P<.000) Differentiated patients fed by tube and no tube on six subscales (food selection, burden, mental health, social functioning, fear, eating desire) (P<.0001) Severity of all subscales aligned with degree of solid food restriction (P<.0001) Severity of two subscales (burden, social functioning) aligned with degree of liquid restriction (P<.000) Severity of all subscales aligned with degree of oral or pharyngeal impairment (P<.0001)

(continued on next page)

Table 1
(continued)

Tools	Outcome	Perspective	Domains (Themes)	Validation Population	Test-Retest Reliability	Validity
Swallowing Quality of Care (SWAL-CARE)[110–112]	Swallowing, quality of care	Items generated by patients and caregivers; Tool completed by patients	Care (clinical information, general advice, patient satisfaction)	386 adult outpatients with mixed etiologies, including cancer (28%), vascular (16%), degenerative neurologic (13%), other neurologic (9%), respiratory (6%), trauma (4%), chronic medical (4%), dementia (1%), other (7%), and unknown (12%)	Clinical subscale: r = 0.83 General: r = 0.60 Satisfaction subscale: r = 0.80	Differentiated patients with dysphagia and no dysphagia on all subscales (P<.000) Did not differentiate patients fed by tube and no tube on any subscale (P>.2) Severity of two subscales (general, satisfaction) aligned with degree of solid food restriction (P<.08) Severity of subscales did not align with degree of liquid restriction (P>1) Severity of all subscales aligned with degree of pharyngeal impairment (P<.02) Severity of one subscale (satisfaction) aligned with degree of oral impairment (P<.03)

[a] Statistic applied unknown.

Recently, the technical feasibility of combining submandibular gland sparing via surgical transfer with IMRT parotid sparing, has been demonstrated in a retrospective planning study.[95] The generalizability of this approach is limited by the need for specialized surgical expertise and its limitation to highly selected, postoperative patients only.

SPEECH AND SWALLOWING

Disordered speech and swallowing are common sequelae of HNC and there is good evidence that they significantly reduce overall QOL.[96] Of HNC patients who undergo surgical treatment, speech will be affected in most patients immediately after surgery[97] and continues to be affected in over one-third (37%) of patients at 3 months after surgery.[98] Likewise, dysphagia is prominent in these surgically treated patients,[99] of which half (50%) continue to have dysphagia at 3 years.[100] Swallowing and speech problems also occur in HNC patients who are treated with nonsurgical organ preservation treatment, such as CRT. In general, radiation has a greater effect on swallowing than on speech,[101] and the addition of chemotherapy can increase acute toxicity of dysphagia.[102] The data are inconclusive about whether the addition of chemotherapy results in increased long-term dysphagia.[102] Patients' perceptions of their swallowing problems are not always consistent with their actual swallowing ability. For example, radiation-induced xerostomia often diminishes patient perception of swallowing abilities, regardless of normal swallow physiology.[103] In contrast, severe dysphagia, such as aspiration leading to pneumonia, was underreported by patients because the aspiration was silent in nature.[104] In another study, eating ability was compromised immediately after treatment and improved over 12 months to near pretreatment levels.[105]

Despite a high prevalence and important impact on QOL, available standardized outcome measures for speech and swallowing outcomes for patients with HNC are rarely used. Often, these impairments are measured using observations that are clinically based and vary across studies, thereby limiting comparison of findings.[106] Currently, there are six available speech- and swallowing-specific outcome measures standardized for HNC patients. Earlier measures target speech, namely the Swedish Self-Evaluation of Communication Experiences after Laryngeal Cancer (S-SECEL)[107] and the Voice Handicap Index (VHI).[108] More recently published measures targeting dysphagia include the MD Anderson Dysphagia Inventory (MDADI),[109] the Swallowing Quality of Life (SWAL-QOL),[110–112] and the Swallowing Quality of Care (SWAL-CARE).[110–112] Only one targets both speech and swallowing consequences, the Performance Status Scale for Head and neck Cancer (PSS-HN).[113] Of all measures specific to speech and swallowing, one measures function,[113] another quality of care,[110–112] and two QOL.[107,110–112] Two measures target both function and QOL.[108,109] The psychometric features of these speech and swallowing outcome measures are detailed in **Table 1**. To date, there is no available measure that targets impairment of either speech or swallowing. Martin-Harris and colleagues[114] have begun development of a comprehensive measure of swallowing impairment using the gold standard videofluoroscopic assessment findings. This tool is titled the MBS Measurement Tool of Swallowing Impairment (MBSImp). At present MBSImp is undergoing reliability and validity analysis for use with the HNC patient population.

A functional limitation, according to the WHO definition, is a restriction in any of the basic core performances of an individual, including communication and swallowing.[31] Social theorists elaborate further to describe functional limitations or disabilities at the societal level, referring to them as limitations in doing socially defined tasks,[115] such as eating in public or tolerating an unrestricted diet texture. According to the social theorists, disability will depend on both the individual's limitations of core functions and also on external factors, such as environmental accommodations. These accommodations, if appropriate, may themselves reduce the disability even though the impairment and the functional limitations remain the same.[116] For example, a patient will not be limited avoiding eating in public provided that the restaurant will accommodate his or her diet texture restriction. Of the available speech and swallowing measures identified that target function, all capture limitations related to core performances,[108,109,113] but none account for the influence of environmental accommodations.

QOL specific to speech and swallowing outcomes represent the patients' perceived disadvantage as it relates to their speech or swallowing impairment and disability. This perceived disadvantage thereby limits or prevents their personal fulfillment and well being.[31] Therefore, the QOL outcome is a construct that can only be captured from the opinion of patients themselves. The patient perspective is critical in generating items for these measures. Of the speech- and swallowing-specific QOL measures identified, all generated items using the patient perspective. A few expanded the patient perspective to also include perspectives from the caregivers[110–112] or clinicians,[109] but no measure included all three.

Speech and swallowing are complex processes that depend on a series of precisely coordinated biomechanical events. If disrupted by the HNC cancer or its treatment, the effects can be seen at any outcome level: impairment, function, and QOL. In HNC patients treated with CRT, the adverse impact of radiation can result in long-term impairments in speech, voice, and swallowing and may increase in severity even years after the completion of radiation therapy.[97] Fortunately, there are data that appropriate swallowing rehabilitation can reduce the dysphagia impairment and successfully return more than 75% of selected patients with dysphagia to oral intake, even years after treatment.[117]

SUMMARY

Despite concerns about the toxicity of treatment intensification, not all recent modifications of HNC treatment have had a negative impact on QOL and functional outcomes. While it is increasingly recognized that organ preservation does not always equate with functional preservation, appropriately selected patients may still benefit by the avoidance of ablative surgery.[101] The advent of IMRT has led to a reduction in xerostomia, and with it, evidence for improved overall QOL and swallowing function compared with conventional RT.[87,118] The development of biologic agents, such as cetuximab, has been exciting, because the drug's use with RT did not produce the intensification of toxicity seen with standard CRT, and QOL was equivalent between the RT and RT-cetuximab arms.[13] An upcoming multicenter Canadian trial (NCIC HN.6) plans to compare an EGFR inhibitor given with accelerated RT versus standard CRT, with outcomes including QOL and swallowing function, in the hope of developing a less toxic alternative therapy.

In addition to improving the toxicity profile of treatments through technology advances and appropriate supportive care, our ongoing challenge is to better select patients for the treatment option that will produce the most favorable combination of local control, overall survival, function, and QOL.

REFERENCES

1. Canadian Cancer Society/National Cancer Institute of Canada. Canadian cancer statistics 2007. Toronto: Canadian Cancer Society; 2007.

2. Bernier J. A multidisciplinary approach to squamous cell carcinomas of the head and neck: an update. Curr Opin Oncol 2008;20(3):249–55.
3. Semrau R, Mueller RP, Stuetzer H, et al. Efficacy of intensified hyperfractionated and accelerated radiotherapy and concurrent chemotherapy with carboplatin and 5-fluorouracil: updated results of a randomized multicentric trial in advanced head-and-neck cancer. Int J Radiat Oncol Biol Phys 2006;64(5):1308–16.
4. National Cancer Institute. Availabe at: http://www.cancer.gov. Accessed June 30, 2008.
5. Pignon JP, le Maitre A, Bourhis J. Meta-analyses of chemotherapy in head and neck cancer (mach-nc): an update. Int J Radiat Oncol Biol Phys 2007; 69(2 Suppl):S112–4.
6. Bonner JA, Harari PM, Giralt J, et al. Radiotherapy plus cetuximab for squamous-cell carcinoma of the head and neck. N Engl J Med 2006;354(6):567–78.
7. Trotti A, Pajak TF, Gwede CK, et al. TAME: development of a new method for summarizing adverse events of cancer treatment by the Radiation Therapy Oncology Group. Lancet Oncol 2007;8(7):613–24.
8. Rogers SN, Ahad SA, Murphy AP. A structured review and theme analysis of papers published on 'quality of life' in head and neck cancer: 2000–2005. Oral Oncol 2007;43(9):843–68.
9. Lipscomb J, Gotay CC, Snyder CF. Patient-reported outcomes in cancer: a review of recent research and policy initiatives. CA Cancer J Clin 2007; 57(5):278–300.
10. Lipscomb J, Reeve BB, Clauser SB, et al. Patient-reported outcomes assessment in cancer trials: taking stock, moving forward. J Clin Oncol 2007;25(32):5133–40.
11. Murphy BA, Ridner SH, Wells N, et al. Quality of life research in head and neck cancer: a review of the current state of the science. Crit Rev Oncol Hematol 2007;62(3):251–67.
12. Chaturvedi SK, Shenoy A, Prasad KM, et al. Concerns, coping and quality of life in head and neck cancer patients. Support Care Cancer 1996;4(3):186–90.
13. Curran D, Giralt J, Harari PM, et al. Quality of life in head and neck cancer patients after treatment with high-dose radiotherapy alone or in combination with cetuximab. J Clin Oncol 2007;25(16):2191–7.
14. Murphy BA, Gilbert J, Cmelak A, et al. Symptom control issues and supportive care of patients with head and neck cancers. Clin Adv Hematol Oncol 2007; 5(10):807–22.
15. Glover JA. The incidence of tonsillectomy in school children. Proc R Soc Med 1938;31:1219–36.
16. Eddy D. Variations in physician practice: the role of uncertainty. Health Aff 1984; 3:75–89.
17. Wennberg J. Dealing with medical practice variations: a proposal for action. Health Aff 1988;7:7–32.
18. Relman AS. Assessment and accountability: the third revolution in medical care. N Engl J Med 1988;319(18):1220–2.
19. Ellwood PM. Shattuck lecture—outcomes management. A technology of patient experience. N Engl J Med 1988;318(23):1549–56.
20. McHorney CA. Ten recommendations for advancing patient-centered outcomes measurement for older persons. Ann Intern Med 2003;139(5 Pt 2):403–9.
21. McDowell I, Jenkinson C. Development standards for health measures. J Health Serv Res Policy 1996;1(4):238–46.
22. Long AF, Dixon P. Monitoring outcomes in routine practice: defining appropriate measurement criteria. J Eval Clin Pract 1996;2(1):71–8.

23. McHorney CA. Health status assessment methods for adults: past accomplishments and future challenges. Annu Rev Public Health 1999;20:309–35.
24. Cleary PD. Future directions of quality of life research. In: Spilker B, editor. Quality of life and pharmacoeconomics in clinical trials. Philadelphia: Lippincott-Raven Publishers; 1996. p. 73–8.
25. Wilson IB, Cleary PD. Linking clinical variables with health-related quality of life. A conceptual model of patient outcomes. JAMA 1995;273(1):59–65.
26. Wood-Dauphinee S. Assessing quality of life in clinical research: from where have we come and where are we going? J Clin Epidemiol 1999;52(4):355–63.
27. McDowell I, Newell C. Measuring health: a guide to rating scales and questionnaires. Toronto: Oxford University Press; 1996.
28. Gill TM, Feinstein AR. A critical appraisal of the quality of quality-of-life measurements. JAMA 1994;272(8):619–26.
29. Andresen EM, Lollar DJ, Meyers AR. Disability outcomes research: why this supplement, on this topic, at this time? Arch Phys Med Rehabil 2000; 81(12 Suppl 2):S1–4.
30. Gray DB, Hendershot GE. The ICIDH-2: developments for a new era of outcomes research. Arch Phys Med Rehabil 2000;81(12 Suppl 2):S10–4.
31. World Health Organization. International classification of impairments, activities and participation: a manual of dimensions of disablement and functioning. Geneva: World Health Organization; 1997.
32. Meyers AR, Andresen EM, Hagglund KJ. A model of outcomes research: spinal cord injury. Arch Phys Med Rehabil 2000;81(12 Suppl 2):S81–90.
33. Bombardier C, Tugwell P. Methodological considerations in functional assessment. J Rheumatol 1987;14(Suppl 15):6–10.
34. Guyatt GH, Kirshner B, Jaeschke R. Measuring health status: what are the necessary measurement properties? J Clin Epidemiol 1992;45(12):1341–5.
35. Feinstein AR. Chapter 2: Nomenclature and functional classification of clinimetric indexes. Clinemetrics. New Haven (CT): Yale University Press; 1987. p. 6–21.
36. Kane RA, Kane RL. Assessing the elderly: a practical guide to measurement. Toronto: Lexington Books; 1981.
37. Kirshner B, Guyatt G. A methodological framework for assessing health indices. J Chronic Dis 1985;38(1):27–36.
38. Williams JI, Naylor CD. How should health status measures be assessed? Cautionary notes on procrustean frameworks. J Clin Epidemiol 1992;45(12):1347–51.
39. McHorney CA, Tarlov AR. Individual-patient monitoring in clinical practice: are available health status surveys adequate? Quality of Life Research 1995;4(4): 293–307.
40. Nunnally JC, Bernstein IH. Psychometric theory. Toronto: McGraw-Hill, Inc.; 1994.
41. Streiner DL, Norman GR. Health measurement scales: a practical guide to their development and use. New York: Oxford University Press; 1995.
42. McHorney CA. Generic health measurement: past accomplishments and a measurement paradigm for the 21st century. Ann Intern Med 1997;127(8 Pt 2): 743–50.
43. Wright JG, Feinstein AR. A comparative contrast of clinimetric and psychometric methods for constructing indexes and rating scales. J Clin Epidemiol 1992; 45(11):1201–18.
44. Marx RG, Bombardier C, Hogg-Johnson S, et al. Clinimetric and psychometric strategies for development of a health measurement scale. J Clin Epidemiol 1999;52(2):105–11.

45. Chambers LW, Macdonald LA, Tugwell P, et al. The McMaster Health index questionnaire as a measure of quality of life for patients with rheumatoid disease. J Rheumatol 1982;9(5):780–4.
46. Feinstein AR. Clinimetrics. New Haven (CT): Yale University Press; 1987.
47. Meyer GJ. Guidelines for reporting information in studies of diagnostic test accuracy: the Stard initiative. J Pers Assess 2003;81(3):191–3.
48. Streiner DL, Norman GR. Health measurement scales: a practical guide to their development and use. New York: Oxford University Press; 2003.
49. World Health Organization. Rehabilitation after cardiovascular diseases, with special emphasis on developing countries. Report of a WHO expert committee. World Health Organ Tech Rep Ser 1993;831:1–122.
50. Juniper E, Guyatt G, Jaeschke R. How to develop and validate a new health-related quality of life instrument. In: Spilker B, editor. Quality of life and pharmacoeconomics in clinical trials. 2nd edition. Philadelphia: Lipppincott-Raven Publishers; 1996. p. 49–56.
51. Scientific Advisory Committee. Assessing health status and quality-of-life instruments: attributes and review criteria. Qual Life Res 2002;11(3):193–205.
52. Gliklich RE, Goldsmith TA, Funk GF. Are head and neck specific quality of life measures necessary? Head Neck 1997;19(6):474–80.
53. Pusic A, Liu JC, Chen CM, et al. A systematic review of patient-reported outcome measures in head and neck cancer surgery. Otolaryngol Head Neck Surg 2007;136(4):525–35.
54. Bjordal K, Kaasa S. Psychometric validation of the EORTC core quality of life questionnaire, 30-item version and a diagnosis-specific module for head and neck cancer patients. Acta Oncol 1992;31(3):311–21.
55. Terrell JE, Nanavati KA, Esclamado RM, et al. Head and neck cancer-specific quality of life: instrument validation. Arch Otolaryngol Head Neck Surg 1997; 123(10):1125–32.
56. Funk GF, Karnell LH, Christensen AJ, et al. Comprehensive head and neck oncology health status assessment. Head Neck 2003;25:561–75.
57. Ringash J, Bezjak A. A structured review of quality of life instruments for head and neck cancer patients. Head Neck 2001;23(3):201–13.
58. Cella DF, Tulsky DS, Gray G, et al. The Functional Assessment of Cancer Therapy Scale: development and validation of the general measure. J Clin Oncol 1993;11(3):570–9.
59. List MA, D'Antonio LL, Cella DF, et al. The Performance Status Scale for head and neck cancer patients and the Functional Assessment of Cancer Therapy-Head and Neck Scale. A study of utility and validity. Cancer 1996;77(11):2294–301.
60. Weymuller EA, Alsarraf R, Yueh B, et al. Analysis of the performance characteristics of the University of Washington quality of life instrument and its modification (UW-QOL-R). Arch Otolaryngol Head Neck Surg 2001;127(5):489–93.
61. Johnson DJ, Casey L, Noriega B. A pilot study of patient quality of life during radiation therapy treatment. Qual Life Res 1994;3(4):267–72.
62. Trotti A, Johnson DJ, Gwede C, et al. Development of a head and neck companion module for the Quality of Life-Radiation Therapy Instrument (QOL-RTI). Int J Radiat Oncol Biol Phys 1998;42(2):257–61.
63. Browman GP, Levine MN, Hodson DI, et al. The Head and Neck Radiotherapy questionnaire: a morbidity/quality-of-life instrument for clinical trials of radiation therapy in locally advanced head and neck cancer. J Clin Oncol 1993;11(5):863–72.
64. Ringash J, O'Sullivan B, Bezjak A, et al. Interpreting clinically significant changes in patient-reported outcomes. Cancer 2007;110(1):196–202.

65. Gotay CC, Kawamoto CT, Bottomley A, et al. The prognostic significance of patient-reported outcomes in cancer clinical trials. J Clin Oncol 2008;26(8): 1355–63.
66. Karvonen-Gutierrez CA, Ronis DL, Fowler KE, et al. Quality of life scores predict survival among patients with head and neck cancer. J Clin Oncol 2008;26(16): 2754–60.
67. Ringash J, Lockwood G, O'Sullivan B, et al. Hyperfractionated, accelerated radiotherapy for locally advanced head and neck cancer: quality of life in a prospective phase I/II trial. Radiother Oncol 2008;87(2):181–7.
68. Siddiqui F, Pajak TF, Watkins-Bruner D, et al. Pretreatment quality of life predicts for locoregional control in head and neck cancer patients: a Radiation Therapy Oncology Group analysis. Int J Radiat Oncol Biol Phys 2008;70(2):353–60.
69. Chandu A, Smith AC, Rogers SN. Health-related quality of life in oral cancer: a review. J Oral Maxillofac Surg 2006;64(3):495–502.
70. Nguyen NP, Sallah S, Karlsson U, et al. Combined chemotherapy and radiation therapy for head and neck malignancies: quality of life issues. Cancer 2002; 94(4):1131–41.
71. Mehanna HM, Morton RP. Deterioration in quality-of-life of late (10-year) survivors of head and neck cancer. Clin Otolaryngol 2006;31(3):204–11.
72. Hammerlid E, Taft C. Health-related quality of life in long-term head and neck cancer survivors: a comparison with general population norms. Br J Cancer 2001;84(2):149–56.
73. Dirix P, Nuyts S, Van den Bogaert W. Radiation-induced xerostomia in patients with head and neck cancer: a literature review. Cancer 2006;107(11):2525–34.
74. Hamlet S, Faull J, Klein B, et al. Mastication and swallowing in patients with post-irradiation xerostomia. Int J Radiat Oncol Biol Phys 1997;37(4):789–96.
75. Rhodus NL, Moller K, Colby S, et al. Articulatory speech performance in patients with salivary gland dysfunction: a pilot study. Quintessence Int 1995;26(11): 805–10.
76. Roesink JM, Schipper M, Busschers W, et al. A comparison of mean parotid gland dose with measures of parotid gland function after radiotherapy for head-and-neck cancer: implications for future trials. Int J Radiat Oncol Biol Phys 2005;63(4):1006–9.
77. LENT-SOMA tables. Radiother Oncol 1995;35:17–60.
78. Cox JD, Stetz J, Pajak TF. Toxicity criteria of the Radiation Therapy Oncology Group (RTOG) and the European Organization for Research and Treatment of Cancer (EORTC). Int J Radiat Oncol Biol Phys 1995;31(5):1341–6.
79. Trotti A, Colevas AD, Setser A, et al. CTCAE v3.0: development of a comprehensive grading system for the adverse effects of cancer treatment. Semin Radiat Oncol 2003;13(3):176–81.
80. Johnson JT, Ferretti GA, Nethery WJ, et al. Oral pilocarpine for post-irradiation xerostomia in patients with head and neck cancer. N Engl J Med 1993;329(6): 390–5.
81. Eisbruch A, Kim HM, Terrell JE, et al. Xerostomia and its predictors following parotid-sparing irradiation of head-and-neck cancer. Int J Radiat Oncol Biol Phys 2001;50(3):695–704.
82. Ringash J, Warde P, Lockwood G, et al. Postradiotherapy quality of life for head-and-neck cancer patients is independent of xerostomia. Int J Radiat Oncol Biol Phys 2005;61(5):1403–7.
83. Sprangers MA, Schwartz CE. Integrating response shift into health-related quality of life research: a theoretical model. Soc Sci Med 1999;48(11):1507–15.

84. Kam MK, Leung SF, Zee B, et al. Prospective randomized study of intensity-modulated radiotherapy on salivary gland function in early-stage nasopharyngeal carcinoma patients. J Clin Oncol 2007;25(31):4873–9.

85. Pow EH, Kwong DL, McMillan AS, et al. Xerostomia and quality of life after intensity-modulated radiotherapy vs. conventional radiotherapy for early-stage nasopharyngeal carcinoma: initial report on a randomized controlled clinical trial. Int J Radiat Oncol Biol Phys 2006;66(4):981–91.

86. Jellema AP, Slotman BJ, Doornaert P, et al. Unilateral versus bilateral irradiation in squamous cell head and neck cancer in relation to patient-rated xerostomia and sticky saliva. Radiother Oncol 2007;85(1):83–9.

87. Yao M, Karnell LH, Funk GF, et al. Health-related quality-of-life outcomes following IMRT versus conventional radiotherapy for oropharyngeal squamous cell carcinoma. Int J Radiat Oncol Biol Phys 2007;69(5):1354–60.

88. Chambers MS, Garden AS, Rosenthal D, et al. Intensity-modulated radiotherapy: is xerostomia still prevalent? Curr Oncol Rep 2005;7(2):131–6.

89. Cannon DM, Lee NY. Recurrence in region of spared parotid gland after definitive intensity-modulated radiotherapy for head and neck cancer. Int J Radiat Oncol Biol Phys 2008;70(3):660–5.

90. Brizel DM, Wasserman TH, Henke M, et al. Phase III randomized trial of amifostine as a radioprotector in head and neck cancer. J Clin Oncol 2000;18(19):3339–45.

91. Wasserman TH, Brizel DM, Henke M, et al. Influence of intravenous amifostine on xerostomia, tumor control, and survival after radiotherapy for head-and-neck cancer: 2-year follow-up of a prospective, randomized, phase III trial. Int J Radiat Oncol Biol Phys 2005;63(4):985–90.

92. Jha N, Seikaly H, McGaw T, et al. Submandibular salivary gland transfer prevents radiation-induced xerostomia. Int J Radiat Oncol Biol Phys 2000;46(1):7–11.

93. Seikaly H, Jha N, Harris JR, et al. Long-term outcomes of submandibular gland transfer for prevention of postradiation xerostomia. Arch Otolaryngol Head Neck Surg 2004;130(8):956–61.

94. Jha N, Seikaly H, Harris J, et al. Prevention of radiation induced xerostomia by surgical transfer of submandibular salivary gland into the submental space. Radiother Oncol 2003;66(3):283–9.

95. Saibishkumar EP, Jha N, Scrimger RA, et al. Sparing the parotid glands and surgically transferred submandibular gland with helical tomotherapy in postoperative radiation of head and neck cancer: a planning study. Radiother Oncol 2007;85(1):98–104.

96. Karnell LH, Funk GF, Hoffman HT. Assessing head and neck cancer patient outcome domains. Head Neck 2000;22(1):6–11.

97. Lewin JS. Speech and swallowing following treatment for oral cancer. In: Werning JW, editor. Oral cancer. New York: Thieme Medical Publishers; 2007. p. 304–8.

98. Perry AR, Shaw MA. Evaluation of functional outcomes (speech, swallowing and voice) in patients attending speech pathology after head and neck cancer treatment(s): development of a multi-centre database. J Laryngol Otol 2000;114(8):605–15.

99. Pauloski BR, Rademaker AW, Logemann JA, et al. Pretreatment swallowing function in patients with head and neck cancer. Head Neck 2000;22(5):474–82.

100. Ward EC, Bishop B, Frisby J, et al. Swallowing outcomes following laryngectomy and pharyngolaryngectomy. Arch Otolaryngol Head Neck Surg 2002;128(2):181–6.

101. Rieger JM, Zalmanowitz JG, Wolfaardt JF. Functional outcomes after organ preservation treatment in head and neck cancer: a critical review of the literature. Int J Oral Maxillofac Surg 2006;35(7):581–7.

102. Lewin JS. Dysphagia after chemoradiation: prevention and treatment. Int J Radiat Oncol Biol Phys 2007;69(2 Suppl):S86–7.

103. Logemann JA, Pauloski BR, Rademaker AW, et al. Xerostomia: 12-month changes in saliva production and its relationship to perception and performance of swallow function, oral intake, and diet after chemoradiation. Head Neck 2003; 25(6):432–7.

104. Nguyen NP, Frank C, Moltz CC, et al. Aspiration rate following chemoradiation for head and neck cancer: an underreported occurrence. Radiother Oncol 2006;80(3):302–6.

105. Rademaker AW, Vonesh EF, Logemann JA, et al. Eating ability in head and neck cancer patients after treatment with chemoradiation: a 12-month follow-up study accounting for dropout. Head Neck 2003;25(12):1034–41.

106. Frowen JJ, Perry AR. Swallowing outcomes after radiotherapy for head and neck cancer: a systematic review. Head Neck 2006;28(10):932–44.

107. Blood GW. Development and assessment of a scale addressing communication needs of patients with laryngectomies. Am J Speech Lang Pathol 1993;2(3):82–90.

108. Jacobson BH, Johnson A, Grywalski C, et al. The Voice Handicap Index (VHI): development and validation. Am J Speech Lang Pathol 1997;6(3):66–70.

109. Chen AY, Frankowski R, Bishop-Leone J, et al. The development and validation of a dysphagia-specific quality-of-life questionnaire for patients with head and neck cancer: the M.D. Anderson dysphagia inventory. Arch Otolaryngol Head Neck Surg 2001;127(7):870–6.

110. McHorney CA, Bricker DE, Kramer AE, et al. The SWAL-QOL outcomes tool for oropharyngeal dysphagia in adults: I. Conceptual foundation and item development. [see comments]. Dysphagia 2000;15(3):115–21.

111. McHorney CA, Bricker DE, Robbins J, et al. The SWAL-QOL outcomes tool for oropharyngeal dysphagia in adults: II. Item reduction and preliminary scaling. [see comments]. Dysphagia 2000;15(3):122–33.

112. McHorney CA, Robbins J, Lomax K, et al. The SWAL-QOL and SWAL-CARE outcomes tool for oropharyngeal dysphagia in adults: III. Documentation of reliability and validity. Dysphagia 2002;17(2):97–114.

113. List MA, Ritter-Sterr C, Lansky SB. A performance status scale for head and neck cancer patients. Cancer 1990;66(3):564–9.

114. Martin-Harris B, Michel Y, Brodsky MB, et al. Standardized MBS assessment of swallowing impairment. [abstract]. Dysphagia 2007;22:355–68.

115. Nagi SZ. Disability concepts revisited: implications for prevention. In: Pope A, Tarlov A, editors. Diability in America: toward a national agenda for prevention. Washington, DC: National Academy Press; 1991. p. 309–27.

116. Jette AM, Badley E. Conceptual issues in the measurement of work disability. In: Wunderlich GS, Rice DP, Amado NL, editors. The dynamics of disability: measuring and monitoring disability for social security program. Washington, DC: National Academies Press; 2002. p. 183–210.

117. Logemann JA, Pauloski BR, Rademaker AW, et al. Super-supraglottic swallow in irradiated head and neck cancer patients. Head Neck 1997;19(6):535–40.

118. Graff P, Lapeyre M, Desandes E, et al. Impact of intensity-modulated radiotherapy on health-related quality of life for head and neck cancer patients: matched-pair comparison with conventional radiotherapy. Int J Radiat Oncol Biol Phys 2007;67(5):1309–17.

Understanding the Results of Meta-Analyses in the Treatment of Head and Neck Squamous Cell Cancer

Sebastien J. Hotte, MD[a,b,*], James R. Wright, MD[a,b]

KEYWORDS

- Review • Meta-analyses • Head and neck cancer
- Squamous cell • Treatment

META-ANALYSES IN HEAD AND NECK SQUAMOUS CELL CANCER

Head and neck squamous cell cancer (HNSCC) is a term typically used to describe a cancer that originates in the oral cavity, oropharynx, hypopharynx, or larynx. In distinction, cancers of the nasopharynx, maxillary and facial sinuses, salivary glands, thyroid, and lips are usually investigated and treated as separate clinical entities. Although cancers from any one of these primary sites are rare, as a group, head and neck cancers comprise approximately 6% of all malignancies.[1] Although emerging evidence may suggest a need to evaluate treatment strategies within smaller, better-defined populations, such as those based on human papilloma virus status, historically, treatment interventions have been studied in larger, more broadly defined groups of patients, such as those who have stage III and IV HNSCC.

Unfortunately, because of age and overlapping risk factors, this population of patients also tends to suffer from numerous concurrent health problems. Thus, the ability to demonstrate an overall survival advantage of a specific treatment strategy in any one clinical trial is often compromised by the fact that patients who have HNSCC are more likely to die from other health issues beyond their underlying head and neck cancer than are patients who have other types of cancers (ie, the challenge of

a Department of Oncology, McMaster University, 699 Concession Street, Hamilton, Ontario L8V 5C2, Canada
b Juravinski Cancer Centre at Hamilton Health Sciences, 699 Concession Street, Hamilton, Ontario L8V 5C2, Canada
* Corresponding author.
E-mail address: sebastien.hotte@jcc.hhsc.ca (S. Hotte).

Hematol Oncol Clin N Am 22 (2008) 1257–1266
doi:10.1016/j.hoc.2008.09.001
0889-8588/08/$ – see front matter © 2008 Elsevier Inc. All rights reserved.

hemonc.theclinics.com

competing risks). This problem is often dealt with by using surrogate clinical outcomes that are thought to be predictive of overall survival, such as local disease control, or progression-free survival. With many clinical trials unable to provide a clear survival signal, HNSCC is a disease site with obvious appeal for combining the results of many smaller clinical trials.

A meta-analysis is a statistical technique used to summarize several independent clinical trials in a systematic fashion.[2–4] Meta-analyses have enjoyed broad acceptance in medicine and, although first described in the early 1900s, it was only after the introduction of more complex statistical modeling in the 1970s that their use increased more notably. This technique of combining clinical trials is used most often to assess quantitatively the clinical effectiveness of an intervention by combining data from two or more randomized trials. Meta-analysis of clinical trials provides a more precise estimate of treatment effects, and typically gives a proportional weighting to the size of the different studies included. The validity of any meta-analysis depends on the quality of the systematic literature review on which it is based.[5] Ideally, a meta-analysis should include all relevant studies and the methodology of selecting studies for inclusion should be published. Measures to determine the presence and level of heterogeneity among trials should be undertaken and the robustness of the main findings should be explored using sensitivity analyses.

Meta-analyses lead to a shift of emphasis from single to multiple studies. They emphasize the practical importance of the effect size instead of the statistical significance of individual studies. The results of a meta-analysis are often shown using a forest plot, where the results of all studies are presented graphically by themselves and as a group.

One weakness of meta-analyses is that sources of bias are hard to control. A good meta-analysis of poorly designed studies will still result in a set of unreliable numbers. One approach to this issue is to exclude any trials that are not methodologically sound or internally valid.[6] However, the inclusion of weaker studies may be supported by adding a study-level predictor variable to reflect the quality of studies included and to examine the effect of study quality on effect size. A second potential weakness of meta-analyses is their heavy reliance on published studies, which may increase the reported effect size. The impact of this publication bias was one of the factors that led to recommendations that all phase III trials be registered in the public domain.

Meta-analyses that rely solely on published clinical trial results can only summarize the data available within the available publication or publications, whereas the use of individual patient data may provide longer follow-up for all patients and may increase the contribution of each patient to the question under review.

Published meta-analyses exist on various topics related to HNSCC, including risk factors,[7] screening,[8] diagnostic tests,[9] second malignancies,[10] and various supportive strategies and therapies.[11,12] The focus of this article is on the primary treatment strategies for locally advanced HNSCC.

ROLE OF CHEMOTHERAPY IN LOCOREGIONAL TREATMENT

The first meta-analysis addressing the role of chemotherapy in the locoregional treatment of patients who have HNSCC was published by Stell[13] in 1992. This publication followed a previous review of phase III trials published in 1990.[14] The analysis included 28 trials, and a total of 3977 patients were included in the survival analysis. As with most early meta-analyses, it was based on published phase III trials, and it included only full papers, not abstracts, published before 1991. The overall use of chemotherapy was reported to have a 2.8% overall survival advantage. With the use of concurrent chemoradiotherapy specifically, the absolute survival advantage was reported to be 7.0%. Only the concurrent use of chemotherapy was a statistically significant improvement in overall survival. Other strategies, such as induction chemotherapy before radiation alone, did not result in measurable survival improvements.

In 1994, Browman[15] published a meta-analysis of 12 studies evaluating the role of neoadjuvant chemotherapy for the routine management of patients who have HNSCC, in which 10 trials totaling 1626 patients could be included in the quantitative meta-analysis. He observed that the weighted median survival was 20.9 months for the control arms compared with 20.0 months for neoadjuvant chemotherapy, with consistent trends for resectable and nonresectable disease and for chemotherapy combinations or single agents. Odds ratios (OR) for death at various time points all favored the control treatment. Therefore, this article strongly recommended not offering neoadjuvant chemotherapy to patients who have stage III and IV HNSCC if improved survival is the primary objective and also noted that its use for organ preservation, although promising, required further evaluation. These recommendations were reiterated in a practice guideline of the Cancer Care Ontario Practice Guideline Initiative, first published online in February 1996 and updated in February 2003.[16] The guideline found three published meta-analyses and 23 randomized trials in the original report, and the updated report included a further three additional published meta-analyses and 12 new or updated reports of randomized trials, and one quality-of-life report. The results of the original report indicated no survival benefit with neoadjuvant chemotherapy, with an OR of 1.07 (95% CI 0.89–1.29) tending to favor the controls. These results did not change substantially in the updated report. For patients in whom it may be technically feasible to preserve organ function to maintain quality of life, neoadjuvant chemotherapy followed by radiotherapy can preserve organ function in a substantial proportion of otherwise resectable patients with improved quality of life, albeit with a non–statistically significant trend toward reduced survival (OR1.19, 95% CI 0.97–1.46). The investigators went on to comment that preliminary evidence from a large organ preservation trial indicated that no differences in overall survival were observed between neoadjuvant chemotherapy and radiotherapy and radiotherapy alone, but that neither treatment was as effective as concomitant chemotherapy and radiation in terms of laryngectomy preservation rate and locoregional control.

In 1995, Munro[17] published a meta-analysis of the 54 identified phase III trials that were published between January 1963 and August 1993. This report included trial results published in abstract form only, and included a total of 7443 patients in the survival analysis. Munro classified the chemotherapy trials as neoadjuvant, synchronous, or postdefinitive. Overall, chemotherapy was found to increase overall survival by 6.5%, a statistically significant improvement. Consistent with Stell's report, an even larger advantage was noted for the use of single-agent chemotherapy given synchronously with radiation therapy, which was reported to show a 12.1% overall survival advantage. This finding was also statistically significant and was reported by Munro to be a clinically significant difference that required further investigation.

In a subsequent letter to the editor, Pignon and Bourhis[18] thanked Munro for his contribution in updating the meta-analysis first published by Stell. They went on to outline their ongoing meta-analysis of chemotherapy in head and neck cancer (MACH-NC), which they stated at the time included 70 trials from the period of Jan 1963 to December 1993. They also outlined the rationale for performing a meta-analysis based on individual patient data.

In 1996, El-Sayed and Nelson[19] published a report of a meta-analysis also based on published phase III trials up to and including 1993. With stricter criteria for inclusion, only 42 trials were included in the analysis and of those, only 25 had sufficient data to be included in the survival analysis. These 25 trials contained 73% of all patients within the 42 trials but the exact number of patients this percentage represented was not reported in the primary publication. Trials were also categorized as induction, maintenance, or concurrent. Survival differences were reported as relative improvements, but when anchored against 50% survival in the control arm, chemotherapy-containing regimens yielded a 4% absolute survival advantage, and concurrent chemotherapy specifically provided an 8% survival advantage, both of which were statistically significant improvements.

In 1999, Bourhis and Pignon[20] published a review of the three previously published meta-analyses evaluating the usefulness of chemotherapy in the management of locoregional HNSCC, and included their own as yet unpublished data from the MACH-NC. The meta-analysis by Browman was not included because it dealt exclusively with neoadjuvant chemotherapy. The MACH-NC included 63 trials at that time, and a total of 10,741 patients. The three previous reports contained several trials, ranging from 28 to 54, and between 4292 and 7828 patients. Despite the differences in the actual trials included in each of the four meta-analyses, the results were found to be consistent. All four analyses suggested a small survival advantage with the use of any chemotherapy, ranging from a low of 2.8% in the Stell report, which was the only one without statistical significance, to a high of 6.5% in the Munro report. The survival benefit was also consistently highest with the use of chemotherapy concomitantly with radiotherapy, ranging from 7.0% to 12.1%, in the Stell and Munro reports, respectively.

In February 2000, the Cancer Care Ontario Practice Guideline Initiative published a systematic review aiming to answer the question as to whether patients who have locally advanced stage III or IV HNSCC in whom radiotherapy is considered the initial modality of choice for cure benefited from improved survival with acceptable toxicity from the addition of concomitant chemotherapy.[21] This review was subsequently published in July 2001 and included results from 18 randomized controlled trials (RCTs) and 20 comparisons involving 3192 patients. In their paper, Browman and colleagues concluded that concomitant chemotherapy with conventional fractionated radiotherapy should be the treatment of choice for patients who have advanced HNSCC and that at that time, data were insufficient to recommend the use of concomitant chemotherapy with altered fractionation schedules. The pooled analysis demonstrated a reduction in mortality for concomitant therapy compared with radiation alone, with an OR of 0.62 (95% CI 0.52–0.74) and absolute risk reduction of 11%. Platinum-based regimens involving 1514 patients from nine trials and 10 comparisons were most effective, with an OR of 0.57 and a 12% absolute risk reduction. This improvement in survival came at the cost of incremental acute toxicity, such as stomatitis, xerostomia, weight loss, and hematologic abnormalities. The investigators went on to qualify that the choice of concomitant therapy should take into account the toxicity produced by various regimens and the convenience of treatment administration, given that an examination of individual trial results and toxicity profiles using concomitant cisplatin-based treatment suggested that reasonable options outside a clinical trial, given all the circumstances, could include either single-agent daily cisplatin or carboplatin with conventional radiotherapy, or alternating split-course radiotherapy with cisplatin plus infusional 5-fluorouracil.

Pignon and colleagues[22] first published the full, and much anticipated, results of the MACH-NC group in *Lancet* in March 2000, and concluded that the small overall survival advantage of 4% at 5 years for the use of chemotherapy made the routine use of chemotherapy debatable. In this publication, the heterogeneity of results from trials evaluating concurrent chemoradiotherapy prohibited the investigators from making any firm conclusions, but the use of concurrent therapy was associated with significant overall survival benefits of 8% at 5 years.

For this article, the investigators updated the data on all patients in randomized trials between 1965 and 1993. The patients required a diagnosis of squamous carcinoma of the oropharynx, oral cavity, larynx, or hypopharynx. The main meta-analysis comprised 63 trials and 10,741 patients who received locoregional treatment with or without chemotherapy. Pooled hazard ratio (HR) of death was 0.90 (95% CI 0.85–0.94), corresponding to an absolute benefit of 4% at 2 and 5 years in favor of the use of chemotherapy. The subgroup of patients who received concomitant chemotherapy at the time of radiation appeared to have had significantly improved survival, with an 8% absolute reduction in the risk for death at 5 years. However, significant heterogeneity of the results prohibited a firm conclusion on the real impact of this modality.

Six trials with 861 patients that evaluated the effects of neoadjuvant chemotherapy plus radiotherapy compared with concomitant or alternating chemoradiotherapy yielded an HR of 0.91 (95% CI 0.79–1.06) in favor of concomitant or alternating chemoradiotherapy. Three larynx-preservation trials randomized 602 patients to radical surgery plus radiotherapy with neoadjuvant chemotherapy or neoadjuvant chemotherapy plus radiotherapy in responders or radical surgery and radiotherapy in nonresponders. Patients in the chemotherapy group appeared to have a non–statistically significant negative effect with an HR of 1.19 (95% CI 0.97–1.46).

Because of the considerable heterogeneity that limited the conclusions of the 2000 publication, an update of the MACH-NC that focused on the concomitant use of chemoradiotherapy was presented at the 2004 annual meeting of the American Society of Clinical Oncology (ASCO).[23] Updated individual data from patients randomized to trials of locoregional radiation with out or without concomitant therapy between 1994 and 2000 were added to the pre-existing database. Twenty-four new trials were included, for an updated total of 87 trials and more than 16,000 patients. The overall pooled HR was 0.88, with an absolute benefit of 5% at 5 years for all chemotherapy treatments, independent of timing. Fifty trials evaluated the effect of concomitant therapy on survival. For this group, the HR was 0.81, with an absolute benefit of 8% at 5 years. For the group of patients receiving cisplatin monotherapy, this benefit was extended to 11% at 5 years. No difference was seen between trials that evaluated one chemotherapy drug (HR of 0.84) or more than one agent (HR of 0.77). The magnitude of benefit was statistically higher ($P < .01$) for platinum-based chemotherapy than for other chemotherapy regimens (HR of 0.75, compared with 0.85). The concomitant addition of chemotherapy had diminishing benefits with advancing age ($P = .01$).

In 2007, Pignon and colleagues published the most recent update of the MACH-NC group.[24] As presented at the 2004 ASCO update, 16,665 patients with a median 5.5 years of follow-up were included. These patients had been recruited to 87 trials, including 50 concomitant, 32 neoadjuvant, and 9 adjuvant trials. (Because some trials had more than two arms, they were counted within two groups of chemotherapy.) The absolute benefit of 8% at 5 years was again reported and is identical for the 1994 to 2000 trials and the 1965 to 1993 trials, but without significant heterogeneity in the more recent group.

Similar results were obtained in the trials with postoperative radiotherapy, conventional radiotherapy, and altered fractionation radiotherapy with HRs of 0.80, 0.83, and 0.73, respectively. Again a significant interaction was the decreasing effect of chemotherapy with increasing age (test for trend, 0.003). For the 692 patients over 70, the HR for survival was 0.97 (95% CI 0.76–1.23), whereas patients in the other age brackets had statistically significant improvements in survival (50 or younger: HR 0.76; 51–60: HR 0.78; 61–70: HR 0.88). The causes of death were available in the recent (1994–2000) trials of the MACH-NC. The proportion of deaths not due to head and neck cancer increased with age, from 15% in patients up to age 50 to 39% in patients older than 70. As for most meta-analyses of chemoradiotherapy in this population (with the exception of the Browman and colleagues systematic review), unfortunately no information was provided about the severity and quantification of the excess acute and long-term toxicity encountered with combined modality treatment in any of the MACH-NC publications.

In summary, platinum-based chemotherapy administered concomitantly with radiation can improve survival estimates by a magnitude of 8% to 11%. These same analyses have shown that chemotherapy currently has little role in a purely neoadjuvant or adjuvant fashion before or after definitive therapy. Furthermore, the efforts of the MACH-NC have been able to demonstrate that most patients older than 70 are unlikely to benefit from the addition of chemotherapy and should only be offered this additional modality on an individual basis after in-depth discussion of the pros and cons. Unfortunately, although all the meta-analyses have provided valuable information as to the benefits of chemoradiotherapy, little has been reported on the impact of the addition of chemotherapy on acute and late toxicity or on quality of life. Future efforts of groups such as the MACH-NC should concentrate on providing practitioners with this information to better inform their patients.

RADIATION FRACTIONATION IN LOCOREGIONAL TREATMENT

One of the first meta-analyses dealing with radiation in HNSCC was published by Stuschke and Thames[25] in 1997. In fact, this report dealt with hyperfractionated radiotherapy versus conventional radiotherapy in several disease sites, but did specifically address the issue of the published trials of HNSCC patients. The investigators reported that the OR for local control and overall survival were significantly improved, at 0.48 and 0.35, respectively, in favor of hyperfractionated radiotherapy. However, only three and four studies, respectively, contributed to these conclusions, and several concerns relating to the validity of the underlying trials have been raised.[26]

In early 2006, Budach and colleagues[27] published a meta-analysis more unique to HNSCC that reviewed not only hyperfractionated but also accelerated radiotherapy, and the combination with chemotherapy. Eligible studies included all phase III randomized trials that evaluated radiation therapy given with curative intent published as a full paper or in abstract form only between 1975 and 2003. A total of 32 trials were identified and they included 10,225 patients. Ten of these trials dealt with standard radiotherapy with or without chemotherapy. Consistent with the reported meta-analyses outlined previously, statistical and clinically significant improvements in overall survival were reported for all radiation fractionation regimens when used along with chemotherapy. No difference was reported in overall survival between accelerated radiotherapy and conventional radiotherapy, but an increase of median survival of more than 14 months ($P > .001$) did occur for the use of hyperfractionated radiotherapy compared with conventional radiotherapy when used as single-treatment modalities (ie, no chemotherapy). The investigators noted, however, that their inclusion criteria for trials evaluating hyperfractionation required at least a 5% increase in total dose, and that previous studies testing hyperfractionation without dose escalation had not demonstrated a consistent survival advantage.

Later that same year (2006), Bourhis and colleagues[28] published a separate meta-analysis on the use of hyperfractionated or accelerated radiotherapy in HNSCC. This article represented work on behalf of the Meta-Analysis of Radiotherapy in

Carcinomas of the Head and Neck (MARCH) Collaborative Group. A total of 15 trials and 6515 patients were included in the report, with a median follow-up of 6 years. Individual patient data were obtained. Trials were grouped into three prespecified categories: hyperfractionated, accelerated, and accelerated with total dose reduction. Seventy-four percent of patients had advanced stage (III-IV) disease. A significant survival benefit, corresponding to an absolute survival advantage of 3.4% at 5 years (HR 0.92, 95% CI 0.86–0.97), was reported for altered fractionated radiotherapy. The benefit was highest with hyperfractionated radiotherapy, which had an 8% survival advantage at 5 years, in comparison to accelerated radiotherapy, which had only a 2% and 1.7% increase for accelerated fractionation without total dose reduction and with a total dose reduction, respectively. Altered fractionation appeared to result in improved locoregional control, particularly at the primary site of disease rather than nodal sites. The benefit appeared to be significantly higher in the youngest patients, particularly those under 50 years of age, where the HR was 0.78 (95% CI 0.65–0.94), versus those 51 to 60, 61 to 70, and over 70, where the HR increased to 0.95 (95% CI 0.83–1.09), 0.92 (95% CI 0.81–1.06), and 1.08 (95% CI 0.89–1.30), respectively. Altered fractionation had no effect on distant metastases.

In summary, these publications support improved tumor control and overall survival with the use of altered fractionation. In part because of the variability of doses with accelerated fractionation, hyperfractionation seems to provide a more consistent survival advantage, which, at least in the Bourhis report (8%), closely approximated the survival advantage reported for the use of concurrent chemotherapy with standard radiotherapy.

POSTOPERATIVE CHEMORADIOTHERAPY

Winquist and colleagues[29] from the Cancer Care Ontario Program for Evidence-Based Care published the results of their systematic review with meta-analysis in 2007. Articles were eligible for inclusion if they were published reports or abstracts of RCTs that only included patients who had newly diagnosed HNSCC who received any combination of postoperative concurrent chemoradiotherapy versus the identical postoperative radiotherapy regimen alone. Practice guidelines, meta-analyses, or systematic reviews were also eligible for inclusion. Four RCTs were considered eligible for inclusion. Two larger trials reported data after target accrual was reached and two smaller trials reported data before target patient accrual. All the trials used conventionally fractionated radiotherapy at total doses of at least 54 Gy in fractions of 170 to 200 cGy/day. Including boost doses, total radiotherapy to target volume was 54 to 70 Gy. Three trials used cisplatin (100 mg/m^2 every 21 days in two trials and 50 mg/m^2 every 7 days in the third) and one study used mitomycin C and bleomycin. All patients entered were younger than 70 years of age, with good performance status and considered to be at "high risk" for postoperative recurrence. These high-risk features included pathologic evidence of residual disease, positive margins, extracapsular tumor spread, or lymphatic, perineural, or vascular invasion.

Pooled data from the four trials found a significant difference in locoregional recurrence in favor of patients who received chemoradiotherapy with a relative risk of 0.59 (95% CI 0.47–0.75), which translated into an absolute improvement of 12.5% or a number needed to treat of 8 in favor of the combined approach. All four trials also reported data on overall survival. The improvement in survival ranged from 10% to 23% across trials, all in favor of chemoradiotherapy. Median survival was also longer. When all four RCTs were pooled, a statistically significant improvement in overall survival was observed, with a relative risk of 0.80 (95% CI 0.71–0.90), translating into a 12.5% absolute improvement and a number needed to treat to prevent one death of 8. As expected, toxicity was greater in patients who received chemoradiation and the most common grade 3 and 4 adverse events were mucositis or dysphagia, hematologic events, and nausea and vomiting. Differences in late adverse events were reported as nonsignificant in three trials and one trial did not report data on that outcome.

In summary, postoperative chemoradiation, preferably with high-dose cisplatin at 100 mg/m^2 every 21 days for three cycles, should be offered to appropriate patients at high risk for recurrence, to maximize the chance of locoregional control and prolongation of overall survival.

ROLE OF CHEMOTHERAPY IN METASTATIC TREATMENT

To the authors' knowledge, the only systematic review that directly evaluated the role of chemotherapy in the metastatic setting was published by Browman and Cronin[30] in 1994. In their review, the investigators sought to evaluate the relative therapeutic efficacy of chemotherapeutic approaches in metastatic and recurrent HNSCC by asking the following comparative research questions: What is the relative therapeutic efficacy of (1) single-agent methotrexate (MTX) versus all other therapies? (2) single agents versus combination chemotherapy? (3) single-agent MTX versus combination chemotherapy? (4) single-agent MTX versus single-agent cisplatin? (5) cisplatin-containing regimens versus other treatments? (6) cisplatin plus fluorouracil (FU) versus single agents? (7) cisplatin plus FU versus other combinations?

Their search yielded 26 potentially eligible articles, but only 15 trials could be included for a meta-analysis related to the comparative research questions. With regards to response rates, the pooled analyses tended to suggest that cisplatin plus infusion FU is superior to other combinations or to single agents. The investigators reported that treatments that were compared with single-agent MTX in randomized trials produced higher response rates than MTX, with an OR of 1.66 (95% CI 1.27–2.18). Combination regimens produced statistically higher response rates than single agents, including MTX, bleomycin, cisplatin, and FU, with an OR of 1.59 (95% CI 1.28–2.01). For the three trials that directly compared single-agent MTX with single-agent cisplatin, a nonstatistically significant trend favored cisplatin, with an OR of 1.38 (95% CI 0.67–2.87). Treatments that involved cisplatin produced response rates that were similar to treatments that did not contain cisplatin, but cisplatin plus infusional FU produced higher response rates compared with single agents and with other combinations (OR of 0.43 and 0.69, respectively).

All of the 15 trials that qualified for analysis included survival data. Pooled median survival times for all treatments were short, ranging from 4.24 to 6.39 months, and the survival differences observed within the comparisons were small, ranging from 0.14 to 0.84 months. Other clinical outcomes, such as quality-of-life domains, weight gain, or pain relief were not addressed because none of the original trials recorded such information. However, all trials addressed side effects related to the treatments themselves and cisplatin-containing regimens and combination regimens were generally associated with more toxicity, such as nausea and vomiting, or hematologic toxicities, when compared with single-agent MTX.

In summary, although a small survival benefit may exist for chemotherapy in the metastatic setting, this benefit was not firmly established. The combination of cisplatin and infusional FU appeared superior to other combinations or to single agents. However, the added toxicity from this regimen and its ability to relieve the symptoms that prompted its use in the first place (which has never been well established) needs to be considered before making treatment decisions. From the results of this systematic review, single-agent MTX and best supportive care alone remain appropriate treatment choices, depending on the patient's wishes and underlying performance status.

SUMMARY

Meta-analyses published over the last 20 years have provided practitioners with valuable insight into the management of HNSCC. Large databases with individual patient data will continue to contribute long-term outcomes. In general, these reports have supported the rationale for treatment intensification with evidence of small survival advantages to support the use of concurrent chemoradiotherapy (primary and postoperative), and altered fractionation radiotherapy.

REFERENCES

1. Argiris A, Karamouzis M, Raben D, et al. Head and neck cancer. Lancet 2008; 371(9625):1695–709.
2. Kassirer J. Clinical trials and meta-analysis: what do they do for us? N Engl J Med 1992;327:273–4.
3. Antman F, Lau J, Kupelnick B, et al. A comparison of results of meta-analyses of randomized control trials and recommendations of clinical experts. JAMA 1992; 268:240–8.
4. Chalmers T, Lau J. Meta-analytic stimulus for changes in clinical trials. Stat Methods Med Res 1993;2:161–72.
5. Jadad A, Cook D, Browman G. A guide to interpreting discordant systematic reviews. CMAJ 1997;156:1411–6.
6. Moher D, Pham B, Jones A, et al. Does quality of reports of randomised trials affect estimates of intervention efficacy reported in meta-analyses? Lancet 1998;352(9128):609–13.
7. Hobbs C, Sterne J, Bailey M, et al. Human papillomavirus and head and neck cancer: a systematic review and meta-analysis. Clin Otolaryngol 2006;31(4): 259–66.
8. Moles D, Downer M, Speight P. Meta-analysis of measures of performance reported in oral cancer and precancer screening studies. Br Dent J 2002; 192(6):340–4.
9. deBondt R, Nelemans P, Hofman P, et al. Detection of lymph node metastases in head and neck cancer: a meta-analysis comparing US, USgFNAC, CT and MR imaging. Eur J Radiol 2007;64(2):266–72.
10. Haughey B, Gates G, Arfken C, et al. Meta-analysis of second malignant tumors in head and neck cancer: the case for an endoscopic screening protocol. Ann Otol Rhinol Laryngol 1992;101:105–12.
11. Sutherland S, Browman G. Prophylaxis of oral mucositis in irradiated head-and-neck cancer patients: a proposed classification scheme of interventions and meta-analysis of randomized controlled trials. Int J Radiat Oncol Biol Phys 2001;49(4):917–30.
12. Worthington H, Clarkson J, Glenny A. Preventive intervention possibilities in radiotherapy-and-chemotherapy-induced oral mucositis: results of meta-analyses. Authors failed to acknowledge the Cochrane review on this topic. J Dent Res 2006;85(12):1085.
13. Stell P. Adjuvant chemotherapy for head and neck cancer. Semin Radiat Oncol 1992;2:195–205.

14. Stell P, Rawson N. Adjuvant chemotherapy in head and neck cancer. Br J Cancer 1990;61:779–87.

15. Browman G. Evidence based recommendations against neoadjuvant chemotherapy for routine management of patients with squamous cell head and neck cancer. Cancer Invest 1994;12:662–71.

16. The role of neoadjuvant chemotherapy in the treatment of locally advanced squamous cell carcinoma of the head and neck (excluding the nasopharynx). Available at: http://www.cancercare.on.ca/pdf/full5_1.pdf. Accessed July 1, 2008.

17. Munro A. An overview of randomized controlled trials of adjuvant chemotherapy in head and neck cancer. Br J Cancer 1995;71:83–91.

18. Pignon J, Bourhis J. Meta-analysis of chemotherapy in head and neck cancer: individual patient data vs literature data. Br J Cancer 1995;72:1062.

19. El Sayed S, Nelson N. Adjuvant and adjunctive chemotherapy in the management of squamous cell carcinoma of the head and neck region: a meta-analysis in cancer. J Clin Oncol 1996;14:838–47.

20. Bourhis J, Pignon. Meta-analyses in head and neck squamous cell carcinoma. What is the role of chemotherapy? Head and Neck Cancer 1999;13(4):769–74.

21. Browman G, Hodson I, Mackenzie R, et al. Choosing a concomitant chemotherapy and radiotherapy regimen for squamous cell head and neck cancer: a systematic review of the published literature with subgroup analysis. Head Neck 2001;23:579–89.

22. Pignon J, Bourhis J, Domenge C, et al. Chemotherapy added to locoregional treatment for head and neck squamous-cell carcinoma: three meta-analyses of updated individual data. Lancet 2000;355(9208):949–55.

23. Bourhis J, Amand C, Pignon J, On behalf of the MACH-NC Collaborative Group. Update of MACH_NC (Meta-Analysis of Chemotherapy in Head & Neck Cancer) database focused on concomitant chemoradiotherapy. Proceedings of the American Society of Clinical Oncology 2004;22:488.

24. Bourhis J, LeMaitre A, Baujat B, et al. Individual patients' data meta-analyses in head and neck cancer. Curr Opin Oncol 2007;19:188–94.

25. Stuschke M, Thames H. Hyperfractionated radiotherapy of human tumours: overview of the randomized clinical trials. Int J Radiat Oncol Biol Phys 1997;37: 259–67.

26. Liertz-Petersen C, Dubben H, Beck-Bornholdt H. Outcome of hyperfractionated radiation therapy in randomized clinical trials. Int J Radiat Oncol Biol Phys 1998;40:257–9.

27. Budach W, Hehr T, Budach V, et al. A meta-analysis of hyperfractionated and accelerated radiotherapy and combined chemotherapy regimens in unresected locally advanced squamous cell carcinoma of the head and neck. BMC Cancer 2006;6:28.

28. Bourhis J, Overgaard J, Audry H, et al. Hyperfractionated or accelerated radiotherapy in head and neck cancer: a meta-analysis. Lancet 2006;368:843–54.

29. Winquist E, Oliver T, Gilbert R. Postoperative chemoradiotherapy for advanced squamous cell carcinoma of the head and neck: a systematic review with meta-analysis. Head Neck 2007;29(1):38–46.

30. Browman G, Cronin L. Standard chemotherapy in squamous cell head and neck cancer: what we have learned from randomized trials. Semin Oncol 1994;21(3): 311–9.

Update on the Management and Therapeutic Monitoring of Advanced Nasopharyngeal Cancer

Herbert H. Loong, MBBS, MRCP[a], Brigette B. Ma, MBBS, FRACP[a,b,*], Anthony T. Chan, MD, FRCP[a,b]

KEYWORDS

- Nasopharyngeal cancer • Chemotherapy
- Chemoradiotherapy • IMRT • Plasma EBV-DNA

Nonkeratinizing nasopharyngeal carcinoma (NPC) is distinguished from the other malignancies of the head and neck with respect to its epidemiology, pathology, clinical presentation, and response to treatment. NPC is endemic to Southeast Asia, North Africa, and parts of the Mediterranean basin, with the highest prevalence in Southern China, where an average of 80 cases per 100,000 population are reported each year.[1] It is the seventh most common cancer in Hong Kong and accounts for more than 50% of newly diagnosed cases of head and neck cancers. Nonkeratinizing NPC is uniquely sensitive to chemotherapy and is almost universally associated with the Epstein-Barr virus (EBV).[1] Plasma-derived EBV DNA has been shown to be an important biomarker of prognosis and response to treatment in large cohort studies conducted in endemic regions.[2,3]

Although patients with American Joint Committee on Cancer (AJCC, 6th edition) stages I and II NPC have a high rate of cure with radiotherapy (RT) alone, those

[a] Department of Clinical Oncology, Prince of Wales Hospital, Shatin, New Territories, Hong Kong SAR
[b] Department of Clinical Oncology, Sir Y K Pao Center for Cancer, Hong Kong Cancer Institute, Li Ka Shing Institute for Health Sciences, State Key Laboratory in Oncology in South China, Chinese University of Hong Kong, Hong Kong
* Corresponding author. Department of Clinical Oncology, Prince of Wales Hospital, Shatin, New Territories, Hong Kong SAR.
E-mail address: brigette@clo.cuhk.edu.hk (B.B. Ma).

Hematol Oncol Clin N Am 22 (2008) 1267–1278
doi:10.1016/j.hoc.2008.08.012   hemonc.theclinics.com

who present with nonmetastatic stages III and IV (or locoregionally advanced) disease have a 5-year overall survival rate of only 50% to 60% after RT alone.[4,5] This is because approximately 30% and 20% of these patients will develop distant and local recurrences after RT, respectively.[5,6] The median overall survival of patients who develop distant metastases is at best 12 to 15 months after treatment with platinum-based chemotherapy in phase II clinical trials.[7] Researchers have focused their efforts on evaluating new treatment strategies, and as a result, the treatment outcome for patients who have NPC has improved substantially in recent years. This article examines some of these therapeutic advances that could have contributed to this improvement.

INTEGRATING CHEMOTHERAPY WITH RADIOTHERAPY IN THE MANAGEMENT OF LOCOREGIONALLY ADVANCED NASOPHARYNGEAL CARCINOMA

Since the early 1990s, more than 15 randomized clinical trials and 3 meta-analyses have been reported on the use of induction and concurrent and adjuvant chemotherapy in the treatment of locoregionally advanced NPC. The predominant finding of these studies is a survival advantage associated with the use of concurrent chemoradiotherapy over RT alone.[4,5,8–11] The magnitude of this benefit was reported in a meta-analysis by the MAC-NPC Collaborative Group,[12] in which the pooled hazard ratio of death was 0.60 (95% confidence interval, 0.48–0.76). This benefit was observed regardless of the type or schedule of concurrent chemotherapy used, which included cisplatin alone,[4,8,9] cisplatin and 5-fluorouracil in combination,[5] or Tegafur and uracil.[11]

The pivotal study is the US Intergroup (0099) trial,[10] in which 147 patients were randomized to either RT alone (70 Gy in 35 fractions) or RT with three cycles of concurrent cisplatin (100 mg/m^2) followed by three cycles of adjuvant cisplatin (80 mg/m^2, day 1) and fluorouracil (100 mg/m^2, days 1–4) repeated every 3 weeks. The 5-year overall survival rate was 37% in the RT alone arm compared with 67% in the combined arm ($P = .001$). Statistically significant advantages in disease-free survival and locoregional and distant failure rates also were reported with the combined arm. The applicability of this result to Asian patients in whom nonkeratinizing NPC is more prevalent had been questioned, however. Consequently, at least five other phase III studies have been completed in Asian populations,[4,5,8,9,11] which confirmed the benefit of concurrent chemoradiotherapy.

To date, little evidence suggests that adjuvant chemotherapy alone without concurrent chemotherapy adds to the benefits of RT in advanced NPC.[11,13,14] In comparison, the contribution of induction chemotherapy to the treatment outcome of patients with advanced NPC has been conflicting in the literature. None of the phase III studies completed to date has identified a clear survival benefit of adding chemotherapy before RT.[15–19] This negative result should be interpreted with caution because some of the studies were underpowered,[4,19] and the toxicities of some of the chemotherapy regimens were significant.[16] A recent updated and pooled analysis of two phase III studies reported a 5% absolute improvement in disease-specific survival with the use of induction chemotherapy.[20] A randomized phase II study that evaluated the role of adding two cycles of cisplatin-docetaxel before chemoradiotherapy recently was completed at our center. Preliminary results suggested that induction chemotherapy was associated with an improved overall survival and a hazard ratio of death of 0.17 (confidence interval 0.04–0.82, $P = .013$).[21] Further evaluation of this approach in a well-powered phase III study is warranted.

Current level 1 evidence supports the use of concurrent chemoradiotherapy in the management of locoregionally advanced NPC. This approach does exacerbate some of the acute and late toxicities of RT in normal tissues,[22] and better RT techniques and higher precision planning are equally important factors that contribute to improving treatment outcome.

IMPROVEMENT IN RADIOTHERAPY TECHNIQUES

Before the 1990s, the delivery of two-dimensional external RT via lateral opposing fields at a dose of 66 to 70 Gy over 6.6 to 7 weeks was the standard of care in many centers. The main drawback of this technique is the incidental irradiation of normal tissues, which increases the risk of treatment complications. Measures that were intended to spare incidental irradiation to vital structures (eg, the central nervous system) could sometimes compromise target coverage and contribute to local failures.[23]

Intensity-modulated radiation therapy (IMRT), by virtue of its dosimetric advantage and its ability to exploit the spatial relationship between targets and organs at risk, has gained increasing popularity in the treatment of head and neck cancers.[24,25] Retrospective studies have suggested that IMRT carries lower morbidity than two-dimensional RT or three-dimensional conformal RT.[23–26] In a prospectively randomized study from our institution,[27] IMRT was found to be better than two-dimensional RT in preserving parotid function. Of the 60 patients recruited, patients treated with IMRT had a lower incidence of late severe xerostomia than patients treated with two-dimensional RT (39.3% versus 82.1%; $P = .001$). There was no difference between the two arms in the incidence of late serious toxicities such as hearing loss, endocrine dysfunction, and temporal lobe necrosis, however.

IMPROVING THE TREATMENT OF LOCALLY RECURRENT NASOPHARYNGEAL CARCINOMA

Local recurrence is an important cause of treatment failure and death from NPC. With the advent of modern RT techniques, the incidence of local failure after primary treatment of NPC has decreased and the 5-year local failure-free rate for all T stages approaches 85%.[8] Despite this development, approximately 20% of patients with T3 to T4 disease still experience local failure after RT.[8] The TNM stage at the time of diagnosis of local recurrence is the most important factor that dictates treatment and prognosis. A thorough evaluation to exclude concomitant metastatic disease is needed because it has been estimated that up to 54% of patients with local recurrence harbor synchronous distant metastases.[28]

Re-irradiation is often the only option that is potentially curative for patients with local failure because most local recurrences tend to be deep-seated at the base of skull, where surgical resection is not feasible. In a population-based evaluation of survival outcome of patients with local failure by the Hong Kong Nasopharyngeal Carcinoma Study Group, 319 of 2915 patients with NPC developed local failure after RT, of whom 50% had stage T3 to T4 disease at recurrence. The treatment distribution for these patients was as follows: 80% had re-irradiation (including external RT, brachytherapy, or both), 11% underwent nasopharyngectomy with or without postoperative RT, and 9% were treated with chemotherapy alone.[29] The 3-year overall survival rate for the entire cohort was 74%, and subgroup analysis showed that salvage treatment only improved survival in patients with stages T1 to T2 disease at recurrence.

Salvage Surgery

The challenge of skull base or nasopharyngeal surgery is to achieve an adequate surgical margin while preserving the neurovascular bundle and restoring critical mucosal barriers. There is a lack of comparative studies in the literature on the different approaches to nasopharyngectomy, and most were retrospective reports from single centers. The more commonly used anterior approaches, such as the "maxillary swing"[30] or mid-face degloving technique, are favored for tumors located in the naso-pharynx or tumors with limited involvement of the parapharyngeal space. In a large surgical series conducted at our hospital,[31] 79 patients underwent nasopharyngec-tomy for recurrent NPC over a 16-year period; the presence of positive surgical margin was found to be an important negative prognostic factor. In another series of 53 patients from Taiwan, margin status was a prognostic factor for local control, whereas the presence of dural or brain invasion and postoperative adjuvant chemotherapy were significant factors for survival.[32]

Re-Irradiation

Re-irradiation poses a therapeutic challenge for recurrent NPC because the tolerance of normal tissues to RT often has been reached in previous treatments of the primary tumor, thereby limiting the amount of radiation dose that can be delivered safely with standard fractionation. This applies especially to recurrent tumors that are located near the spinal cord or brainstem or have bilateral parapharyngeal extension. Although brachytherapy can deliver a high dose to a tumor with smaller volume, it is applicable only to tumors confined to the nasopharyngeal cavity and away from the skull base.[33] Using interstitial implants with radioactive gold grains, Kwong and colleagues[34] re-ported a 5-year local relapse-free rate of 63%. Complications included headache (28%), palatal fistula (19%), and mucosal necrosis (16%). Law and colleagues[35] used iridium mold in their series and achieved an excellent local salvage rate of 89% but had a complication rate of 53%. Stereotactic radiosurgery has been used to treat recurrent NPC,[36] but this technique can be problematic for larger tumors and is restricted by the fact that only relatively large doses in single fractions can be used. Three-dimensional conformal RT can overcome these problems by conforming dose distributions around complex-shaped targets, improving target coverage, and reducing radiation dose to the surrounding normal tissues. Several retrospective series have compared the toxicities and disease control rate of three-dimensional RT and two-dimensional RT. Chang and colleagues[37] found that temporal lobe necro-sis occurred in 14% of patients who were re-irradiated with a two-dimensional tech-nique, compared with 0% in patients treated with three-dimensional RT. A local salvage rate of 71% was reported in another series of 86 patients who were treated with three-dimensional RT, but the respective 5-year rates of grades 3 to 4 late toxic-ities were high at 100% and 49%, respectively.[38]

Reports on using IMRT in the treatment of recurrent NPC have shown encouraging early results. Chua and colleagues[39] gave IMRT at a median dose of 54 Gy to 31 patients with or without the use of concomitant induction chemotherapy and stereo-tactic boost. The group reported 1-year locoregional progression-free and overall sur-vival rates at 56% and 63%, respectively. A subgroup analysis revealed that patients with recurrent T1 to T3 tumors had significantly better 1-year local progression-free rates than patients with T4 tumors, and longer follow-up is warranted.

IMPROVING THE TREATMENT OUTCOME OF METASTATIC NASOPHARYNGEAL CARCINOMA

Platinum-based chemotherapy has been a cornerstone in the management of meta-static NPC, and phase II studies have reported response rates ranging from 50% to 90% and median overall survival of 12 to 15 months.[40–43] Multidrug combinations (three or more agents) also have been investigated within the last two decades. In a European study of a three-drug regimen of cisplatin, bleomycin, and 5-fluorouracil,[44] the overall response rate was found to be 80% in some phase II studies, with a complete response rate of 20%. A subsequently reported Asian study of a similar regimen failed to reproduce this result, however,[45] and was complicated by significant hematologic toxicities and septic deaths. Four- and five-drug combinations have been investigated but were associated with a high incidence of grade 3 to 4 neutropenia (>80% in 1 study) and excessive treatment-related deaths (up to 9%).[46–48] Platinum-based doublet should remain the standard of care for metastatic NPC until newer and less toxic agents are available.

Incorporating Modern Agents in Metastatic Nasopharyngeal Carcinoma

Gemcitabine, taxanes, capecitabine, irinotecan, and vinorelbine are some of the modern cytotoxic agents that have shown activity in the first-line and refractory setting in phase II studies of metastatic NPC. Gemcitabine has been used to treat recurrent or metastatic NPC, with reported response rates of 34% as a single agent and 78% when combined with cisplatin in phase II clinical trials.[42,49] The combination of gemcitabine and cisplatin resulted in an overall response rate of 73% (20% complete response), a median time to progression of 10.6 months, and a median overall survival of 15 months.

Paclitaxel is active alone or in combination with platinum in the first-line or refractory setting. When used in combination with carboplatin, response rates of 60% to 72% have been reported in phase II studies, with a median time to progression of approximately 7 months.[43,50,51] Phase II studies have evaluated the combination of docetaxel with platinum in the treatment of recurrent NPC.[20,52] Chua and colleagues[20] reported a response rate of 62.5% when docetaxel (75 mg/m^2) was combined with cisplatin (60 mg/m^2) in the first-line setting. Grade 4 neutropenia was reported in 79% of patients and febrile neutropenia was reported in 42% of patients, however. A Canadian study[52] was terminated prematurely because of modest activity and high incidence of grades 3 to 4 neutropenia.

Capecitabine is an orally available pro-drug of fluoropyrimidine that has a single agent activity of approximately 37% in previously treated patients with recurrent NPC.[53] A recent study of cisplatin and capecitabine of 48 patients with untreated recurrent NPC reported an overall response rate of 62.5% and a median time to progression of 7.7 months.[54] This regimen was well tolerated, and grades 3 to 4 toxicities were uncommon. These initial results suggested that capecitabine may be a suitable substitute for infusional 5-fluorouracil in the management of NPC. Several studies of capecitabine-based combinations are ongoing. Vinorelbine[55] and irinotecan[56] have been shown to be active in platinum-refractory recurrent NPC. When combined with gemcitabine, vinorelbine has an overall response rate of 36%, whereas irinotecan has a reported response rate of 14% as a single agent in heavily treated patients.

Incorporating Molecular Targeted Therapy

The epidermal growth factor receptor has been the most studied therapeutic target in NPC to date. At least two retrospective studies have demonstrated that epidermal growth factor receptor overexpression can be found in more than 80% of cases of NPC[57,58] and was associated with inferior survival in locoregionally advanced NPC. The monoclonal antibody cetuximab is the first anti–epidermal growth factor receptor agent that has been investigated in NPC. In a multicenter study of cetuximab and carboplatin in patients with multiply treated and platinum-refractory recurrent NPC,[59] an overall response rate of 12% and disease stabilization rate of 48% were reported. Toxicities were manageable, with acneform rash being the most common cetuximab-related effect. In view of the encouraging results of combining cetuximab and RT with advanced nonnasopharyngeal squamous carcinoma of the head and neck cancer,[60] cetuximab has been evaluated in combination with a weekly schedule of cisplatin and IMRT in patients with advanced NPC at our hospital.[61] Preliminary reports suggested that this strategy is feasible, although there is an increased incidence of acute mucositis and dermatitis.

Gefitinib is a small molecule inhibitor of the epidermal growth factor receptor tyrosine kinase that has been evaluated in heavily pretreated patients with recurrent NPC.[62] No objective response was seen, and three patients had stable disease for up to 8.5 months. The study was terminated prematurely at the first stage after 15 patients were accrued. Studies on other agents that target vascular endothelial growth factor receptors have been reported or are ongoing. In a study of sorafenib,[63] a multitargeted kinase inhibitor, no activity was observed among the seven patients with poorly or undifferentiated NPC who were treated.

EPSTEIN-BARR VIRUS DNA: ROLE IN PROGNOSTICATION AND THERAPEUTIC MONITORING

EBV infection is ubiquitous in endemic NPC and is involved in its carcinogenesis.[64] Lo and colleagues[65] pioneered the technique of real-time quantitative polymerase chain reaction, which enabled the quantitative analysis of circulating tumor-derived EBV DNA in patients who have NPC. This technology has created a new way of monitoring disease activity in NPC in an accurate and minimally invasive manner. Based on the initial finding that plasma EBV DNA was associated with disease stage and recurrence after RT,[66] this biomarker has been validated prospectively in an Asian study of 170 patients who had locoregionally advanced NPC.[2] This study showed that plasma EBV DNA is a powerful prognostic marker with a relative risk for recurrence of 11.9 in patients with elevated levels after RT and positive and negative predictive values of 87% and 83%, respectively. This study was subsequently confirmed by another prospective study in Taiwan.[3] Other studies have found an association between tumor burden and the level of plasma EBV DNA in patients undergoing nasopharyngectomy[67] or palliative chemotherapy for NPC.[68] This finding was subsequently confirmed in studies that found correlation between plasma EBV DNA and tumor volume in animal models[69] and radiologically derived tumor volume in humans.[70] Pretreatment plasma EBV DNA has been shown to be a better discriminator of prognosis than conventional TNM staging in stage II NPC.[71]

Plasma EBV DNA is an important biomarker for EBV-associated NPC, and further prospective studies are warranted in the evaluation of its role in several clinical areas: (1) as an identifier of patients at high risk for distant recurrence after RT for adjuvant therapy and (2) as a surrogate biomarker of early drug response in early phase clinical trials. It should be borne in mind, however, that plasma EBV DNA in itself is relatively insensitive in detecting new cases of NPC or detecting local recurrence after RT.

IMPROVING THE STAGING AND MONITORING OF NASOPHARYNGEAL CARCINOMA USING POSITRON EMISSION TOMOGRAPHY

Several studies have suggested the superiority of ^{18}F-fluoro-2-deoxy-D-glucose (^{18}F-FDG) positron emission tomography (PET) with or without fusion CT (PET-CT), over conventional imaging (eg, CT scan, nuclear bone scan) in various clinical indications. These studies included the determination of nodal stage and M-stage before treatment,[72,73] diagnosis of residual or recurrent NPC,[74] identification of bone metastases,[73] and ascertainment of response to treatment.[75,76] Most of these studies were conducted prospectively with large sample size of approximately 200 to 300 patients.

The use of ^{18}FDG-PET-CT in T staging is more controversial. MRI has been the modality of choice in staging primary tumors.[77,78] In a recent study conducted at our center on 52 patients who had NPC,[79] the T stages and N stages determined by MRI and ^{18}FDG-PET/CT scans were discordant in 28 patients (54%). The study found that MRI was more able to define and detect the extent of tumor involvement of the nasopharynx, skull base, brain, and the orbits than PET-CT, whereas the use of PET-CT did not affect the overall M-stage or change the management in any of the patients. This study is relatively small compared with some larger prospective studies that found that PET-CT is more sensitive than other imaging modalities in determining the N stage and M stage of NPC at diagnosis.[72,73]

In the foreseeable future, PET-CT is likely to play a more significant role in the staging of NPC at diagnosis and at recurrence and in the monitoring of response treatment. Further studies are warranted in the evaluation of tumoral FDG uptake as a prognostic factor and early predictor of treatment response in NPC.

SUMMARY

Throughout the last decade, important advances have been made with regard to the management and monitoring of NPC. Several prospective clinical trials have unanimously confirmed the efficacy of concurrent chemoradiotherapy. New developments in RT planning and techniques have allowed a more precise delivery of radiation with less toxicity and long-term morbidity. Improvements in the techniques of re-irradiation and nasopharyngectomy have contributed to a better treatment outcome of patient subgroups with locally recurrent NPC. The development of newer cytotoxic and molecular targeted agents has shown promise in extending survival and improving palliation in those with incurable recurrences. Further advancements in imaging techniques are vital in improving the staging of NPC. Finally, further evaluation of tumoral FDG uptake as a prognostic and predictor of response to treatment and prospective validation of plasma EBV DNA as a biomarker of drug response are warranted.

REFERENCES

1. Chan AT, Teo PM, Johnson PJ. Nasopharyngeal carcinoma. Ann Oncol 2002; 13(7):1007–15.
2. Chan AT, Lo YM, Zee B, et al. Plasma Epstein-Barr virus DNA and residual disease after radiotherapy for undifferentiated nasopharyngeal carcinoma. J Natl Cancer Inst 2002;94(21):1614–9.
3. Lin JC, Wang WY, Chen KY, et al. Quantification of plasma Epstein-Barr virus DNA in patients with advanced nasopharyngeal carcinoma. N Engl J Med 2004; 350(24):2461–70.
4. Chan AT, Leung SF, Ngan RK, et al. Overall survival after concurrent cisplatin-radiotherapy compared with radiotherapy alone in locoregionally advanced nasopharyngeal carcinoma. J Natl Cancer Inst 2005;97(7):536–9.
5. Lin JC, Jan JS, Hsu CY, et al. Phase III study of concurrent chemoradiotherapy versus radiotherapy alone for advanced nasopharyngeal carcinoma: positive effect on overall and progression-free survival. J Clin Oncol 2003;21(4):631–7.
6. Lee AW, Foo W, Mang O, et al. Changing epidemiology of nasopharyngeal carcinoma in Hong Kong over a 20-year period (1980-99): an encouraging reduction in both incidence and mortality. Int J Cancer 2003;103(5):680–5.
7. Ma BB, Chan AT. Systemic treatment strategies and therapeutic monitoring for advanced nasopharyngeal carcinoma. Expert Rev Anticancer Ther 2006;6(3): 383–94.

8. Lee AW, Sze WM, Au JS, et al. Treatment results for nasopharyngeal carcinoma in the modern era: the Hong Kong experience. Int J Radiat Oncol Biol Phys 2005; 61(4):1107–16.

9. Wee J, Tan EH, Tai BC, et al. Randomized trial of radiotherapy versus concurrent chemoradiotherapy followed by adjuvant chemotherapy in patients with American Joint Committee on Cancer/International Union against cancer stage III and IV nasopharyngeal cancer of the endemic variety. J Clin Oncol 2005; 23(27):6730–8.

10. Al-Sarraf M, LeBlanc M, Giri PG, et al. Chemoradiotherapy versus radiotherapy in patients with advanced nasopharyngeal cancer: phase III randomized Intergroup study 0099. J Clin Oncol 1998;16(4):1310–7.

11. Kwong DL, Sham JS, Au GK, et al. Concurrent and adjuvant chemotherapy for nasopharyngeal carcinoma: a factorial study. J Clin Oncol 2004;22(13):2643–53.

12. Baujat B, Audry H, Bourhis J, et al. Chemotherapy in locally advanced nasopharyngeal carcinoma: an individual patient data meta-analysis of eight randomized trials and 1753 patients. Int J Radiat Oncol Biol Phys 2006;64(1):47–56.

13. Chi KH, Chang YC, Guo WY, et al. A phase III study of adjuvant chemotherapy in advanced nasopharyngeal carcinoma patients. Int J Radiat Oncol Biol Phys 2002;52(5):1238–44.

14. Rossi A, Molinari R, Boracchi P, et al. Adjuvant chemotherapy with vincristine, cyclophosphamide, and doxorubicin after radiotherapy in local-regional nasopharyngeal cancer: results of a 4-year multicenter randomized study. J Clin Oncol 1988;6(9):1401–10.

15. Chan AT, Teo PM, Leung TW, et al. A prospective randomized study of chemotherapy adjunctive to definitive radiotherapy in advanced nasopharyngeal carcinoma. Int J Radiat Oncol Biol Phys 1995;33(3):569–77.

16. International Nasopharynx Cancer Study Group. Preliminary results of a randomized trial comparing neoadjuvant chemotherapy (cisplatin, epirubicin, bleomycin) plus radiotherapy vs. radiotherapy alone in stage IV(> or = N2, M0) undifferentiated nasopharyngeal carcinoma: a positive effect on progression-free survival. VUMCA I trial. Int J Radiat Oncol Biol Phys 1996;35(3):463–9.

17. Chua DT, Sham JS, Choy D, et al. Preliminary report of the Asian-Oceanian Clinical Oncology Association randomized trial comparing cisplatin and epirubicin followed by radiotherapy versus radiotherapy alone in the treatment of patients with locoregionally advanced nasopharyngeal carcinoma. Asian-Oceanian Clinical Oncology Association Nasopharynx Cancer Study Group. Cancer 1998; 83(11):2270–83.

18. Ma J, Mai HQ, Hong MH, et al. Results of a prospective randomized trial comparing neoadjuvant chemotherapy plus radiotherapy with radiotherapy alone in patients with locoregionally advanced nasopharyngeal carcinoma. J Clin Oncol 2001;19(5):1350–7.

19. Hareyama M, Sakata K, Shirato H, et al. A prospective, randomized trial comparing neoadjuvant chemotherapy with radiotherapy alone in patients with advanced nasopharyngeal carcinoma. Cancer 2002;94(8):2217–23.

20. Chua DT, Ma J, Sham JS, et al. Long-term survival after cisplatin-based induction chemotherapy and radiotherapy for nasopharyngeal carcinoma: a pooled data analysis of two phase III trials. J Clin Oncol 2005;23(6):1118–24.

21. Hui EP, Leung SF, King A, et al. Efficacy of neoadjuvant docetaxel and cisplatin followed by concurrent cisplatin-radiotherapy in locally advanced nasopharyngeal carcinoma (NPC): a randomized phase II study. Presented at the ASCO Annual Meeting. Chicago, May 29–June 2, 2007.

22. Lee AW, Lau WH, Tung SY, et al. Preliminary results of a randomized study on therapeutic gain by concurrent chemotherapy for regionally-advanced nasopharyngeal carcinoma: NPC-9901 Trial by the Hong Kong Nasopharyngeal Cancer Study Group. J Clin Oncol 2005;23(28):6966–75.

23. Kam MK, Chau RM, Suen J, et al. Intensity-modulated radiotherapy in nasopharyngeal carcinoma: dosimetric advantage over conventional plans and feasibility of dose escalation. Int J Radiat Oncol Biol Phys 2003;56(1):145–57.

24. Kam MK, Teo PM, Chau RM, et al. Treatment of nasopharyngeal carcinoma with intensity-modulated radiotherapy: the Hong Kong experience. Int J Radiat Oncol Biol Phys 2004;60(5):1440–50.

25. Wolden SL, Chen WC, Pfister DG, et al. Intensity-modulated radiation therapy (IMRT) for nasopharynx cancer: update of the Memorial Sloan-Kettering experience. Int J Radiat Oncol Biol Phys 2006;64(1):57–62.

26. Lee N, Xia P, Fischbein NJ, et al. Intensity-modulated radiation therapy for head-and-neck cancer: the UCSF experience focusing on target volume delineation. Int J Radiat Oncol Biol Phys 2003;57(1):49–60.

27. Kam MK, Leung SF, Zee B, et al. Prospective randomized study of intensity-modulated radiotherapy on salivary gland function in early-stage nasopharyngeal carcinoma patients. J Clin Oncol 2007;25(31):4873–9.

28. Lee AW, Law SC, Foo W, et al. Retrospective analysis of patients with nasopharyngeal carcinoma treated during 1976–1985: survival after local recurrence. Int J Radiat Oncol Biol Phys 1993;26(5):773–82.

29. Yu KH, Leung SF, Tung SY, et al. Survival outcome of patients with nasopharyngeal carcinoma with first local failure: a study by the Hong Kong Nasopharyngeal Carcinoma Study Group. Head Neck 2005;27(5):397–405.

30. Wei WI, Ho CM, Yuen PW, et al. Maxillary swing approach for resection of tumors in and around the nasopharynx. Arch Otolaryngol Head Neck Surg 1995;121(6): 638–42.

31. Vlantis AC, Tsang RK, Yu BK, et al. Nasopharyngectomy and surgical margin status: a survival analysis. Arch Otolaryngol Head Neck Surg 2007;133(12): 1296–301.

32. Hao SP, Tsang NM, Chang KP, et al. Nasopharyngectomy for recurrent nasopharyngeal carcinoma: a review of 53 patients and prognostic factors. Acta Otolaryngol 2008;128(4):473–81.

33. Lu JJ, Shakespeare TP, Tan LK, et al. Adjuvant fractionated high-dose-rate intracavitary brachytherapy after external beam radiotherapy in TI and T2 nasopharyngeal carcinoma. Head Neck 2004;26(5):389–95.

34. Kwong DL, Wei WI, Cheng AC, et al. Long term results of radioactive gold grain implantation for the treatment of persistent and recurrent nasopharyngeal carcinoma. Cancer 2001;91(6):1105–13.

35. Law SC, Lam WK, Ng MF, et al. Reirradiation of nasopharyngeal carcinoma with intracavitary mold brachytherapy: an effective means of local salvage. Int J Radiat Oncol Biol Phys 2002;54(4):1095–113.

36. Chua DT, Sham JS, Kwong PW, et al. Linear accelerator-based stereotactic radiosurgery for limited, locally persistent, and recurrent nasopharyngeal carcinoma: efficacy and complications. Int J Radiat Oncol Biol Phys 2003;56(1):177–83.

37. Chang JT, See LC, Liao CT, et al. Locally recurrent nasopharyngeal carcinoma. Radiother Oncol 2000;54(2):135–42.

38. Zheng XK, Ma J, Chen LH, et al. Dosimetric and clinical results of three-dimensional conformal radiotherapy for locally recurrent nasopharyngeal carcinoma. Radiother Oncol 2005;75(2):197–203.

39. Chua DT, Sham JS, Leung LH, et al. Re-irradiation of nasopharyngeal carcinoma with intensity-modulated radiotherapy. Radiother Oncol 2005;77(3):290–4.
40. Au E, Ang PT. A phase II trial of 5-fluorouracil and cisplatinum in recurrent or metastatic nasopharyngeal carcinoma. Ann Oncol 1994;5(1):87–9.
41. Wang TL, Tan YO. Cisplatin and 5-fluorouracil continuous infusion for metastatic nasopharyngeal carcinoma. Ann Acad Med Singap 1991;20(5):601–3.
42. Ngan RK, Yiu HH, Lau WH, et al. Combination gemcitabine and cisplatin chemotherapy for metastatic or recurrent nasopharyngeal carcinoma: report of a phase II study. Ann Oncol 2002;13(8):1252–8.
43. Yeo W, Leung TW, Chan AT, et al. A phase II study of combination paclitaxel and carboplatin in advanced nasopharyngeal carcinoma. Eur J Cancer 1998;34(13):2027–31.
44. Boussen H, Cvitkovic E, Wendling JL, et al. Chemotherapy of metastatic and/or recurrent undifferentiated nasopharyngeal carcinoma with cisplatin, bleomycin, and fluorouracil. J Clin Oncol 1991;9(9):1675–81.
45. Su WC, Chen TY, Kao RH, et al. Chemotherapy with cisplatin and continuous infusion of 5-fluorouracil and bleomycin for recurrent and metastatic nasopharyngeal carcinoma in Taiwan. Oncology 1993;50(4):205–8.
46. Taamma A, Fandi A, Azli N, et al. Phase II trial of chemotherapy with 5-fluorouracil, bleomycin, epirubicin, and cisplatin for patients with locally advanced, metastatic, or recurrent undifferentiated carcinoma of the nasopharyngeal type. Cancer 1999;86(7):1101–8.
47. Siu LL, Czaykowski PM, Tannock IF. Phase I/II study of the CAPABLE regimen for patients with poorly differentiated carcinoma of the nasopharynx. J Clin Oncol 1998;16(7):2514–21.
48. Hasbini A, Mahjoubi R, Fandi A, et al. Phase II trial combining mitomycin with 5-fluorouracil, epirubicin, and cisplatin in recurrent and metastatic undifferentiated carcinoma of nasopharyngeal type. Ann Oncol 1999;10(4):421–5.
49. Foo KF, Tan EH, Leong SS, et al. Gemcitabine in metastatic nasopharyngeal carcinoma of the undifferentiated type. Ann Oncol. 2002;13(1):150–6.
50. Tan EH, Khoo KS, Wee J, et al. Phase II trial of a paclitaxel and carboplatin combination in Asian patients with metastatic nasopharyngeal carcinoma. Ann Oncol 1999;10(2):235–7.
51. Airoldi M, Pedani F, Marchionatti S, et al. Carboplatin plus taxol is an effective third-line regimen in recurrent undifferentiated nasopharyngeal carcinoma. Tumori 2002;88(4):273–6.
52. McCarthy JS, Tannock IF, Degendorfer P, et al. A phase II trial of docetaxel and cisplatin in patients with recurrent or metastatic nasopharyngeal carcinoma. Oral Oncol 2002;38(7):686–90.
53. Chua D, Wei WI, Sham JS, et al. Capecitabine monotherapy for recurrent and metastatic nasopharyngeal cancer. Jpn J Clin Oncol 2008;38(4):244–9.
54. Li YH, Wang FH, Jiang WQ, et al. Phase II study of capecitabine and cisplatin combination as first-line chemotherapy in Chinese patients with metastatic nasopharyngeal carcinoma. Cancer Chemother Pharmacol 2008;62(3):539–44.
55. Wang CC, Chang JY, Liu TW, et al. Phase II study of gemcitabine plus vinorelbine in the treatment of cisplatin-resistant nasopharyngeal carcinoma. Head Neck 2006;28(1):74–80.
56. Poon D, Chowbay B, Cheung YB, et al. Phase II study of irinotecan (CPT-11) as salvage therapy for advanced nasopharyngeal carcinoma. Cancer 2005;103(3):576–81.
57. Ma BB, Poon TC, To KF, et al. Prognostic significance of tumor angiogenesis, Ki 67, p53 oncoprotein, epidermal growth factor receptor and HER2 receptor

protein expression in undifferentiated nasopharyngeal carcinoma: a prospective study. Head Neck 2003;25(10):864–72.

58. Chua DT, Nicholls JM, Sham JS, et al. Prognostic value of epidermal growth factor receptor expression in patients with advanced stage nasopharyngeal carcinoma treated with induction chemotherapy and radiotherapy. Int J Radiat Oncol Biol Phys 2004;59(1):11–20.

59. Chan AT, Hsu MM, Goh BC, et al. Multicenter, phase II study of cetuximab in combination with carboplatin in patients with recurrent or metastatic nasopharyngeal carcinoma. J Clin Oncol 2005;23(15):3568–76.

60. Bonner JA, Harari PM, Giralt J, et al. Radiotherapy plus cetuximab for squamous-cell carcinoma of the head and neck. N Engl J Med 2006;354(6):567–78.

61. Ma BB, Hui EP, King AD, et al. A phase II study of concurrent cetuximab-cisplatin and intensity-modulated radiotherapy (IMRT) in locoregionally advanced nasopharyngeal carcinoma (NPC) with correlation using dynamic contrast-enhanced magnetic resonance imaging (DCE-MRI) [abstract 6055]. In Programs and Abstracts of the 2008 ASCO Annual Meeting Proceedings. Chicago, May 30–June 3, 2008.

62. Ma B, Hui EP, King A, et al. A phase II study of patients with metastatic or locoregionally recurrent nasopharyngeal carcinoma and evaluation of plasma Epstein-Barr virus DNA as a biomarker of efficacy. Cancer Chemother Pharmacol 2008;62(1):59–64.

63. Elser C, Siu LL, Winquist E, et al. Phase II trial of sorafenib in patients with recurrent or metastatic squamous cell carcinoma of the head and neck or nasopharyngeal carcinoma. J Clin Oncol 2007;25(24):3766–73.

64. Lo KW, Huang DP. Genetic and epigenetic changes in nasopharyngeal carcinoma. Semin Cancer Biol 2002;12(6):451–62.

65. Lo YM, Chan LY, Chan AT, et al. Quantitative and temporal correlation between circulating cell-free Epstein-Barr virus DNA and tumor recurrence in nasopharyngeal carcinoma. Cancer Res 1999;59(21):5452–5.

66. Lo YM, Chan AT, Chan LY, et al. Molecular prognostication of nasopharyngeal carcinoma by quantitative analysis of circulating Epstein-Barr virus DNA. Cancer Res 2000;60(24):6878–81.

67. To E, Leung SF, Chan LYS, et al. Rapid clearance of plasma Epstein-Barr Virus DNA after surgical treatment of nasopharyngeal carcinoma. Clin Cancer Res 2003;9:3254–9.

68. Ngan RK, Lau WH, Yip TT, et al. Remarkable application of serum EBV EBER-1 in monitoring response of nasopharyngeal cancer patients to salvage chemotherapy. Ann N Y Acad Sci 2001;945:73–9.

69. Chan KC, Zhang J, Chan AT, et al. Molecular characterization of circulating EBV DNA in the plasma of nasopharyngeal carcinoma and lymphoma patients. Cancer Res 2003;63(9):2028–32.

70. Ma BB, King A, Lo YM, et al. Relationship between pretreatment level of plasma Epstein-Barr virus DNA, tumor burden, and metabolic activity in advanced nasopharyngeal carcinoma. Int J Radiat Oncol Biol Phys 2006;66(3):714–20.

71. Leung SF, Zee B, Ma BB, et al. Plasma Epstein-Barr viral deoxyribonucleic acid quantitation complements tumor-node-metastasis staging prognostication in nasopharyngeal carcinoma. J Clin Oncol 2006;24(34):5414–8.

72. Chang JT, Chan SC, Yen TC, et al. Nasopharyngeal carcinoma staging by (18)F-fluorodeoxyglucose positron emission tomography. Int J Radiat Oncol Biol Phys 2005;62(2):501–7.

73. Liu FY, Lin CY, Chang JT, et al. 18F-FDG PET can replace conventional work-up in primary M staging of nonkeratinizing nasopharyngeal carcinoma. J Nucl Med 2007;48(10):1614–9.

74. Chan SC, Ng SH, Chang JT, et al. Advantages and pitfalls of 18F-fluoro-2-deoxy-D-glucose positron emission tomography in detecting locally residual or recurrent nasopharyngeal carcinoma: comparison with magnetic resonance imaging. Eur J Nucl Med Mol Imaging 2006;33(9):1032–40.

75. Yen RF, Chen TH, Ting LL, et al. Early restaging whole-body (18)F-FDG PET during induction chemotherapy predicts clinical outcome in patients with locoregionally advanced nasopharyngeal carcinoma. Eur J Nucl Med Mol Imaging 2005;32(10):1152–9.

76. Yen TC, Lin CY, Wang HM, et al. 18F-FDG-PET for evaluation of the response to concurrent chemoradiation therapy with intensity-modulated radiation technique for stage T4 nasopharyngeal carcinoma. Int J Radiat Oncol Biol Phys 2006;65(5):1307–14.

77. Olmi P, Fallai C, Colagrande S, et al. Staging and follow-up of nasopharyngeal carcinoma: magnetic resonance imaging versus computerized tomography. Int J Radiat Oncol Biol Phys 1995;32(3):795–800.

78. King AD, Teo P, Lam WW, et al. Paranasopharyngeal space involvement in nasopharyngeal cancer: detection by CT and MRI. Clin Oncol (R Coll Radiol) 2000;12(6):397–402.

79. King AD, Ma BB, Yau YY, et al. The impact of 18F-FDG PET/CT on assessment of nasopharyngeal carcinoma at diagnosis. Br J Radiol 2008;81(964):291–8.

New Agents in the Treatment for Malignancies of the Salivary and Thyroid Glands

Ranee Mehra, MD, Roger B. Cohen, MD*

KEYWORDS

- Malignant • Salivary gland tumors
- Thyroid cancer • Tyrosine kinase inhibitors

The treatment of relatively rare malignancies, such as those of the salivary glands and iodine refractory thyroid cancer, has been invigorated by the development of novel molecular targeting agents. Accrual to clinical trials for these disease sites continues to be limited by their relatively low incidence. Nonetheless, multicenter collaborations have contributed greatly to the development of a number of emerging systemic therapies. This article briefly summarizes the epidemiology and pathogenesis of salivary gland and thyroid cancer, and then describes some of the new drugs under evaluation for these malignancies.

MALIGNANT SALIVARY GLAND TUMORS

Malignant salivary gland tumors (MSGT) are relatively rare and encompass a diverse group of histologies and natural histories. The incidence per year is about 1 to 3 per 100,000 people, accounting for about 6% of head and neck cancers.[1] Surgery is the primary modality for cure of local disease. Treatment for metastatic disease is usually palliative. MSGT often exhibit a notably indolent course, especially the low grade, more differentiated histologies. Thus, given the potential for an unusually long natural history and prolonged periods of stable disease, appropriate endpoints in clinical trials need to be chosen. Because of these factors, clinical investigation for this disease group continues to present some unique challenges.

Malignancies in the salivary gland can arise in either the major or minor glands, with about 70% of cases arising in the parotid gland. Unlike squamous cell head and neck

Department of Medical Oncology, Fox Chase Cancer Center, 333 Cottman Avenue, Philadelphia, PA 19111, USA
* Corresponding author.
E-mail address: rb_cohen@fccc.edu (R.B. Cohen).

Hematol Oncol Clin N Am 22 (2008) 1279–1295
doi:10.1016/j.hoc.2008.08.010
0889-8588/08/$ – see front matter © 2008 Elsevier Inc. All rights reserved.

malignancies, smoking and tobacco have not been associated with an increased risk of MSGTs. A history of radiation exposure, however, is associated with the development of benign and malignant SGTs.[2,3] Because of the common risk factor of radiation exposure, there can also be coincident MSGTs and thyroid cancers, although the molecular pathogenesis of the two diseases varies.[4,5] Another potential risk factor for the lymphoepithelial salivary gland carcinoma variant includes Epstein-Barr virus exposure, which has especially been noted in East Asia, similar to the epidemiology of nasopharyngeal lymphoepithelioma.[6–9] The exact mechanism for pathogenesis remains unknown, but mutations in the LMP1 gene, associated with aberrant transcriptional regulation, have been detected.[10]

The histology and clinical course of salivary gland tumors vary greatly.[11] For the purposes of this article, the authors will focus on salivary gland carcinomas rather than benign tumors that do not have malignant potential and thus do not require systemic therapy. The classification of carcinomas according to the World Health Organization (WHO) histologic classification is presented in **Table 1**. It should be noted that this is a histologic classification; it does not provide insight into the molecular pathogenesis of each variant. The more indolent carcinomas include acinic cell carcinoma, low-grade mucoepidermoid carcinomas, and epithelial-myoepithelial carcinoma. By contrast, the more aggressive histologies include adenoid cystic carcinoma, high-grade mucoepidermoid carcinomas, salivary duct carcinoma, invasive carcinoma in pleomorphic adenoma, and small cell carcinoma.

Management of localized salivary gland tumors primarily involves surgical resection. At times, adjuvant radiation is offered, depending on risk factors such as positive surgical margins and perineural invasion, but unlike squamous cell carcinoma of the head and neck, there is no role for adjuvant chemoradiotherapy. The use of systemic therapy is reserved for patients with unresectable, locally advanced, or metastatic disease. Even in patients with unresectable locally advanced disease there is a major palliative role for local radiation therapy. Given the often indolent disease course (for instance, the median survival for metastatic adenoid cystic carcinoma is 3 years and can be up to 10 years), it is important to consider the benefit of routine systemic cytotoxic chemotherapy in the management of this metastatic disease.[12] Therefore, watchful waiting is often an appropriate strategy for many, if not the majority of patients with asymptomatic, indolent disease. For those with rapidly progressing, symptomatic disease, on the other hand, therapeutic options include monotherapy with traditional cytotoxic agents, such as monotherapy with cisplatin, vinorelbine, or paclitaxel (mucoepidermoid and adenocarcinoma), but the benefits are very modest and the potential for toxicity considerable.[13–15] Combination regimens appear to have higher response rates at the expense of greater toxicity, but there are no randomized comparisons to assess a survival benefit versus monotherapy. Combinations with antitumor activity include CAP (cyclophosphamide, doxorubicin, cisplatin), which has been shown to have a modest response rate of 27% in a phase 2 setting.[16] Cisplatin/vinorelbine (ORR 44%) and carboplatin/paclitaxel are other combination regimens with antitumor activity, again with unproven impact on survival.[14,17]

Molecular Pathogenesis and Novel Targets

With the availability of novel agents directed at molecular targets commonly over-expressed or altered in cancer, including MSGT, most interest to date has focused on the following markers: c-kit, vascular endolethial growth factor (VEGF)/VEGFR, epidermal growth factor receptor (EGFR), and Her-2/neu. High c-kit expression detected by immunohistochemistry (IHC) has been observed in adenoid cystic, acinic cell, polymorphous low-grade adenocarcinoma, epithelial-myoepithelial carcinoma, and

Table 1
WHO classification of salivary gland tumors

Carcinomas	Features
Low grade, favorable prognosis	
Acinic cell carcinoma	Low grade and low malignant potential
	Lymphoid infiltrate in supporting stroma
Low-grade mucoepidermoid carcinoma	Low grade: cystic, mucous producing cells
Polymorphous low-grade adenocarcinoma	Arises in minor salivary glands
	Good prognosis
Epithelial—myoepithelial carcinoma	Predominately in parotid gland
	Higher incidence in females
Basal cell adenocarcinoma	Low grade with regional recurrence
	Predominantly in parotid
Sebaceous carcinoma	–
Papillary cystadenocarcinoma	–
Mucinous adenocarcinoma	–
Oncocytic carcinoma	–
High grade, poor prognosis	
Salivary duct carcinoma	High grade, poor prognosis
High-grade mucoepidermoid carcinoma	High grade: solid, with hemorrhage and necrosis
Adenoid cystic carcinoma	Biologically aggressive
Adenocarcinoma	–
Malignant myoepithelioma	–
Carcinoma in pleomorphic adenoma (mixed malignant tumor)	Degree of invasiveness determines prognosis
Squamous cell carcinoma	–
Small cell carcinoma	Poor prognosis similar to small cell carcinoma of the lung and other anatomic sites
Undifferentiated carcinoma	Histologically similar to lymphoepithelial carcinoma of the nasopharynx

Data from Seifert G, Sobin LH. The World Health Organization's histological classification of salivary gland tumors. A commentary on the second edition. Cancer 1992;70(2):380.

carcinosarcoma.[18–21] Two phase 2 studies were conducted to assess the antitumor activity of imatinib, an inhibitor of the c-kit tyrosine kinase, in patients with adenoid cystic carcinoma that over-expressed c-kit.[22,23] No objective responses were observed in either study. Other preclinical work has suggested that loss of c-kit is associated with high malignant grade and decreased survival.[20] In a third small clinical study, rapid disease progression was observed with imatinib treatment.[24]

Increased VEGF expression by IHC has also been noted in small preclinical studies and seems to correlate with lymph node metastases, advanced clinical stage, high risk of recurrence, and inferior cause-specific survival.[25,26] Adenoid cystic carcinoma cell lines with high metastatic potential have demonstrated increased angiogenic ability.[27] AEE788, a dual inhibitor of EGFR and VEGFR, has inhibited growth and induced apoptosis in adenocystic carconoma (ACC) cell lines.[28] Multikinase inhibitors, such as sorafenib and sunitinib, and the monoclonal antibody bevacizumab, have been studied widely in oncology and are Food and Drug Administration (FDA)-approved in a variety of solid tumors. The use of these agents remains investigational for salivary gland tumors, and their effectiveness in for this disease is unknown. Currently, phase 2 trials specifically studying the efficacy of one of these agents in salivary gland malignancies are not available, and appropriate phase 1 studies are reasonable treatment options.

The finding of elevated EGFR/HER1 and Her2/neu expression in MSGTs has logically led to preclinical investigation of EGFR and Her2/neu targeting agents. For instance, the malignant component of carcinoma in pleomorphic adenoma had increased expression of these receptors in comparison to the benign component.[29] The more aggressive variant of mucoepidermoid carcinoma has been associated with increased Her-2/neu expression as well.[30] In addition to increased protein expression by IHC, increased amplification of the Her-2/neu gene by fluorescence in situ hybridization (FISH) has been detected in salivary duct carcinomas, but it is not clear if this phenomenon correlates with outcome.[31,32] By contrast, Her-2/neu overexpression was only noted in a small number of adenoid cystic carcinoma specimens.[33]

To attempt to exploit these findings therapeutically, a salivary gland adenocarcinoma cell line was treated with the small molecule tyrosine kinase inhibitor of the EGFR, gefitinib, and resulted in cytostasis with down-regulation of cyclin D1, STAT3, and MAPK.[34] In the clinic, however, treatment with gefitinib yielded no responses in 29 patients with MSGT (19 ACC, 2 mucoepidermoid).[35] Ten patients did have stabilization of disease, but the significance of this will remain unclear in a relatively indolent disease process. A phase 2 trial studying the EGFR targeting monoclonal antibody cetuximab in salivary gland tumors has also been presented.[36] Histologies that were treated included predominantly adenoid cystic carcinoma, in addition to mucoepidermoid, myoepithelial, and acinic cell. Half of the 22 evaluable patients had stable disease (SD), seven of which had durable stability lasting over 6 months. There were no partial or complete responses. Clinical benefit (duration of SD) did not correlate with the classic EGFR inhibitor associated rash or with EGFR amplification by FISH, although several patients with increased EGFR expression by IHC had prolonged SD. This study indicated potential activity of this agent in a selected population but again, the finding of prolonged stable SD is hard to interpret in such an indolent disease.

Given the preclinical data regarding Her-2/neu expression, there was interest in testing trastuzumab in the clinical setting. A phase 2 study was initiated in which subjects with 2+ and 3+ Her-2/neu IHC staining were to be treated with trastuzumab monotherapy.[37] To screen potentially eligible patients for this study, 137 tumor specimens were screened. Only 14 subjects were enrolled before the study was terminated because of generally low levels of Her-2 expression in most screened patients. The median time-to-progression for all subjects treated was only 4.2 months.[38] The overall frequency of Her-2/neu over-expression was 17%, but among the adenoid cystic tumors the frequency of over-expression was only 4%. Salivary duct tumors, on the other hand, had a higher rate of over-expression of Her-2/neu of 83%. These findings led to a study that was conducted by the Southwest Oncology Group, in which patients with Her-2/neu over-expression or gene amplification were selected for treatment. Adenoid cystic carcinomas were specifically excluded (www.clinicaltrials.gov). Unfortunately, a poor funding climate led to withdrawal of financial support and further accrual was discontinued. Thus, there is a lack of clinical data to suggest which criteria might select patients with MSGTs that would respond to trastuzumab.

Lapatinib is a small molecule tyrosine kinase inhibitor that binds to the ATP binding site of both EGFR and Her-2/neu. Given the known potential for cross-talk between these two tyrosine kinase receptors, dual targeting has been of interest. In a recent study of MSGTs, patients were stratified and enrolled according to ACC and non-ACC histologies.[39] In the ACC treatment arm, at least one objective response was required after the first 12 subjects in order for enrollment to continue. Eligibility criteria included measurable disease with evidence of disease progression and positive IHC staining for EGFR and Her-2/neu. As in prior studies, there were no partial responses in either group. However, tumor stabilization was noted in 75% of the subjects with ACC, and in 47% of non-ACC subjects. Stable disease lasting over 6 months was noted in 45% and 21% of subjects in the two groups, respectively, which is greater than what would be expected based on historical controls. Serial biopsies were done to assess possible biologic markers of activity, but there were none that correlated with response, with the possible exception of a suggestion that increased EGFR and Her-2/neu expression might serve as markers for patients who would benefit from lapatinib therapy.

Currently, most of the clinical efforts for the study of MSGTs have focused on EGFR and Her-2/neu targeting agents. Future trials will likely incorporate antiangiogenesis agents, especially multitargeted tyrosine kinase inhibitors, into treatment regimens as well. Based on recent studies of these agents in other more common cancers, the expectation for outcome must be disease stabilization rather than objective responses.

To increase the chance of detecting a clinical benefit, it will be important to develop studies that take into account the different histologies and molecular profiles of MSGTs. Given the rarity of these tumors, however, this will continue to present a major challenge and will require multi-institutional collaborations and study designs based on preclinical data of target expression and sensitivity to the selected molecular therapeutics.

THYROID CANCER

Thyroid cancers, while relatively uncommon with an annual incidence of 34,000 cases, have been increasing in incidence at a rate of 3% per year, for reasons that remain unclear.[1,40,41] Known risk factors include prior radiation exposure, reduced iodine intake, lymphocytic thyroiditis, and a family history of thyroid cancer.[42] In addition, those exposed to nuclear fall-out as a result of nuclear disasters are known to have a higher risk of papillary thyroid cancer.[43] The rising incidence of thyroid cancer seems to be mainly a result of increased rates of papillary thyroid cancer, as opposed to the other histologies, and appears driven in part by an increase in the detection of small cancers via ultrasound and other imaging technologies.[41] There are two distinct cellular origins: papillary, follicular, and anaplastic thyroid cancers arise from the follicular cells, while medullary cancers arise from the parafollicular C-cells. The majority of thyroid cancers are the differentiated histologies (DTC), with papillary thyroid cancer (PTC) accounting for 80%, follicular cancer/Hürthle cell variant (FTC) accounting for 15%, and anaplastic (ATC) accounting for 2% of diagnoses. The mainstay of treatment for thyroid malignancies is surgical resection. The differentiated thyroid cancers are often amenable to adjuvant treatment for cure with radioactive iodine (I)-131, and this modality is also the initial preferred treatment for metastatic disease that is iodine-avid. This group of thyroid cancers is also sensitive to thyroid stimulating hormone and they produce thyroglobulin. In contrast, medullary thyroid cancers (MTC) do not have any of these features.

Doxorubicin is currently the only FDA-approved systemic agent for the treatment of advanced, incurable thyroid cancer. Doxorubicin has been shown to induce apoptosis in thyroid cancer cell lines.[44,45] While the clinical experience with doxorubicin in thyroid cancer has spanned decades, in practice there has been little enthusiasm to use it as a routine, first-line option. Historically, numerous small phase 2 studies of doxorubicin, with sample sizes ranging from 2 to 19 subjects, have shown response rates ranging from 22% to 90%.[46–52] It is widely believed that the small subject numbers and varying criteria for assessing response, especially among the older studies that pre-dated spiral CT scans and consensus criteria for response assessment such as RECIST (response evaluation criteria in solid tumors), exaggerated the effectiveness of this agent. Even a small phase 2 study of the combination of cisplatin and doxorubicin only resulted in a response rate of 9%.[53] Doxorubicin has been studied in two relatively contemporary trials. In one trial, 17 subjects were treated with doxorubicin in combination with interferon alpha.[54] Only one patient had a partial response and 10 had stable disease, with a median time to progression of 5.9 months. In another study, doxorubicin monotherapy (either given weekly or once every 3 weeks) was administered.[55] Among the subjects with papillary or follicular cancer, there was a partial response (PR) rate of 5%, with 42% of patients showing SD. Among patients with MTC, the rates of PR and SD were both 11%. Thus, while doxorubicin has single agent activity, there is an obvious need for a more effective, less toxic therapy.

Molecular Pathogenesis of Thyroid Cancer

Iodine-refractory thyroid cancer arises as a result of tumor cell de-differentiation and accounts for about 2% to 5% of all thyroid cancers. High-risk features for developing eventual iodine refractory disease include tumor necrosis, extrathyroidal extension, older age, male gender, and high-grade histology. The majority of deaths from differentiated thyroid cancer occur in patients with iodine refractory disease. In the past, treatment options for this unfortunate group of patients have included surgery or external beam radiation for localized disease in the neck and upper thorax, doxorubicin for systemic disease, or referral for experimental therapy, usually phase 1 trials.

Novel molecular therapies are having a potentially dramatic impact on the course of incurable, iodine-refractory thyroid cancer, as well as MTC, and are likely to change our treatment paradigms. An understanding of the pathogenesis of thyroid cancer is necessary to understand why responses are occurring and also to determine how best to use the multi-kinase inhibitors that are currently under evaluation in the clinic. This involves an understanding of the initiating genetic lesions responsible for these diseases, as well as and those transformation events that lead to the progressive de-differentiation that results in undifferentiated and anaplastic cancers.

The molecular events associated with the development of PTC mainly appear to involve alterations of genes encoding effectors of the MAPK pathway. This typically includes nonoverlapping activating mutations in one of the following four genes, which are detectable in 70% of papillary thyroid cancers: RET/PTC rearrangements, BRAF, NTRK1 (neutrotrophic tyrosine kinase receptor 1) rearrangements, or RAS.[56,57] RET and NTRK1 are both tyrosine kinase receptors, and Raf is a serine/threonine kinase. Numerous RET/PTC rearrangements have been identified in sporadic and radiation exposure related papillary thyroid cancers, with RET/PTC1 and RET/PTC3 being more common.[58] A somatic mutation in BRAF (V600E) is one of the more common mutations identified (36%–69%), while RAS mutations are more rare in papillary cancers and appear to be more common in follicular cancers.[57,59] RAF mutations correlate with adverse clinical features, such as extrathyroidal invasion, lymph node metastases, advanced stage, risk of recurrence, and loss of I-131 avidity.[60,61] In one series, RAF point mutations have been detected in 38% of papillary carcinomas, 13% of poorly differentiated carcinomas, and 10% of anaplastic carcinomas, but not in follicular or Hürthle cell malignancies.[61] In addition, BRAF mutation has been shown to correlate with low expression of the sodium iodide symporter (NIS), which could provide a molecular explanation of the dedifferentiated, noniodine-avid phenotype of these cancers.[62] Interestingly, the RET/PTC alteration was not associated with NIS expression. Inhibition of the MAPK pathway therefore becomes an obvious therapeutic approach for iodine refractory thyroid cancers. Preclinical data from cell lines with either BRAF, RAS, or RET mutations indicate that only the BRAF mutation predicts for sensitivity to MEK inhibition, the downstream effector of all of these pathways.[63] Raf kinase inhibitors also inhibited the growth of thyroid cancer cells with BRAF- or RET/PTC-activating mutations.[64]

FTCs differ molecularly from papillary cancers and are characterized by RAS mutations and PAX8-PPARγ rearrangements (t(2;3)(q13;p25)). The fusion of the thyroid transcription factor PAX8 and the steroid nuclear hormone receptor PPARγ has been detected in up to 50% of FTCs, but not follicular adenomas nor PTCs, and results in a distinct gene expression profile.[65,66] The rearrangement likely inhibits cell differentiation while stimulating growth, functioning as a dominant negative inhibitor of the wild-type PPARγ receptor, the latter probably serving as a tumor suppressor.[67] In vitro, PPARγ agonists led to reduced growth of follicular carcinoma tumor cells, and thus the clinical study of PPARγ modulators in follicular cancers, such as the thiazolidenediones (pioglitazone and rosiglitazone), is warranted.[68]

RAS mutations and PAX8-PPARγ rearrangements are rarely found in the same tumor, suggesting two separate molecular pathogenic pathways for this disease.[69] Point mutations in H-RAS and N-RAS have been detected in FTCs.[70,71] As RAS mutations are also seen in papillary carcinomas, it is possible that these mutations contribute to tumorigenesis in conjunction with other oncogenes, and thus are not specific to follicular carcinomas serving as the primary instigators of malignancy.

While the genes discussed above have been implicated in the initial pathogenesis of thyroid cancers, other growth factor receptors appear to play a role in the progression and behavior of thyroid carcinomas. For instance, VEGF is detected at increased levels in papillary and follicular thyroid cancers compared with hyperplastic or benign thyroid tissue, and is associated with increased risk for recurrence and metastatic disease.[72–75] Targeting angiogenesis in this disease is thus another area of extensive research. The growth of tumors in ATC mouse xenografts, for example, was curtailed by AZD2171, a potent inhibitor of the VEGFR.[76]

EGFR is also expressed and phosphorylated in thyroid cancer cell lines and tissue.[77] It is over-expressed in human thyroid cancer as well, and is associated with a worse prognosis.[78] EGFR activation may also result in activation of c-met signaling.[79] There are provocative interactions between the EGFR and the RET/PTC fusion protein. It is known that the RET/PTC oncogene dimerizes, resulting in autophosphorylation of tyrosine kinase motifs and constitutive activation of downstream signaling.[80] Inhibition of EGFR decreases RET autophosphorylation, and the two proteins co-immunoprecipitate from cell lysates and thus appear to form a complex.[81] In vitro, a role for EGFR activation in thyroid cancer is also supported by the finding that the EGFR and multi-kinase inhibitors, gefitinib, PKI1166, and AEE788 had growth inhibitory effects in cell lines with the RET-activating mutation. AEE788 also has activity against VEGFR, and this compound also had inhibitory effects on ATC xenografts.[82] The agent ZD6474 (vandetanib), which targets RET, VEGFR, and EGFR, is another attractive compound to explore in this setting, and in preclinical studies does limit the growth of thyroid cancer cells with the RET/PTC activating rearrangement.[83]

Activation of Akt, a downstream effector of PI3kinase, has been observed in follicular and papillary thyroid cancer cells.[84] Inhibition of Akt did result in decreased cell proliferation and increased apoptosis in thyroid carcinoma cell lines in vitro. It is also well known that patients with Cowden's syndrome, who have a loss of PTEN resulting in activation of the Akt pathway, are at increased risk of developing thyroid cancer. A mouse model of follicular thyroid adenoma has been generated by engineering a loss of PTEN in the thyroid follicular cells, but another genetic event is likely required for malignant transformation.[85]

Anaplastic and undifferentiated thyroid cancers are aggressive malignancies that are not responsive to radioactive iodine or other systemic cytotoxic therapies. It is felt that originally differentiated thyroid cancers undergo additional molecular changes, resulting in clonal evolution to a less differentiated variant. One such genetic event includes p53 mutations, which have been detected in anaplastic carcinoma cell lines but not in the more differentiated histologies.[86,87] In one series, evidence of p53 mutations was noted in cells which also harbored BRAF mutations, suggesting that both events are important to malignant transformation.[87] Mutations in the catalytic subunit of PI3K, PIK3CA, have also been observed in ATC cell lines.[88] Modification of the extracellular matrix likely influences malignant progression and metastatic potential as well. For instance, E-cadherin expression is low in recurrent metastic thyroid carcinomas, but is present in less advanced, well-differentiated cancers.[89,90] In addition, β-catenin, which associates with cadherins, was found to have low expression, with increased nuclear localization of this molecule.[91] In the future, further delineation of the molecular events associated with the undifferentiated histologies will aid greatly in the development of more effective therapies for this aggressive and notoriously refractory group of carcinomas.

MTC is characterized by activating mutations in the RET proto-oncogene, with constitutive activity of this tyrosine kinase receptor. The majority (75%) of MTCs are sporadic, with mutations in RET detected in up to 25% to 66% of this population.[92] Most of these somatic mutations are in exon 16. In contrast, of the remaining 25% of MTCs that are familial as part of the multiple endocrine neoplasia type 2 syndrome nearly all carry RET mutations, often in exons 10 or 11.[93,94]

Systemic Therapy for Metastatic Disease

Novel multikinase small molecule inhibitors are being actively studied in I-131 nonavid papillary and follicular carcinomas (DTC), as well as MTCs, with encouraging early results. **Table 2** lists these agents, the targets they act upon, and the subtypes of thyroid cancer in which they have been studied. It is clear from **Table 2** that a shared mechanism of action for most of the agents is to inhibit angiogenesis, with most of these molecules binding to VEGF or VEGFRs. In addition, RET is an obvious target, given its role as an initiating factor in papillary and medullary thyroid cancer. **Table 3** summarizes the numerous phase 2 studies that have been conducted in recent years with these agents, several of which will be discussed further below.

Motesanib is an oral inhibitor of the VEGF receptors 1, 2, and 3, PDGF (platelet derived growth factor), KIT, and RET. An open-label, single-arm, multicenter phase 2 study was conducted in subjects with locally advanced or metastatic differentiated thyroid cancers that were refractory to radioactive iodine therapy.[95] In total, 93 subjects (61% PTC) were treated with 125 mg of motesanib once daily; 83% had not received prior chemotherapy. Tumor genotyping was conducted, but was not performed in 52% of samples; 30% had the BRAF(V600E) mutation and 18% had RAS mutations, but neither finding was clearly associated with response. The objective response rate was 14%, with SD observed in 67% of subjects. The median duration of response was 32 weeks, with a median progression free survival (PFS) of 40 weeks. Grade 3 toxicities occurred in 55% of subjects, including diarrhea, hypertension, fatigue, nausea, and anorexia. Of note, 12 subjects discontinued treatment because of adverse events and 5 developed cholecystitis.

| Table 2 | | |
| Current small molecule inhibitors in trials for thyroid cancer and their targets | | |
	Subtypes	Targets
Motesanib	DTC	VEGFR 1,2,3, PDGF, KIT, RET
Lenalidomide	DTC	Antiangiogenic properties, anti-tumor necrosis factor-α, immunomodulator
Axitinib	DTC, MTC	VEGFR-1, 2, 3; PDGFR- α, β; KIT (but not RET)
Sunitinib	DTC, MTC	VEGFR, PDGFR, c-kit, RET
Sorafenib	DTC, MTC	VEGFR-2, VEGFR-3, PDGFR-β, Flt-3, C-Kit, RET, RAF and FGFR-1
Vandetanib	MTC	RET, VEGFR, EGFR
XL184	MTC	MET, VEGFR2, and RET
AZD6244	DTC	MEK

Axitinib is also a potent oral antiangiogenesis agent, with selective inhibition of VEGF receptors 1, 2, 3. An open-label phase 2, single-arm, multicenter study enrolled 60 subjects.[96] All histologies were included (papillary, 50%; follicular, 25%; anaplastic, 3%; and medullary, 18%) as long as the disease was not appropriate for treatment with I-131. Therapy was started at a dose of 5 mg orally twice daily, with an option to increase to 7 mg and 10 mg twice daily if there were minimal toxicities. Only 15% of subjects had received prior chemotherapy. The objective response rate was 30%, with disease stability greater than 16 weeks in an additional 38%, and a median PFS of 18.1 months. Treatment benefit and response was noted in all histologies. Because of adverse events, eight subjects discontinued therapy. Grade 3 and 4 toxicities occurred in 19 subjects (32%) and 3 subjects, respectively, and included hypertension, diarrhea, proteinuria, and fatigue. A decrease in soluble VEGFR levels was noted in response to treatment, but no conclusions could be made in regards to how this correlated with response.

Sunitinib, an oral tyrosine kinase inhibitor that inhibits RET, PDFGR, and VEGFR is an attractive agent to study given its dual actions as an antiangiogenic agent and a RET inhibitor. A recently presented phase 2 study treated 43 subjects with all

| Table 3 | | | |
| Response rates in recent phase 2 studies in thyroid cancer | | | |
	No. of Patients	Partial Response	Stable Disease
Motesanib (S. Sherman, 2007)	93 DTC	14%	67%
Axitinib (E. Cohen, 2007)	45 DTC	31% DTC	44% DTC
	12 MTC	25% MTC	33% MTC
Sorafenib (Brose, 2008)	42	21%	59%
Sunitinib (E. Cohen, 2008)	37 DTC	13% DTC	68% DTC
	6 MTC		83% MTC
Gefitinib (Pennell, 2007)	25	0%	48%
Lenalidomide (Ain, 2008)	18 DTC	22%	44%
Vandetanib (Haddad, 2008)	19 MTC	16%	63%
Vandetanib (Wells, 2007)	30 MTC	17%	50%
XL184 (Salgia, 2008)	22 MTC	47%	53%

histologies of thyroid cancer (37 DTC, 6 MTC) with sunitinib at a dose of 50 mg orally, daily for 4 weeks, followed by 2 weeks off.[97] Response assessments were as follows: in DTC the PR was 13%, SD 68%; and in MTC the SD rate was 83%. Grade 3 to 4 toxicities included neutropenia (26%), thrombocytopenia (16%), hypertension (16%), fatigue (14%), palmar-plantar erythrodysesthesia (14%), and gastrointestinal tract events (14%). Preliminary results from two other phase 2 studies with this agent were reported at the 2008 American Society of Clinical Oncology meeting. In the first, 17 subjects have been enrolled so far, with a PR in 1 and SD in 12.[98] In another phase 2 trial, a schedule of sunitinib 37.5 mg orally, daily was used to treat DTC and MTC. After enrollment of 18 subjects, preliminary results indicate 44% of subjects had a PET response after 7 days, but further efficacy data are not mature.[99]

Sorafenib, another multikinase inhibitor against Raf, VEGFR, and PDGFR has also been studied in several phase 2 studies. One open-label phase 2 study has treated 36 subjects with iodine refractory disease (papillary 61%, follicular 28%, anaplastic 5.5%) and MTC (5.5%).[100] Seven subjects had a PR, and an additional 20 had SD. Grade 3 toxicities reported to date include hypertension and palmar-plantar erythrodysesthesia. Early correlative studies show a decrease of pERK and pAKT in posttreatment tissue.[101] An additional study has been reported in which 18 subjects (10 MTC, 8 DTC) were treated, but it is too early to draw conclusions about response.[102]

Additional agents that have been evaluated include gefitinib and lenalidomide. In a phase 2 study of gefitinib, there were no objective responses noted in the 25 subjects treated. Thus, while there are preclinical data regarding EGFR activation in thyroid cancer, EGFR inhibitors may have limited single agent activity.[103] Preliminary results with the antiangiogenic agent lenalidomide showed favorable activity in DTC, with a PR of 22% and SD in 44% of the first evaluable 18 subjects. However, this is a small number of patients, with only short-term follow-up. Grade 3 toxicities were primarily hematologic.[104]

Vandetanib, an oral agent that targets RET, VEGFR, and EGFR, has been studied predominantly in hereditary MTC, which would harbor a RET mutation. In one study, vandetanib was administered at a dose of 100 mg orally, daily to 19 subjects.[105] Of the subjects in this study, 16% had a confirmed PR and 63% had SD. Three subjects withdrew because of adverse events, and six subjects had grade 3 to 4 events. An earlier study had treated 30 subjects with hereditary MTC with a higher dose of 300 mg daily. A PR was noted in 17%, with SD in 50%.[106]

Finally, another interesting agent, XL184, is in the process of being studied for MTC. This inhibitor of RET, MET, and VEGFR2 was evaluated in a phase 1 study in advanced solid tumor patients. In this study, 22 subjects with MTC were treated; of interest, this number included patients who had received prior tyrosine kinase inhibitor therapy with either motesanib, vandetanib, or sorafenib. Nearly all the MTC subjects treated had a treatment benefit with 47% PR and 53% SD. Grade 3 toxicities included low rates of nausea, diarrhea, mucositis, and increased liver function tests. This drug is currently being studied further in an ongoing trial in patients with MTC.

DISCUSSION

Many of the agents that were discussed above are still being evaluated in ongoing studies for advanced thyroid malignancies. Additional agents, such as the MEK inhibitor AZD6244 and the anti-angiogenesis small molecule pazopanib, are in trials now. There are a number of obvious challenges. One is patient selection. The authors have reviewed the principal genetic lesions driving the development and evolution of thyroid cancer. What the authors do not know is how well any of these lesions predicts response to a given agent or class of agents. For instance, based on preclinical data, a BRAF mutation may predict for responsiveness to agents that target MEK, but this needs to be studied prospectively in clinical trials. In addition, the mechanisms of resistance, primary and acquired, to these drugs need to be studied further to optimize their use.

A second challenge is to be able to determine when a patient should begin treatment with one of these agents. Although less toxic than traditional cytotoxic therapies (including doxorubicin), these drugs nevertheless have a number of very significant toxicities. One must also consider that many patients might end up being treated for prolonged periods of time, if not the rest of their lives. Clinical trial designs must therefore consider that advanced thyroid cancer, even when destined to be fatal, is an indolent metastatic cancer compared with many malignancies. Stable disease is an obvious endpoint that has already emerged from the ongoing trials, but the clinical significance of stable disease remains a matter of ongoing scientific and regulatory debate. With so many potentially active agents for a relatively rare disease, designing feasible (completable) phase 3 studies to eventually merit FDA registration will also require an evaluation of patient resources and the creation of effective, likely international, research consortia. An additional relevant question is whether or not these agents need to be or should be compared with a current approved FDA drug, doxorubicin, knowing that this approval occurred many years ago in a different therapeutic and regulatory environment. An international registration study for axitinib for patients who had formally failed doxorubicin was planned, but accrual was poor because of the requirement for prior doxorubicin treatment that patients and physicians were hesitant to consider.

While the data to date are preliminary, it is clear that we are in a new era in the treatment of advanced thyroid cancer. The new drugs will provide significant insight into the disease itself and likely alter the natural history of what had previously been an untreatable medical illness. The next steps are clear, namely to validate the clinical utility of these agents in well-designed clinical trials, and understand the determinants of clinical response and resistance.

REFERENCES

1. Jemal A, Siegel R, Ward E, et al. Cancer statistics, 2008. CA Cancer J Clin 2008; 58(2):71–96.
2. Beal KP, Singh B, Kraus D, et al. Radiation-induced salivary gland tumors: a report of 18 cases and a review of the literature. Cancer J 2003;9(6):467–71.
3. Schneider AB, Lubin J, Ron E, et al. Salivary gland tumors after childhood radiation treatment for benign conditions of the head and neck: dose-response relationships. Radiat Res 1998;149(6):625–30.
4. Mihailescu D, Shore-Freedman E, Mukani S, et al. Multiple neoplasms in an irradiated cohort: pattern of occurrence and relationship to thyroid cancer outcome. J Clin Endocrinol Metab 2002;87(7):3236–41.
5. Sun EC, Curtis R, Melbye M, et al. Salivary gland cancer in the United States. Cancer Epidemiol Biomarkers Prev 1999;8(12):1095–100.
6. Kim KI, Kim YS, Kim HK, et al. The detection of Epstein-Barr virus in the lesions of salivary glands. Pathol Res Pract 1999;195(6):407–12.
7. Leung SY, Chung LP, Yuen ST, et al. Lymphoepithelial carcinoma of the salivary gland: in situ detection of Epstein-Barr virus. J Clin Pathol 1995;48(11):1022–7.

8. Larbcharoensub N, Tubtong N, Praneetvatakul V, et al. Epstein-Barr virus associated lymphoepithelial carcinoma of the parotid gland; a clinicopathological report of three cases. J Med Assoc Thai 2006;89(9):1536–41.

9. Saku T, Cheng J, Jen KY, et al. Epstein-Barr virus infected lymphoepithelial carcinomas of the salivary gland in the Russia-Asia area: a clinicopathologic study of 160 cases. Arkh Patol 2003;65(2):35–9.

10. Jen KY, Cheng J, Li J, et al. Mutational events in LMP1 gene of Epstein-Barr virus in salivary gland lymphoepithelial carcinomas. Int J Cancer 2003;105(5):654–60.

11. Seifert G, Sobin LH. The World Health Organization's Histological Classification of Salivary Gland Tumors. A commentary on the second edition. Cancer 1992; 70(2):379–85.

12. Spiro RH. Distant metastasis in adenoid cystic carcinoma of salivary origin. Am J Surg 1997;174(5):495–8.

13. Licitra L, Marchini S, Spinazze S, et al. Cisplatin in advanced salivary gland carcinoma. A phase II study of 25 patients. Cancer 1991;68(9):1874–7.

14. Airoldi M, Pedani F, Succo G, et al. Phase II randomized trial comparing vinorelbine versus vinorelbine plus cisplatin in patients with recurrent salivary gland malignancies. Cancer 2001;91(3):541–7.

15. Gilbert J, Li Y, Pinto HA, et al. Phase II trial of taxol in salivary gland malignancies (E1394): a trial of the Eastern Cooperative Oncology Group. Head Neck 2006; 28(3):197–204.

16. Licitra L, Cavina R, Grandi C, et al. Cisplatin, doxorubicin and cyclophosphamide in advanced salivary gland carcinoma. A phase II trial of 22 patients. Ann Oncol 1996;7(6):640–2.

17. Airoldi M, Fornari G, Pedani F, et al. Paclitaxel and carboplatin for recurrent salivary gland malignancies. Anticancer Res 2000;20(5C):3781–3.

18. Andreadis D, Epivatianos A, Poulopoulos A, et al. Detection of C-KIT (CD117) molecule in benign and malignant salivary gland tumours. Oral Oncol 2006; 42(1):57–65.

19. Edwards PC, Bhuiya T, Kelsch RD. C-kit expression in the salivary gland neoplasms adenoid cystic carcinoma, polymorphous low-grade adenocarcinoma, and monomorphic adenoma. Oral Surg Oral Med Oral Pathol Oral Radiol Endod 2003;95(5):586–93.

20. Ettl T, Schwarz S, Kuhnel T, et al. [Prognostic value of immunohistochemistry in salivary gland cancer]. HNO 2008;56(2):231–8 [in German].

21. Seethala RR, Barnes EL, Hunt JL. Epithelial-myoepithelial carcinoma: a review of the clinicopathologic spectrum and immunophenotypic characteristics in 61 tumors of the salivary glands and upper aerodigestive tract. Am J Surg Pathol 2007;31(1):44–57.

22. Hotte SJ, Winquist EW, Lamont E, et al. Imatinib mesylate in patients with adenoid cystic cancers of the salivary glands expressing c-kit: a Princess Margaret Hospital phase II consortium study. J Clin Oncol 2005;23(3):585–90.

23. Pfeffer MR, Talmi Y, Catane R, et al. A phase II study of Imatinib for advanced adenoid cystic carcinoma of head and neck salivary glands. Oral Oncol 2007; 43(1):33–6.

24. Lin CH, Yen RF, Jeng YM, et al. Unexpected rapid progression of metastatic adenoid cystic carcinoma during treatment with imatinib mesylate. Head Neck 2005;27(12):1022–7.

25. Lequerica-Fernandez P, Astudillo A, de Vicente JC. Expression of vascular endothelial growth factor in salivary gland carcinomas correlates with lymph node metastasis. Anticancer Res 2007;27(5B):3661–6.

26. Lim JJ, Kang S, Lee MR, et al. Expression of vascular endothelial growth factor in salivary gland carcinomas and its relation to p53, Ki-67 and prognosis. J Oral Pathol Med 2003;32(9):552–61.
27. Zhang J, Peng B. In vitro angiogenesis and expression of nuclear factor kappaB and VEGF in high and low metastasis cell lines of salivary gland adenoid cystic carcinoma. BMC Cancer 2007;7:95–101.
28. Younes MN, Park YW, Yazici YD, et al. Concomitant inhibition of epidermal growth factor and vascular endothelial growth factor receptor tyrosine kinases reduces growth and metastasis of human salivary adenoid cystic carcinoma in an orthotopic nude mouse model. Mol Cancer Ther 2006;5(11): 2696–705.
29. Matsubayashi S, Yoshihara T. Carcinoma ex pleomorphic adenoma of the salivary gland: an immunohistochemical study. Eur Arch Otorhinolaryngol 2007; 264(7):789–95.
30. Nguyen LH, Black MJ, Hier M, et al. HER2/neu and Ki-67 as prognostic indicators in mucoepidermoid carcinoma of salivary glands. J Otolaryngol 2003;32(5): 328–31.
31. Skalova A, Starek I, Vanecek T, et al. [Amplification and overexpression of HER-2/neu in parotid gland salivary duct carcinoma. Immunohistochemical study and fluorescence in situ hybridization]. Cesk Patol 2002;38(Suppl 1):27–34 [in Czech].
32. Cornolti G, Ungari M, Morassi ML, et al. Amplification and overexpression of HER2/neu gene and HER2/neu protein in salivary duct carcinoma of the parotid gland. Arch Otolaryngol Head Neck Surg 2007;133(10):1031–6.
33. Dori S, Vered M, David R, et al. HER2/neu expression in adenoid cystic carcinoma of salivary gland origin: an immunohistochemical study. J Oral Pathol Med 2002;31(8):463–7.
34. Piechocki MP, Yoo GH, Dibbley SK, et al. Iressa induces cytostasis and augments Fas-mediated apoptosis in acinic cell adenocarcinoma overexpressing HER2/neu. Int J Cancer 2006;119(2):441–54.
35. Laurie SA, Licitra L. Systemic therapy in the palliative management of advanced salivary gland cancers. J Clin Oncol 2006;24(17):2673–8.
36. Licitra LF, Locati LD, Potepan P, et al. Cetuximab (C225) in recurrent and/or metastatic salivary gland carcinomas (RMSGCs): a monoinstitutional phase II study. Presented at: ASCO. Atlanta, GA, 2006.
37. Haddad R, Colevas AD, Krane JF, et al. Herceptin in patients with advanced or metastatic salivary gland carcinomas. A phase II study. Oral Oncol 2003;39(7): 724–7.
38. Glisson B, Colevas AD, Haddad R, et al. HER2 expression in salivary gland carcinomas: dependence on histological subtype. Clin Cancer Res 2004;10(3): 944–6.
39. Agulnik M, Cohen EW, Cohen RB, et al. Phase II study of lapatinib in recurrent or metastatic epidermal growth factor receptor and/or erbB2 expressing adenoid cystic carcinoma and non adenoid cystic carcinoma malignant tumors of the salivary glands. J Clin Oncol 2007;25(25):3978–84.
40. Ries L, Eisner M, Kosary C, et al. SEER Cancer Statistics Review. 1975–2002. Available at: seer.cancer.gov/csr/1975_2002/.
41. Davies L, Welch HG. Increasing incidence of thyroid cancer in the United States, 1973–2002. JAMA 2006;295(18):2164–7.
42. Fagin J. Epidemiology of thyroid cancer. In: Thyroid Cancer. Boston: Kluwer Academic Publishers; 1998.

43. Kazakov VS, Demidchik EP, Astakhova LN. Thyroid cancer after Chernobyl. Nature 1992;359(6390):21.

44. Massart C, Barbet R, Genetet N, et al. Doxorubicin induces Fas-mediated apoptosis in human thyroid carcinoma cells. Thyroid 2004;14(4):263–70.

45. Rho JH, Kang DY, Park KJ, et al. Doxorubicin induces apoptosis with profile of large-scale DNA fragmentation and without DNA ladder in anaplastic thyroid carcinoma cells via histone hyperacetylation. Int J Oncol 2005;27(2):465–71.

46. Benker G, Reinwein D [Results of chemotherapy in thyroid cancer]. Dtsch Med Wochenschr 1983;108(11):403–6 [in German].

47. Droz JP, Rougier P, Goddefroy V, et al [Chemotherapy for medullary cancer of the thyroid. Phase II trials with adriamycin and cis-platinum administered as monochemotherapy]. Bull Cancer 1984;71(3):195–9 [in French].

48. Gottlieb JA, Hill CS Jr. Chemotherapy of thyroid cancer with adriamycin. Experience with 30 patients. N Engl J Med 1974;290(4):193–7.

49. Gottlieb JA, Hill CS Jr, Ibanez ML, et al. Chemotherapy of thyroid cancer. An evaluation of experience with 37 patients. Cancer 1972;30(3):848–53.

50. Kolaric K, Maricic Z, Nola P, et al. Modified administration schedule of adriamycin in solid tumors. Z Krebsforsch Klin Onkol Cancer Res Clin Oncol 1977;88(3):255–60.

51. Ravry MJ. Response of medullary thyroid carcinomas and carcinoid tumors to adriamycin. Cancer Treat Rep 1977;61(1):106–7.

52. Shimaoka K, Schoenfeld DA, DeWys WD, et al. A randomized trial of doxorubicin versus doxorubicin plus cisplatin in patients with advanced thyroid carcinoma. Cancer 1985;56(9):2155–60.

53. Williams SD, Birch R, Einhorn LH. Phase II evaluation of doxorubicin plus cisplatin in advanced thyroid cancer: a Southeastern Cancer Study Group Trial. Cancer Treat Rep 1986;70(3):405–7.

54. Argiris A, Agarwala SS, Karamouzis MV, et al. A phase II trial of doxorubicin and interferon alpha 2b in advanced, non-medullary thyroid cancer. Invest New Drugs 2008;26(2):183–8.

55. Matuszczyk A, Petersenn S, Bockisch A, et al. Chemotherapy with doxorubicin in progressive medullary and thyroid carcinoma of the follicular epithelium. Horm Metab Res 2008;40(3):210–3.

56. Frattini M, Ferrario C, Bressan P, et al. Alternative mutations of BRAF, RET and NTRK1 are associated with similar but distinct gene expression patterns in papillary thyroid cancer. Oncogene 2004;23(44):7436–40.

57. Kimura ET, Nikiforova MN, Zhu Z, et al. High prevalence of BRAF mutations in thyroid cancer: genetic evidence for constitutive activation of the RET/PTC-RAS-BRAF signaling pathway in papillary thyroid carcinoma. Cancer Res 2003;63(7):1454–7.

58. Tallini G, Asa SL. RET oncogene activation in papillary thyroid carcinoma. Adv Anat Pathol 2001;8(6):345–54.

59. Soares P, Trovisco V, Rocha AS, et al. BRAF mutations and RET/PTC rearrangements are alternative events in the etiopathogenesis of PTC. Oncogene 2003;22(29):4578–80.

60. Xing M, Westra WH, Tufano RP, et al. BRAF mutation predicts a poorer clinical prognosis for papillary thyroid cancer. J Clin Endocrinol Metab 2005;90(12):6373–9.

61. Nikiforova MN, Kimura ET, Gandhi M, et al. BRAF mutations in thyroid tumors are restricted to papillary carcinomas and anaplastic or poorly differentiated carcinomas arising from papillary carcinomas. J Clin Endocrinol Metab 2003;88(11):5399–404.

62. Romei C, Ciampi R, Faviana P, et al. BRAFV600E mutation, but not RET/PTC rearrangements, is correlated with a lower expression of both thyroperoxidase and sodium iodide symporter genes in papillary thyroid cancer. Endocr Relat Cancer 2008;15(2):511–20.

63. Leboeuf R, Baumgartner JE, Benezra M, et al. BRAFV600E mutation is associated with preferential sensitivity to mitogen-activated protein kinase kinase inhibition in thyroid cancer cell lines. J Clin Endocrinol Metab 2008;93(6):2194–201.

64. Ouyang B, Knauf JA, Smith EP, et al. Inhibitors of Raf kinase activity block growth of thyroid cancer cells with RET/PTC or BRAF mutations in vitro and in vivo. Clin Cancer Res 2006;12(6):1785–93.

65. Kroll TG, Sarraf P, Pecciarini L, et al. PAX8-PPARgamma1 fusion oncogene in human thyroid carcinoma [corrected]. Science 2000;289(5483):1357–60.

66. Lui WO, Foukakis T, Liden J, et al. Expression profiling reveals a distinct transcription signature in follicular thyroid carcinomas with a PAX8-PPAR(gamma) fusion oncogene. Oncogene 2005;24(8):1467–76.

67. McIver B, Grebe SK, Eberhardt NL. The PAX8/PPAR gamma fusion oncogene as a potential therapeutic target in follicular thyroid carcinoma. Curr Drug Targets Immune Endocr Metabol Disord. 2004;4(3):221–34.

68. Martelli ML, Iuliano R, Le Pera I, et al. Inhibitory effects of peroxisome poliferator-activated receptor gamma on thyroid carcinoma cell growth. J Clin Endocrinol Metab 2002;87(10):4728–35.

69. Nikiforova MN, Lynch RA, Biddinger PW, et al. RAS point mutations and PAX8-PPAR gamma rearrangement in thyroid tumors: evidence for distinct molecular pathways in thyroid follicular carcinoma. J Clin Endocrinol Metab 2003;88(5):2318–26.

70. Karga H, Lee JK, Vickery AL Jr, et al. Ras oncogene mutations in benign and malignant thyroid neoplasms. J Clin Endocrinol Metab 1991;73(4):832–6.

71. Lemoine NR, Mayall ES, Wyllie FS, et al. High frequency of ras oncogene activation in all stages of human thyroid tumorigenesis. Oncogene 1989;4(2):159–64.

72. Soh EY, Duh QY, Sobhi SA, et al. Vascular endothelial growth factor expression is higher in differentiated thyroid cancer than in normal or benign thyroid. J Clin Endocrinol Metab 1997;82(11):3741–7.

73. Klein M, Picard E, Vignaud JM, et al. Vascular endothelial growth factor gene and protein: strong expression in thyroiditis and thyroid carcinoma. J Endocrinol 1999;161(1):41–9.

74. Katoh R, Miyagi E, Kawaoi A, et al. Expression of vascular endothelial growth factor (VEGF) in human thyroid neoplasms. Hum Pathol 1999;30(8):891–7.

75. Lennard CM, Patel A, Wilson J, et al. Intensity of vascular endothelial growth factor expression is associated with increased risk of recurrence and decreased disease-free survival in papillary thyroid cancer. Surgery 2001;129(5):552–8.

76. Gomez-Rivera F, Santillan-Gomez AA, Younes MN, et al. The tyrosine kinase inhibitor, AZD2171, inhibits vascular endothelial growth factor receptor signaling and growth of anaplastic thyroid cancer in an orthotopic nude mouse model. Clin Cancer Res 2007;13(15 Pt 1):4519–27.

77. Mitsiades CS, Kotoula V, Poulaki V, et al. Epidermal growth factor receptor as a therapeutic target in human thyroid carcinoma: mutational and functional analysis. J Clin Endocrinol Metab 2006;91(9):3662–6.

78. Schiff BA, McMurphy AB, Jasser SA, et al. Epidermal growth factor receptor (EGFR) is overexpressed in anaplastic thyroid cancer, and the EGFR inhibitor gefitinib inhibits the growth of anaplastic thyroid cancer. Clin Cancer Res 2004;10(24):8594–602.

79. Bergstrom JD, Westermark B, Heldin NE. Epidermal growth factor receptor signaling activates met in human anaplastic thyroid carcinoma cells. Exp Cell Res 2000;259(1):293–9.

80. Santoro M, Melillo RM, Carlomagno F, et al. Molecular mechanisms of RET activation in human cancer. Ann N Y Acad Sci 2002;963:116–21.

81. Croyle M, Akeno N, Knauf JA, et al. RET/PTC-induced cell growth is mediated in part by epidermal growth factor receptor (EGFR) activation: evidence for molecular and functional interactions between RET and EGFR. Cancer Res 2008; 68(11):4183–91.

82. Kim S, Schiff BA, Yigitbasi OG, et al. Targeted molecular therapy of anaplastic thyroid carcinoma with AEE788. Mol Cancer Ther 2005;4(4):632–40.

83. Carlomagno F, Vitagliano D, Guida T, et al. ZD6474, an orally available inhibitor of KDR tyrosine kinase activity, efficiently blocks oncogenic RET kinases. Cancer Res 2002;62(24):7284–90.

84. Mandal M, Kim S, Younes MN, et al. The Akt inhibitor KP372-1 suppresses Akt activity and cell proliferation and induces apoptosis in thyroid cancer cells. Br J Cancer. 2005;92(10):1899–905.

85. Yeager N, Brewer C, Cai KQ, et al. Mammalian target of rapamycin is the key effector of phosphatidylinositol-3-OH-initiated proliferative signals in the thyroid follicular epithelium. Cancer Res 2008;68(2):444–9.

86. Fagin JA, Matsuo K, Karmakar A, et al. High prevalence of mutations of the p53 gene in poorly differentiated human thyroid carcinomas. J Clin Invest 1993; 91(1):179–84.

87. Quiros RM, Ding HG, Gattuso P, et al. Evidence that one subset of anaplastic thyroid carcinomas are derived from papillary carcinomas due to BRAF and p53 mutations. Cancer 2005;103(11):2261–8.

88. Garcia-Rostan G, Costa AM, Pereira-Castro I, et al. Mutation of the PIK3CA gene in anaplastic thyroid cancer. Cancer Res 2005;65(22):10199–207.

89. Brabant G, Hoang-Vu C, Cetin Y, et al. E-cadherin: a differentiation marker in thyroid malignancies. Cancer Res 1993;53(20):4987–93.

90. Scheumman GF, Hoang-Vu C, Cetin Y, et al. Clinical significance of E-cadherin as a prognostic marker in thyroid carcinomas. J Clin Endocrinol Metab 1995; 80(7):2168–72.

91. Garcia-Rostan G, Tallini G, Herrero A, et al. Frequent mutation and nuclear localization of beta-catenin in anaplastic thyroid carcinoma. Cancer Res 1999;59(8): 1811–5.

92. Marsh DJ, Learoyd DL, Andrew SD, et al. Somatic mutations in the RET proto-oncogene in sporadic medullary thyroid carcinoma. Clin Endocrinol (Oxf) 1996;44(3):249–57.

93. Mulligan LM, Eng C, Healey CS, et al. Specific mutations of the RET proto-oncogene are related to disease phenotype in MEN 2A and FMTC. Nat Genet 1994; 6(1):70–4.

94. Eng C, Clayton D, Schuffenecker I, et al. The relationship between specific RET proto-oncogene mutations and disease phenotype in multiple endocrine neoplasia type 2. International RET mutation consortium analysis. JAMA 1996; 276(19):1575–9.

95. Sherman SI, Wirth LJ, Droz JP, et al. Motesanib diphosphate in progressive differentiated thyroid cancer. N Engl J Med 2008;359(1):31–42.

96. Cohen EE, Rosen LS, Vokes EE, et al. Axitinib is an active treatment for all histologic subtypes of advanced thyroid cancer: results from a phase II study. J Clin Oncol 2008;26(24).

97. EE Cohen, Needles BM, Cullen KJ, et al. Phase 2 study of sunitinib in refractory thyroid cancer. Presented at: ASCO. Chicago, IL, 2008.
98. Ravaud A, Fouchardière C, Courbon F, et al. Sunitinib in patients with refractory advanced thyroid cancer: the THYSU phase II trial. Presented at: ASCO. Chicago, IL, 2008.
99. Goulart B, Carr L, Martins RG, et al. Phase II study of sunitinib in iodine refractory, well-differentiated thyroid cancer (WDTC) and metastatic medullary thyroid carcinoma (MTC). Presented at: ASCO. Chicago, IL, 2008.
100. Brose MS, Nellore A, Paziana K, et al. A phase II study of sorafenib in metastatic thyroid carcinoma. Presented at: ASCO. Chicago, IL, 2008.
101. Gupta V, Puttaswamy K, Lassoued W, et al. Sorafenib targets BRAF and VEGFR in metastatic thyroid carcinoma. Presented at: ASCO. Chicago, IL, 2007.
102. Ahmed M, Barbachano Y, Riddell AM, et al. Preliminary results of an open labelled phase 2 study evaluating the safety and efficacy of sorafenib in metastatic advanced thyroid cancer. Presented at: ASCO. Chicago, IL, 2008.
103. Pennell NA, Daniels GH, Haddad RI, et al. A phase II study of gefitinib in patients with advanced thyroid cancer. Presented at: ASCO. Chicago, IL, 2007.
104. Ain KB, Lee C, Holbrook KM, et al. Phase II study of lenalidomide in distantly metastatic, rapidly progressive, and radioiodine-unresponsive thyroid carcinomas: preliminary results. Presented at: ASCO. Chicago, IL, 2008.
105. Haddad RI, Krebs AD, Vasselli J, et al. A phase II open-label study of vandetanib in patients with locally advanced or metastatic hereditary medullary thyroid cancer. Presented at: ASCO. Chicago, IL, 2008.
106. Wells SA, Gosnell JE, Gagel RF, et al. Vandetanib in metastatic hereditary medullary thyroid cancer: Follow-up results of an open-label phase II trial. Presented at: ASCO. Chicago, IL, 2007.

Sinonasal Malignancies of Neuroendocrine Origin

Danny Rischin, MBBS, MD, FRACP[a,b,*], Andrew Coleman, MBBS, MSc, FRANZCR[c]

KEYWORDS

- Sinonasal malignancies • Neuroendocrine tumors
- Esthesioneuroblastoma • Sinonasal undifferentiated carcinoma
- Small cell carcinoma

It has been argued that per cubic millimeter the sinonasal tract gives rise to a greater diversity of neoplasms than any other site in the body.[1] Malignancies arising in the sinonasal tract frequently cause considerable diagnostic and management difficulties. This article focuses on uncommon malignancies of the head and neck arising in the sinonasal tract that are putatively of neuroendocrine origin. In particular, we discuss esthesioneuroblastoma (ENB), sinonasal undifferentiated carcinoma (SNUC), neuroendocrine carcinoma (SNEC), and small cell carcinoma. Other tumors that arise in the sinonasal tract include squamous cell carcinomas, adenocarcinomas, salivary gland tumors, sarcomas, melanomas, and lymphomas. Nasopharyngeal carcinomas can involve the sinonasal, tract, but they almost always arise in the nasopharynx.

Progress in understanding and improving outcomes in these uncommon sinonasal malignancies has been hampered by difficulties in pathologic diagnosis and the rarity of these malignancies. One of the entities, SNUC, was first described only 20 years ago,[2] and there remains controversy about the diagnostic criteria, overlap with other diagnoses, and uncertainty about whether this tumor is of neuroendocrine origin. The uncertainty about consistency of pathologic classification between series combined with almost all the available data coming from small retrospective series makes drawing definitive conclusions about management difficult.

---

[a] Department of Medical Oncology, Peter MacCallum Cancer Centre, Locked Bag No 1, A'Beckett Street, Melbourne 8006, Australia
[b] University of Melbourne, Victoria 3010, Australia
[c] Division of Radiation Oncology, Peter MacCallum Cancer Centre, Locked Bag No 1, A'Beckett Street, Melbourne 8006, Australia
* Corresponding author.
E-mail address: danny.rischin@petermac.org (D. Rischin).

Hematol Oncol Clin N Am 22 (2008) 1297–1316
doi:10.1016/j.hoc.2008.08.008
0889-8588/08/$ – see front matter © 2008 Elsevier Inc. All rights reserved.

hemonc.theclinics.com

ESTHESIONEUROBLASTOMA

ENB is an uncommon malignancy, with a reported incidence rate of 0.4 cases per million inhabitants per year.[3] The first cases were described by Berger and Luc[4] in 1924. The only meta-analysis on the diagnosis, staging, and treatment of EBN was published by Dulguerov and colleagues[5] in 2001. At that time the authors recognized that in addition to the problems created by the relative rarity of ENB, the following three specific factors had allowed controversies to emerge over its optimum management.

ENB showed varying biologic activity, ranging from indolent growth, with patients surviving with known tumor for more than 20 years, to a highly aggressive neoplasm, capable of rapid widespread metastasis with survival limited to a few months.

ENB was easily confused with other poorly differentiated neoplasms of the nasal cavity.

No universally accepted staging system was available.

Pathology

Until recently the exact cell of origin of ENB was the source of some controversy. The presence of neurofilaments in ENB suggested it originated from neuronal or neural crest tissues. An earlier proposal that ENB may have been part of the Ewing sarcoma family of tumors or the primitive neuroectodermal tumors was not sustained when fluorescence in situ hybridization and reverse transcriptase polymerase chain reaction did not confirm the translocation t (11:22) in ENB.

The currently available evidence links ENB with the basal progenitor cells of the olfactory epithelium. These basal cells express neural cell adhesion molecule 87 and the mammalian homolog of *Drosophila* achaete-scute (MASH) gene. ENB tumors have been found to express HASH, the human homolog of the MASH gene.[6] No clear etiologic agent has been documented in human beings. ENB can be consistently induced by nitrosamine compounds in rodents, whereas in cats and mice retroviral particles identified as feline and murine leukemia viruses have been implicated. The role of retroviral sequences in human ENB remains unclear.

Under light microscopy, well-differentiated ENB is composed of homogeneous small- to medium-size cells with uniform round to oval nuclei, rosette or pseudorosette formation, and eosinophilic fibrillary intercellular background material. Under electron microscopy fibrils can be seen and have been shown to represent cellular cytoplasmic processes. These features are used in the most commonly used histopathologic grading system, described by Hyams (**Table 1**).[7] The small number of patients reported in most series means that useful results can only obtained by combining the Hyams histopathologic grades I/II and III/IV into two larger groupings.[5] Even then this system can be difficult to apply and has not always been found to divide cases into prognostically significant groups.[8]

When the tumor is poorly differentiated, differentiation from other small cell nasal neoplasms by light microscopy becomes difficult. The differential diagnosis includes amelanotic malignant melanoma, embryonal rhabdomyosarcoma, malignant lymphoma, extramedullary plasmocytoma, and in particular, sinonasal undifferentiated carcinoma and sinonasal neuroendocrine carcinoma. In these instances, immunohistochemical staining and electron microscopy have become increasingly important in establishing the diagnosis even though there is no specific immunohistochemical stain for ENB.

Table 1
Histopathologic grading, according to Hyams

Grade	Lobular Architecture Preservation	Mitotic Index	Nuclear Polymorphism	Fibrillary Matrix	Rosettes	Necrosis
I	+	None	None	Prominent	HW rosettes	None
II	+	Low	Moderate	Present	HW rosettes	None
III	±	Moderate	Prominent	Low	FW rosettes	Rare
IV	±	High	Marked	Absent	None	Frequent

Abbreviations: FW, Flexner-Wintersteiner; HW, Homer Wright.
Data from Hyams V, Batsakis J, Michaels L. Atlas of tumor pathology. Washington, DC: Armed Forces Institute of Pathology; 1988. p. 240.

ENB is often positive for chromogranin, synaptophysin, and S-100, but most cases are negative for cytokeratin, desmin, vimentin, actin, glial fibrillary acidic protein, UMB45, and leucocyte common antigen. If immunohistochemistry stains are not helpful, electron microscopy can be reliable in visualizing uniform round nuclei, dense core neurosecretory granules with diameters of 125 to 350 nm, neuronal processes containing microtubules and neurofilaments, and rare synapses.[5] Several recent studies have addressed the diagnostic features of ENB.[1,9,10] Despite this, disagreement among pathologists can be common in this uncommon tumor. Cohen reviewed the cases referred to the M.D. Anderson Cancer Center and confirmed the diagnosis in only 2 of 12 patients.[11] Haas[12] reviewed 11 cases of ENB, 7 of SNEC, and 1 of SNUC and despite extensive diagnostic steps it was not possible to exclude a different histopathologic diagnosis in 10 of 19 cases. It is likely that some cases of Grade IV ENB as originally described by Hyams and colleagues[7] may in fact be better classified as SNUC.[13]

The molecular cytogenetic profile of ENB is also being investigated. Analysis by Comparative Genomic Hybridization has shown a characteristic pattern of deletions and overrepresentations in up to 100% of cases in a small series of primary tumors and metastases.[14]

Clinical Presentation

ENB affects male and female patients with similar frequency and can be found in all age groups, although some authors have reported a bimodal pattern with peaks between 11 and 20 years and 40 to 60 years, and other authors report a single peak in the sixth decade.

Symptoms at presentation are usually nonspecific and often cause a long delay between onset of symptoms and diagnosis. The most frequent symptoms are unilateral nasal obstruction, epistaxis, headache, nasal discharge, and anosmia.[15–17] This delay in diagnosis results in many cases presenting with advanced local disease. Most large series report around two thirds of new cases presenting with Kadish stage C disease,[5,18] often with intracranial extension and direct invasion of the orbits or optic pathways. Involvement of these structures has also been reported with the rare but distinct primary sellar ENB, which does not have any involvement of the olfactory apparatus.[19,20] The rate of regional disease at presentation is about 5%, whereas the rate of systemic disease is generally believed to be about 6%. The most common sites are lung and bone.

Radiologic Investigations

CT, MRI, and positron emission tomography (PET) scanning play complementary rolls in the locoregional staging of ENB. T2-weighted or gadolinium-enhanced MRI images are more sensitive than CT in differentiating sinusitis from tumors.[21] Local bone destruction and regional metastasis are best seen with CT. Systemic staging requires at least CT chest and metabolic bone imaging. Fluorine-18 fluorodeoxyglucose PET is being increasingly used because it has been shown to reveal otherwise occult systemic metastasis.[22] In the setting of possible skull base recurrence, octreotide nuclear medicine scans have been reported to be the most sensitive means of distinguishing between skull base tumor and postoperative scarring.[23]

Staging

Kadish[24] and coworkers were the first to propose a staging classification, of three categories, for ENB (**Table 2**). There have been attempts to update this classification,[25,26] with the most frequently used modification being the one proposed by Morita.[26] In addition, Dulguerov[27] proposed a classification based on the more familiar TNM system but this has not achieved widespread acceptance. In general the original Kadish classification continues to be widely used and remains useful in predicting outcome.[8,28]

Treatment

The only meta-analysis, published by Dulguerov[5] in 2001, included 26 studies that reported on 390 patients who had ENB.

Their analysis divided treatment modalities into the following groups:

Surgery alone
Surgery and radiotherapy
Radiotherapy alone
Combined surgery, radiotherapy, and chemotherapy
Combined radiotherapy and chemotherapy
Combined surgery and chemotherapy
Chemotherapy alone

Within these groupings the sequence of treatments was not taken into account given the small number of patients. Overall survival at 5 years was extracted from 25 studies, with the mean being 45% and extremes of 86% and zero. In the meta-analysis local recurrence was found in 29% (SD 16) of patients, with successful salvage in a third of these cases. Regional recurrence occurred in 16% (SD 15) of

Table 2 Kadish staging system	
Stage	**Definition**
A	Tumor confined to the nasal cavity
B	Tumor extension beyond the nasal cavity to the paranasal sinuses
C	Tumor spread beyond the nasal cavity and paranasal sinuses

Data from Kadish S, Goodman M, Wang CC. Olfactory neuroblastoma. A clinical analysis of 17 cases. Cancer 1976;37:1571.

patients, with successful salvage in 27%. Distant metastases eventually occurred in 17% (SD 14) of patients.[5] For patients who had recurrent disease 5-year survival was 45%.

These results are all derived from retrospective studies, and hence are subject to selection bias (eg, one could speculate that patients who had advanced disease would be more likely to receive radiotherapy or chemotherapy and less likely to undergo surgery). Nevertheless, these results suggest that the combination of surgery (generally craniofacial resection) and radiotherapy is a reasonable standard of care for all resectable cases other than for a small tumor located well below the cribriform plate (**Table 3**).

Rosenthal and colleagues[29] have reported the experience of the M.D. Anderson Cancer Center of all sinonasal malignancies with neuroendocrine differentiation treated between 1982 and 2002. After expert pathology review, 31 of 72 cases were assessed as having ENB. Twenty were males, 15 had American Joint Committee on Cancer (AJCC) stage IV disease, and only 2 patients had cervical nodal involvement. For the ENB subset, treatment was predominantly local therapy, with only 5 patients receiving chemotherapy and only 3 patients receiving radiation to regional nodes. They have reported excellent results with 5-year overall survival of 93.1%, and 5-year local, regional, and distant failure rates of 3.8%, 8.7%, and 0%, respectively. They concluded that ENB had a much better prognosis than other neuroendocrine carcinomas of the sinonasal tract, with excellent survival, local control, and distant control rates with local treatment only, typically surgery and postoperative radiotherapy. Other series published since 2000 have not matched the results of Rosenthal and colleagues[29] but have confirmed high rates of local control with surgery and radiotherapy. Lund and colleagues[30] reported on 42 patients treated with craniofacial resection (57% also received radiotherapy). The 5- and 10-year overall survival was 61% and 42%, respectively, and the local failure rate was 17%. Intracranial extension and orbital involvement were independent adverse prognostic factors. Chao and colleagues[15] reported on a series of 25 patients, with 5-year overall survival of 66%. The 5-year local failure rate was 27%, but in patients treated with surgery and radiotherapy it was 12.5%, and 49% for patients treated with radiation alone. Selection bias makes such comparisons problematic, but nevertheless high rates of local control can be achieved in patients suitable for surgery and radiotherapy. Other recent series have reported local failure rates of 17% to 38%.[31–33] There is considerable variability in

Table 3
Survival by treatment modality

Modality	No. of Patients	Frequency (%)	Survival (%)	OR	CI
Surgery alone	87	20 ± 22	48 ± 40	1.9	0.7 to 4.9
Surgery + radiation	169	44 ± 20	65 ± 25	1	—
Radiation only	49	13 ± 19	37 ± 33	2.5	1.02 to 6.0
Surgery + radiation + chemotherapy	48	13 ± 16	47 ± 37	2.1	0.91 to 4.8
Radiation + chemotherapy	26	7 ± 16	51 ± 45	3.4	0.68 to 16.5
Surgery + chemotherapy	1	0 ± 1	0	—	—
Chemotherapy	6	2 ± 4	40 ± 55	—	—

Abbreviation: OR, odds ratio relative to surgery plus radiation.
Data from Dulguerov P, Allal AS, Calcaterra TC. Esthesioneuroblastoma: a meta-analysis and review. Lancet Oncol 2001;2:683.

types of treatment given even within individual series, and there are likely to be significant differences in extent of disease and pathologic interpretation between series.

The University of Virginia group has reported on 50 consecutive patients diagnosed with esthesioneuroblastoma who were treated with a standardized protocol over a 28-year period.[18,34] The stage distribution was almost the same as that included in the meta-analysis with Kadish stage A in 4 patients (8%), stage B in 14 (28%), and stage C in 32 (64%). Patients who had tumors staged Kadish A or B received preoperative radiotherapy followed by craniofacial resection, whereas patients who had Kadish stage C disease were treated with preoperative sequential chemotherapy and radiotherapy followed by a craniofacial resection. The mean follow-up at the time of the latest update was 93 months (range, 1–330 months) and impressively, the series reported a 15-year survival of 82.6%. Seventeen patients (34%) developed recurrent disease, most of which was locoregional (12 patients [24%]). There was a long interval to relapse (mean, 6 years), with the longest time to regional recurrence being 10 years. Distant relapses occurred sooner, with poorer outcomes. Of these 17 patients, 7 (41%) underwent successful salvage surgery, whereas 3 remain alive with disease. The authors concluded that excellent outcomes for ENB are achievable with their triple modality regimen. They also provided strong evidence for continuing long-term follow-up given the extended interval for recurrent disease and that surgical salvage is possible, unlike most other sinonasal malignancies.

Fitzek and colleagues[35] have reported their results with a nonsurgical approach. Patients were treated with two cycles of cisplatin and etoposide followed by high-dose proton-photon radiotherapy to 69.2 cobalt-Gy equivalents, followed by two additional cycles of chemotherapy to responders. Nineteen patients were treated, 9 ENB and 10 neuroendocrine carcinoma. With a median follow-up of 45 months, 15 patients were alive without disease. Thirteen patients had a complete or partial response to the initial chemotherapy. Only 2 patients experienced a local recurrence and both were salvaged with surgery. Four patients died of distant metastases. Rastogi and colleagues[36] reported on a small series from India in which patients were treated with non-craniofacial resection surgery followed by sequential chemotherapy and radiotherapy. They reported a 71% 3-year overall survival, with a 3-year locoregional failure rate of 37%.

ENB also occurs in the pediatric population. The Surveillance Epidemiology and End Results database has shown that ENB is the second most common cause of a malignant nasal cavity mass (25%) following rhabdomyosarcoma (37%).[37] The presentation is similar to that in adults, with nonspecific signs and symptoms, making a high index of suspicion necessary for a timely diagnosis. The principles of therapy developed in the adult population seem to be valid in the pediatric group.[38]

Surgery

A craniotomy is probably not justified for T1 tumors in which there is clear radiologic evidence of a normal cribriform plate and no involvement of the upper ethmoidal cells, but this clinical picture is seldom seen. The intimate relationship between the olfactory epithelium and the cribriform niche allows for early macroscopic and microscopic spread to the olfactory bulbs and tracts that may not be apparent, even on detailed imaging. It is often only confirmed on detailed histologic examination following en bloc resection of the tumor by craniofacial resection.[39] Failure to deal with this intracranial extension before the advent of craniofacial resection was reflected in the poor results achieved with lateral rhinotomy and radiotherapy. Resto and colleagues[40] reported a correlation between survival and extent of surgery with complete resection being predictive of improved disease-free survival and decreased rate of distant metastasis.

Increasing experience with the endoscopic treatment of sinonasal inflammatory disease provided the basis for increasing the use of endoscopes in the effective management of malignant sinonasal pathologies. There is a growing body of series reporting promising results from endoscopic and combined endoscopic and cranial resection of ENB.[33,41–45] The reported benefits are excellent exposure and adequate visualization while avoiding an external facial incision, without compromising the oncological outcome. Given the long natural history of this disease extended follow-up is required to fully define the efficacy of this approach.

Management of the Neck

Approximately 5% of patients present with cervical lymph node metastases. From the cases included in the meta-analysis only 29% of node-positive patients were treated successfully, compared with 64% of N0 patients, a significant difference (odds ratio 5.1 [95% CI 1.6–17.0]) showing that node stage has important prognostic implications.[5] Koka[46] found that cervical metastasis at diagnosis was the only significant risk factor for distant failure.

Macroscopic disease is treated typically by neck dissection and adjuvant radiotherapy. The role of prophylactic treatment to regional nodes in patients who present with local disease is controversial. Regional recurrence has been reported in 15% to 25% of patients[28,15,16,47] and is more common in Kadish stage C.[16] The incidence of isolated neck recurrence is lower, however, at approximately 9%.[15] Some authors have suggested that there is a potential role for elective neck treatment.[15,48,49] Monroe and colleagues[49] reported on 20 patients who had N0 necks, with no recurrences in the 11 patients who had elective neck irradiation, whereas there were 4 out of 9 (44%) neck recurrences in patients who did not receive elective radiation. Others have argued that adding prophylactic regional treatment to an aggressive, multimodality treatment regimen may add considerable morbidity and have instead adopted a policy of observation, reserving neck dissection with or without radiotherapy for salvage.[16,18,30]

Radiotherapy

The available evidence does not support the use of radiotherapy as single-modality therapy for patients treated with radical intent (see **Table 3**).[5] Evidence from the meta-analysis and case series suggests that radiotherapy improves survival when used in combination with surgery.[5,15,17,26,50–52] In the meta-analysis it did not seem that the timing of the radiotherapy altered outcome.[5] Most published series favor the use of radiotherapy as adjuvant postoperative treatment.[16,28,50,53,54] Preoperative radiotherapy has been used in advanced cases, attempting to reduce an unresectable tumor to a resectable size, although an improvement in the rate of clear margins has never been clearly demonstrated.[5]

Traditional radiotherapy techniques have included the use of external megavoltage beams in a three-field technique. The typical prescribed dose ranges from 55 Gy to 65 Gy. In most cases it is greater than 60 Gy with a dose reduction around the critical visual and neurologic pathways to stay within their accepted tolerances. A boost dose to 66 Gy is usually attempted at sites of residual disease.[5] More recently, the use of highly conformal intensity modulated radiotherapy (IMRT) techniques is increasing. Although IMRT does not seem to lead to significant improvements in disease control, it seems to result in a lower incidence of complications.[55] Proton beam therapy may also have potential advantages.[56]

Chemotherapy

Although the use of chemotherapy has been arbitrary in most institutions, the University of Virginia group has consistently treated patients with Kadish stage C disease with chemotherapy as part of a multimodality protocol.[18] They have reported ENB to be sensitive to the preoperative regimen of cyclophosphamide and vincristine. They have achieved good long-term results, but it is not possible to determine the contribution of chemotherapy. Other groups have reported relatively low response rates to neoadjuvant chemotherapy in small series.[15–17] Patients were predominantly treated with cyclophosphamide and vincristine with or without doxorubicin or cisplatin and etoposide. In contrast, Fitzek[35] reported that 6 out of 10 patients who had ENB responded to cisplatin and etoposide. Kim and colleagues[57] reported that 9 out of 11 patients (82%) responded to etoposide, ifosfamide, and cisplatin. Despite this high response rate they reported poor overall survival with a median survival of 18 months. The role of chemotherapy in locoregionally advanced ENB that is amenable to craniofacial resection and radiotherapy remains uncertain. In patients who have distant metastases chemotherapy has a role, and prolonged survival has been reported.[58]

Summary

Esthesioneuroblastoma has a better prognosis than other neuroendocrine sinonasal carcinomas. Good results have been achieved with the combination of craniofacial resection and radiotherapy. In patients who have locoregionally advanced resectable disease, the role of chemotherapy remains uncertain. In patients who have unresectable disease, radiotherapy and chemotherapy may have a role.

SINONASAL UNDIFFERENTIATED CARCINOMA
Pathology

SNUC was first described by Frierson and colleagues[2] in 1986. The etiology of SNUC is unknown. SNUC is not associated with the presence of the Epstein-Barr virus (EBV).[59]

SNUCs are usually large tumors involving the nasal cavity and paranasal sinuses with a propensity to extend into the periorbital tissues and the central nervous system. These tumors are composed of sheets, large nests, trabeculae, and ribbons of pleomorphic intermediate to large cells with frequent necrosis and without any light microscopic evidence of differentiation. As originally described no areas of squamous or glandular differentiation are permitted. The cells often contain large ovoid nuclei and nucleoli may be prominent. Other features include high mitotic activity with atypical mitoses, and lymph-vascular invasion.[2,13,60]

Immunohistochemical studies do not contribute much to the diagnosis, but help to exclude other diagnoses. It has been suggested that SNUCs may exhibit some evidence of neuroendocrine differentiation based on neuron-specific enolase staining in some cases, and occasional neurosecretory granules on electron microscopy.[13] In general, synaptophysin and chromogranin staining is negative.[59] SNUCs are strongly cytokeratin positive.

Although some authors classify SNUC as a neuroendocrine carcinoma,[13,29] others highlight the limited neuroendocrine features and considerable heterogeneity, with many SNUCs showing no features of neuroendocrine differentiation.[61] It has been proposed that SNUC arises in Schneiderian epithelium, but there remains considerable uncertainty about the cell of origin of this malignancy. Ejaz and Wenid[60] have proposed that the histologic definition of SNUC be extended to include tumors with limited foci (<5%) of squamous differentiation provided the clinical picture and most of the histologic features are consistent with a diagnosis of SNUC. The original description of this tumor specifically excluded such cases, however,[2] and most reports have adhered to these criteria.

Recently, it has been reported that some tumors classified as SNUCs may in fact be nuclear protein in testis (NUT) midline carcinomas.[62] NUT midline tumors are aggressive carcinomas that frequently involve the upper aerodigestive tract and are characterized by translocations that involve NUT, a novel gene on chromosome 15. In about two thirds of cases NUT is fused to BRD4 on chromosome 19. These tumors are undifferentiated, but may have focal squamous differentiation and previously had been reported to occur in young adults and children. The authors identified 31 patients who had undifferentiated carcinomas of the upper aerodigestive tract that were not associated with EBV. Twenty-five had been previously diagnosed as SNUC, and there were 2 additional sinonasal tumors that had been classified as undifferentiated carcinomas with focal squamous differentiation. Five of 28 (18%) cases with interpretable FISH results showed rearrangement of NUT and BRD4. Four were sinonasal tumors, 2 originally SNUC, and 2 undifferentiated with squamous differentiation. None of the 5 cases had evidence of neuroendocrine differentiation, and all showed nuclear reactivity with antibodies to p63. The patients who had the sinonasal tumors had an age range of 31 to 47 years. The authors suggest that these tumors may be of squamous origin.

Clinical Presentation

SNUC generally presents with a short (weeks to months) history of symptoms related to an extensive mass involving multiple sites in the sinonasal tract. Symptoms may include nasal obstruction, epistaxis, proptosis, diplopia, altered visual acuity, and facial pain. In most series it seems to be more common in males with median ages of 50 to 57 years and age range 20 to 84 years.[63–66] In most series 10% to 15% of patients have cervical nodal involvement at diagnosis (**Table 4**). Although SNUC has a propensity to also develop distant metastases, this is uncommon at diagnosis.

Imaging

SNUCs require detailed imaging of the primary, which is best delineated with MRI (**Fig. 1**A). Regional lymphadenopathy is best demonstrated on CT. Distant metastases should be excluded with a CT chest/upper abdomen and a bone scan if there are any bone symptoms. Increasingly, PET-CT can be performed to confirm the extent of locoregional disease and exclude distant metastases (**Fig. 1**B).

Staging

Patients are staged according to the AJCC staging system for nasal cavity and ethmoid sinus.[67] The N stage and M stage criteria are the same as for cancers of the oral cavity, pharynx, and larynx, and the T stage and overall stage are outlined in **Box 1**. The Kadish[24] staging system, as originally devised for ENB, can also be used (see **Table 2**).

Treatment

The original reports of SNUC highlighted the aggressive nature of this newly recognized entity and poor prognosis.[68] Subsequent progress has been limited by the rarity of this malignancy, resulting in the available literature consisting of small single-institution retrospective series. Furthermore, the treatment has not been uniform within series, let alone between series. Comparisons of treatment efficacy have been further compounded by major differences in the extent of disease in

Table 4
Patient characteristics—sinonasal undifferentiated carcinoma

	Univ. Florence[63]	Univ. Cincinatti[65]	Univ. Virginia[18]	PMCC[66]	MDAH[29]	Univ. Florida[71]	UCSF[69]
No. patients	13	14	15	10	16	15	21
Age, median (range)	65 (20–82)	49 (22–83)	61 (31–82)	49 (39–84)	—	57 (23–82)	47 (33–71)
Males	54%	93%	93%	80%	50%	67%	67%
AJCC stage 4	62%	(71% Kadish Stage C)	(73% Kadish Stage C)	90%	69%	100%	81%
Positive cervical nodes	15%	14%	13%	30%	0%	13%	10%
Orbital involvement	31%	—	40%	60%	—	—	29%
Intracranial extension	8%	—	53%	60%	—	—	19%

Abbreviations: MDAH, M.D. Anderson Hospital; PMCC, Peter MacCallum Cancer Center; UCSF, University of California San Francisco.

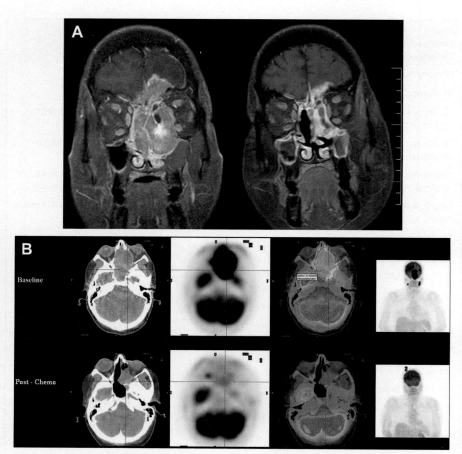

Fig. 1. A 62-year-old woman who had a sinonasal undifferentiated carcinoma presented with a short history of loss of vision left eye, nasal discharge, headaches, and anosmia. (*A*) Baseline MRI (*left image*), coronal T1-weighted postcontrast fat-suppressed sequences demonstrating large left sinonasal mass with extensive intracranial extension and orbital invasion. MRI post three cycles carboplatin and 5-fluorouracil chemotherapy (*right image*) shows a good partial response. (*B*) Baseline PET-CT (*top row*) confirms large left sinonasal mass with intracranial extension into frontal lobe and demonstrates bilateral neck lymphadenopathy. PET-CT post three cycles chemotherapy (*bottom row*) demonstrates near complete metabolic response.

retrospective series (eg, the number of patients who have orbital or intracranial extension). Nevertheless, subsequent series have demonstrated superior results to the initial reports.

Because SNUCs frequently present with locally advanced disease with multiple sinus involvement, orbital and periorbital invasion, and intracranial extension, surgical resection is challenging. Advances in craniofacial resection have led to improved outcomes, but there seems to be considerable variation between treating centers in determining where the boundary is between a resectable and unresectable SNUC.

Reports of radiation alone have generally yielded poor results.[63,68] Improved results have been reported with multimodality therapy, but there is no consensus about which modalities to use and the best sequence. Most of the larger series have included

Box 1
American Joint Committee on Cancer definition of tumor-node-metastasis: nasal cavity and ethmoid sinus

Primary tumor

T1, Tumor restricted to any one subsite, with or without bony invasion

T2, Tumor invading two subsites in a single region or extending to involve adjacent region within the nasoethmoidal complex, with our without bony invasion

T3, Tumor extends to invade the medial wall or floor of the orbit, maxillary sinus, palate, or cribriform plate

T4a, Tumor invades any of the following: anterior orbital contents, skin of nose or cheek, minimal extension to anterior cranial fossa, pterygoid plates, sphenoid, or frontal sinuses

T4b, Tumor invades any of the following: orbital apex, dura, brain, middle cranial fossa, cranial nerves other than (V_2), nasopharynx, or clivus

Stage grouping

Stage 0

   Tis, N0, M0

Stage I

   T1, N0, M0

Stage II

   T2, N0, M0

Stage III

   T3, N0, M0

   T1, N1, M0

   T2, N1, M0

   T3, N1, M0

Stage IVA

   T4a, N0, M0

   T4a, N1, M0

   T1, N2, M0

   T2, N2, M0

   T3, N2, M0

   T4a, N2, M0

Stage IVB

   T4b, Any N, M0

   Any T, N3, M0

Stage IVC

   Any T, Any N, M1

From Greene F, Page D, Fleming I, et al, editors. American Joint Committee on Cancer. Nasal cavity and paranasal sinuses. AJCC cancer staging manual. New York: Springer-Verlag; 2002. p. 61–2; with permission. Used with the permission of the American Joint Committee on Cancer (AJCC), Chicago, IL. The original source for this material is the AJCC cancer staging manual. 6th edition. Springer Science and Business Media LLC; 2002. Available at: http://www.springerlink.com.

craniofacial resection as part of multimodality treatment for patients who have resectable disease.[29,65,69–71] Within each series, it is difficult to compare outcomes in patients who had surgery and radiotherapy vs. patients who received radiation with or without chemotherapy without surgery because of selection bias. In the five larger series wherein the intent was generally to offer surgery for patients who had potentially resectable disease, 55% to 90% had surgery (median 64%) (**Table 5**). In these series, almost all patients also received radiotherapy, and 43% to 80% received some chemotherapy. Although it is difficult to compare outcomes between these retrospective series, these studies report 2-year survival of 45% to 67% and where available in two studies, 5-year survival of 43% and 63%. Differences in outcome may at least partly be accounted for by differences in extent of disease (see **Table 4**). With multimodality therapy many patients achieve complete remission and prolonged survival, with a significant number potentially cured.

The University of Virginia has reported improved results with sequential treatment with neoadjuvant chemotherapy predominantly with cyclophosphamide, doxorubicin, and vincristine, followed by radiotherapy (50–54 Gy), followed by surgical resection when feasible.[70,72] Three out of 10 patients who proceeded to surgery had documented pathologic complete responses.

Based on the University of Virginia experience,[70] the propensity for both locoregional recurrence and distant metastases and that at least a third of patients are unresectable at diagnosis, we have investigated a primary chemoradiation approach. We have reported our experience with three cycles of platinum (cisplatin or carboplatin) and infusional 5-fluorouracil followed by radiotherapy (60 Gy) with two cycles of concurrent cisplatin.[66] Seven patients (all T4) treated with this approach without surgery had a 2-year survival of 64% and 2-year progression-free survival of 43%. Patients had particularly advanced disease: 6 out of 7 had intracranial extension, 6 out of 7 had orbital involvement, and 3 had cervical nodes. These patients had more advanced disease than in many of the other series (see **Table 4**).

For patients who have resectable disease the largest experience with reasonable results has been with surgical resection and radiotherapy. In many series this has been initial resection followed by postoperative radiation with or without concurrent platinum chemotherapy. The University of Florida group has argued that one advantage of the surgery and postoperative radiation sequence is that it may be possible to reduce the radiation dose and thus reduce the risk for radiation-induced optic

Table 5
Treatment outcomes in sinonasal undifferentiated carcinoma

	Univ. Cincinatti[65]	Univ. Virginia[18]	PMCC[66]	MDAH[29]	Univ. Florida[71]	UCSF[69]
No. patients	14	20	10	16	15	21
Surgery	64	55	20	63	73	90
Radiotherapy	86	95	100	—	100	100
Chemotherapy	43	80	70	63	47	62
Alive, disease-free	36% (3–195 m)	20% (24–164 m)	50% (8–62 m)	—	40% (12–128 m)	33% (6–86 m)
2-yr survival	45%	47%	64%	—	67% (3 yr)	65%
5-yr survival	—	—	—	63%	—	43%

Abbreviations: MDAH, M.D. Anderson Hospital; PMCC, Peter MacCallum Cancer Center; UCSF, University of California San Francisco.

neuropathy.[71] They have also used hyperfractionated radiation to reduce the risk of this toxicity. The University of Virginia experience has demonstrated that it is feasible to give neoadjuvant chemotherapy and radiation before surgery.[70] Adjuvant chemotherapy following surgery and radiotherapy has been given in an ad hoc fashion in some series. We believe that our approach of neoadjuvant chemotherapy followed by concurrent chemoradiation represents an alternative approach for patients who have resectable disease, with surgery reserved for patients who have residual disease as determined on MRI and PET. However, our results with this primary chemotherapy and radiation strategy need to be confirmed by other centers. Kramer and colleagues[73] reported a review of published cases of SNUC comparing patients treated with surgery plus radiotherapy with or without chemotherapy to patients who received radiotherapy and chemotherapy without surgery. Not surprisingly the group who underwent surgery had less advanced disease and appeared to have better survival. There was no apparent difference after adjusting for differences in disease extent, however. These results should be interpreted with caution because of the small numbers, the inclusion of older series, and that this analysis precedes publication of some of the more recent larger series of patients.

Management of the uninvolved neck is controversial. The University of Florida has recommended elective neck irradiation based on findings of regional control in seven out of seven (100%) who received elective neck irradiation vs. four out of six (66%) in patients who did not receive elective neck irradiation.[71]

For patients who have unresectable disease, we recommend our combined induction chemotherapy and concurrent chemoradiation approach. Radiation alone, or sequential chemotherapy and radiotherapy, have generally yielded poor results.[63,68] In the University of Florida series, five patients were deemed unresectable and were treated with a primary radiation approach.[71] Four out of five patients received concurrent chemoradiation, but only one patient also received induction chemotherapy, and this patient is the only patient who remained alive without recurrence.

In the M.D. Anderson series 8 out of 16 patients had induction chemotherapy before surgery or radiation with or without concurrent chemotherapy, with 10 out of 16 patients having surgery as part of their treatment.[29] Although the patients in this series may have been less advanced than in some series, they have reported impressive results with 5-year overall survival rate of 62.5%, local failure rate 21.4%, regional failure rate 15.6%, and distant metastasis rate of 25.4%.

Although it is difficult to prove a role for induction chemotherapy in this rare disease, the chemosensitivity of SNUC (**Fig. 1**) suggests a potential role in improving locoregional control and decreasing distant metastases. Induction chemotherapy before radiation may contribute to local control by reducing tumor bulk juxtaposed to vital dose-limiting critical structures, such as the optic chiasm before radiation. Although planning target volumes should not be reduced on the basis of chemotherapy-induced response, the tumor bulk reduction following induction chemotherapy increases the probability that gross residual disease receives the full radiation dose. Concerns about accelerated repopulation following induction chemotherapy are less likely to be relevant in an undifferentiated tumor, such as SNUC.

Summary

SNUC usually presents with locally advanced disease. Despite the aggressive nature of this malignancy with a propensity for locoregional invasion and distant metastases, a nihilistic approach to management is not warranted because good results have been achieved with multimodality therapy. Although the optimal sequence of treatments cannot easily be resolved in this rare disease, treatment approaches that have been successful in the larger series can be used in clinical practice. For patients who have resectable disease, surgery and radiotherapy with or without chemotherapy is the most commonly used approach, but induction chemotherapy followed by concurrent chemoradiation warrants further study. For patients who have unresectable disease, induction chemotherapy followed by concurrent chemoradiation is the most promising strategy.

NEUROENDOCRINE CARCINOMA

The term neuroendocrine carcinoma of the sinonasal tract has caused considerable confusion. Silva[74] identified sinonasal neuroendocrine tumors (SNEC) that he differentiated from ENB. In general, neuroendocrine tumors elsewhere in the body range from the well-differentiated carcinoid tumors to small cell carcinoma at the other end of the spectrum. Within the sinonasal tract, ENB can be regarded as a more differentiated neuroendocrine tumor, whereas SNECs are less differentiated. SNECs are morphologically distinct from small cell carcinoma and immunohistochemically distinct from SNUC, which has questionable features of neuroendocrine differentiation. SNEC are analogous to large cell neuroendocrine carcinomas of other sites (eg, lung). Some authors have argued that these tumors should be classified as SNUCs,[13] but others believe that they are a related but distinct entity.[29,61]

SNEC is a more cellular tumor than ENB without evidence of rosette formation. Cells are larger with more cytoplasm and larger nucleoli than ENB. There is evidence of neurosecretory granules, but no neurofibrillary background. In general, immunohistochemical expression of neuroendocrine markers can be used to distinguish SNEC from SNUC.[61] SNECs are frequently positive for chromogranin, synaptophysin, and S100 in contrast to SNUC.[13,59-61] Some authors have included tumors with chromogranin staining in reports of SNUC, however.[69] Even authors who believe SNUC and SNEC are distinct entities acknowledge that there are cases in which a distinction between SNUC and SNEC is impossible.[61]

The largest series with pathology review is from the M.D. Anderson Cancer Center.[29] There were 18 SNEC cases; 10 were T4 and only 2 were node positive. Fourteen had surgery, and 12 received chemotherapy. SNEC appeared to have been treated in a similar fashion to SNUC, and had an almost identical outcome. Five-year survival was 64%, 5-year local failure rate was 21.4%, regional failure rate was 12.9%, and distant metastasis rate was 14.1%.

Based on the M.D. Anderson experience, the paucity of series of SNEC, and the controversy about whether SNEC should be distinguished from SNUC, it is reasonable to apply similar treatment principles to the two malignancies. The only difference in our approach has been to use platinum and etoposide rather than platinum and 5-fluorouracil when using induction chemotherapy for patients who have unresectable disease. Fitzek and colleagues[35] have reported good results with an initial nonsurgical approach using chemotherapy and radiotherapy. Seven out of nine patients who had SNEC responded to the initial two cycles of cisplatin and etoposide.

SMALL CELL CARCINOMA

Small cell carcinoma of the sinonasal tract has also been called small cell undifferentiated (neuroendocrine) carcinoma, and poorly differentiated neuroendocrine carcinoma, small cell type.[1] In view of the inconsistent use of the term neuroendocrine carcinoma in the sinonasal malignancy literature and that it is morphologically identical to small cell carcinoma of the lung, we believe that it is preferable to use the term small cell carcinoma. Small cell carcinoma can be distinguished from ENB, SNUC, and SNEC on light microscopy features.[61]

Small cell carcinoma of the sinonasal tract is a rare malignancy, with the reported series all having fewer than 10 patients.[75] In the M.D. Anderson series of neuroendocrine tumors there were only 7 cases of small cell carcinoma.[29] Three had nodal disease and 6 were stage IV. Five out of 7 were treated with chemotherapy and radiotherapy. Although there were only 7 patients, the outcome of these patients was inferior to ENB, SNUC, and SNEC. Only 1 patient was a long-term survivor. The local failure rate was 33%, the regional failure rate 44%, and the distant failure rate was 75%. These results are consistent with the expected outcome of small cell carcinoma arising at other sites.[76] Galanis[76] reported that 4 out of 5 patients treated with surgery alone developed distant metastases. In view of the propensity for distant metastases, early introduction of chemotherapy is essential. Our approach has been to treat sinonasal small cell carcinomas using the same treatment principles that are applicable to small cell carcinoma arising in the lung. Currently we treat with four cycles of cisplatin and etoposide, with early introduction of concurrent radiation (with first or second cycle of chemotherapy) for patients who do not have evidence of distant metastases. Our current policy is to exclude distant metastases with a CT chest and upper abdomen and a PET scan. Although few patients are cured, most patients respond well to initial treatment. One other issue to consider when treating small cell carcinomas of the sinonasal tract is the role of prophylactic cranial irradiation. It has been argued that sequential chemotherapy and radiotherapy may be advantageous compared with concurrent chemoradiation, because it permits the incorporation of the prophylactic cranial irradiation into the primary radiation fields without excessive toxicity.[29,77]

SUMMARY

The sinonasal malignancies of putative neuroendocrine origin—ENB, SNEC, SNUC, and small cell carcinoma—usually present with locally advanced disease. They cannot generally be distinguished on clinical or radiologic criteria and hence require expert pathologic diagnosis. Although SNUC and SNEC may be managed along similar lines, it is particularly important to distinguish ENB and small cell carcinomas from SNUC and to exclude other malignancies that can arise in this region.

In view of the rarity of these tumors, the difficulties in establishing the correct diagnosis, and the complexity of multimodality treatment, these patients should be managed by multidisciplinary teams in major centers with expertise in sinonasal malignancies. Although randomized trials in these rare diseases are not feasible, collaboration between major centers to investigate uniform protocols is desirable. Agreement about pathologic diagnostic criteria and central pathology review is essential to ensure that any promising results could be translated into clinical practice.

ACKNOWLEDGMENTS

We thank Robin Cassumbhoy and Rod Hicks for assistance with the figures.

REFERENCES

1. Iezzoni JC, Mills SE. Undifferentiated small round cell tumors of the sinonasal tract: differential diagnosis update. Am J Clin Pathol 2005;124(Suppl):S110–21.
2. Frierson HF Jr, Mills SE, Fechner RE, et al. Sinonasal undifferentiated carcinoma. An aggressive neoplasm derived from schneiderian epithelium and distinct from olfactory neuroblastoma. Am J Surg Pathol 1986;10:771–9.

3. Theilgaard SA, Buchwald C, Ingeholm P, et al. Esthesioneuroblastoma: a Danish demographic study of 40 patients registered between 1978 and 2000. Acta Otolaryngol 2003;123:433–9.

4. Berger L, Luc R. L'esthesioneuropitheliome olfactif. Bull Assoc Fr Etud Cancer 1924;13:410–21.

5. Dulguerov P, Allal AS, Calcaterra TC. Esthesioneuroblastoma: a meta-analysis and review. Lancet Oncol 2001;2:683–90.

6. Carney ME, O'Reilly RC, Sholevar B, et al. Expression of the human Achaete-scute 1 gene in olfactory neuroblastoma (esthesioneuroblastoma). J Neurooncol 1995;26:35–43.

7. Hyams V, Batsakis J, Michaels L. Atlas of tumor pathology. Armed Forces Institute of Pathology 1988;25:240–8.

8. Ingeholm P, Theilgaard SA, Buchwald C, et al. Esthesioneuroblastoma: a Danish clinicopathological study of 40 consecutive cases. Apmis 2002;110:639–45.

9. Bellizzi AM, Bourne TD, Mills SE, et al. The cytologic features of sinonasal undifferentiated carcinoma and olfactory neuroblastoma. Am J Clin Pathol 2008;129: 367–76.

10. Emerson LL, Layfield LJ, Frame R. Pleomorphic olfactory neuroblastoma (esthesioneuroblastoma): histopathological findings and clinical course. Histopathology 2007;51:430–2.

11. Cohen ZR, Marmor E, Fuller GN, et al. Misdiagnosis of olfactory neuroblastoma. Neurosurg Focus 2002;12:e3.

12. Haas I, Ganzer U. Does sophisticated diagnostic workup on neuroectodermal tumors have an impact on the treatment of esthesioneuroblastoma? Onkologie 2003;26:261–7.

13. Mills SE. Neuroectodermal neoplasms of the head and neck with emphasis on neuroendocrine carcinomas. Mod Pathol 2002;15:264–78.

14. Bockmuhl U, You X, Pacyna-Gengelbach M, et al. CGH pattern of esthesioneuroblastoma and their metastases. Brain Pathol 2004;14:158–63.

15. Chao KS, Kaplan C, Simpson JR, et al. Esthesioneuroblastoma: the impact of treatment modality. Head Neck 2001;23:749–57.

16. Diaz EM Jr, Johnigan RH III, Pero C, et al. Olfactory neuroblastoma: the 22-year experience at one comprehensive cancer center. Head Neck 2005;27:138–49.

17. Resto VA, Eisele DW, Forastiere A, et al. Esthesioneuroblastoma: the Johns Hopkins experience. Head Neck 2000;22:550–8.

18. Loy AH, Reibel JF, Read PW, et al. Esthesioneuroblastoma: continued follow-up of a single institution's experience. Arch Otolaryngol Head Neck Surg 2006;132: 134–8.

19. Mariani L, Schaller B, Weis J, et al. Esthesioneuroblastoma of the pituitary gland: a clinicopathological entity? Case report and review of the literature. J Neurosurg 2004;101:1049.

20. Sajko T, Rumboldt Z, Talan-Hranilovic J, et al. Primary sellar esthesioneuroblastoma. Acta Neurochir (Wien) 2005;147:447–8.

21. Iio M, Homma A, Furuta Y, et al. [Magnetic resonance imaging of olfactory neuroblastoma]. Nippon Jibiinkoka Gakkai Kaiho 2006;109:142 [in Japanese].

22. Nguyen BD, Roarke MC, Nelson KD, et al. F-18 FDG PET/CT staging and posttherapeutic assessment of esthesioneuroblastoma. Clin Nucl Med 2006;31: 172–4.

23. Rostomily RC, Elias M, Deng M, et al. Clinical utility of somatostatin receptor scintigraphic imaging (Octreoscan) in esthesioneuroblastoma: a case study and survey of somatostatin receptor subtype expression. Head Neck 2006;28:305–12.

24. Kadish S, Goodman M, Wang CC. Olfactory neuroblastoma. A clinical analysis of 17 cases. Cancer 1976;37:1571–6.

25. Irish J, Dasgupta R, Freeman J, et al. Outcome and analysis of the surgical management of esthesioneuroblastoma. J Otolaryngol 1997;26:1–7.

26. Morita A, Ebersold MJ, Olsen KD, et al. Esthesioneuroblastoma: prognosis and management. Neurosurgery 1993;32:706.

27. Dulguerov P, Calcaterra T. Esthesioneuroblastoma: the UCLA experience 1970–1990. Laryngoscope 1992;102:843–9.

28. Jethanamest D, Morris LG, Sikora AG, et al. Esthesioneuroblastoma: a population-based analysis of survival and prognostic factors. Arch Otolaryngol Head Neck Surg 2007;133:276–80.

29. Rosenthal DI, Barker JL Jr, El-Naggar AK, et al. Sinonasal malignancies with neuroendocrine differentiation: patterns of failure according to histologic phenotype. Cancer 2004;101:2567–73.

30. Lund VJ, Howard DJ, Wei WI, et al. Craniofacial resection for tumors of the nasal cavity and paranasal sinuses—a 17-year experience. Head Neck 1998;20: 97–105.

31. Constantinidis J, Steinhart H, Koch M, et al. Olfactory neuroblastoma: the University of Erlangen-Nuremberg experience 1975-2000. Otolaryngol Head Neck Surg 2004;130:567–74.

32. McLean JN, Nunley SR, Klass C, et al. Combined modality therapy of esthesioneuroblastoma. Otolaryngol Head Neck Surg 2007;136:998.

33. Zafereo ME, Fakhri S, Prayson R, et al. Esthesioneuroblastoma: 25-year experience at a single institution. Otolaryngol Head Neck Surg 2008;138:452–8.

34. Polin RS, Sheehan JP, Chenelle AG, et al. The role of preoperative adjuvant treatment in the management of esthesioneuroblastoma: the University of Virginia experience. Neurosurgery 1998;42:1029–37.

35. Fitzek MM, Thornton AF, Varvares M, et al. Neuroendocrine tumors of the sinonasal tract. Results of a prospective study incorporating chemotherapy, surgery, and combined proton-photon radiotherapy. Cancer 2002;94:2623–34.

36. Rastogi M, Bhatt M, Chufal K, et al. Esthesioneuroblastoma treated with non-craniofacial resection surgery followed by combined chemotherapy and radiotherapy: An alternative approach in limited resources. Jpn J Clin Oncol 2006;36:613–9.

37. Benoit MM, Bhattacharyya N, Faquin W, et al. Cancer of the nasal cavity in the pediatric population. Pediatrics 2008;121:e141–5.

38. Eich HT, Muller RP, Micke O, et al. Esthesioneuroblastoma in childhood and adolescence. Better prognosis with multimodal treatment? Strahlenther Onkol 2005; 181:378–84.

39. Bradley PJ, Jones NS, Robertson I. Diagnosis and management of esthesioneuroblastoma. Curr Opin Otolaryngol Head Neck Surg 2003;11:112–8.

40. Resto VA, Chan AW, Deschler DG, et al. Extent of surgery in the management of locally advanced sinonasal malignancies. Head Neck 2008;30:222–9.

41. Dave SP, Bared A, Casiano RR. Surgical outcomes and safety of transnasal endoscopic resection for anterior skull tumors. Otolaryngol Head Neck Surg 2007;136:920.

42. Liu JK, O'Neill B, Orlandi RR, et al. Endoscopic-assisted craniofacial resection of esthesioneuroblastoma: minimizing facial incisions—technical note and report of 3 cases. Minim Invasive Neurosurg 2003;46:310–5.

43. Podboj J, Smid L. Endoscopic surgery with curative intent for malignant tumors of the nose and paranasal sinuses. Eur J Surg Oncol 2007;33:1081–6.

44. Poetker DM, Toohill RJ, Loehrl TA, et al. Endoscopic management of sinonasal tumors: a preliminary report. Am J Rhinol 2005;19:307–15.

45. Suriano M, De Vincentiis M, Colli A, et al. Endoscopic treatment of esthesioneuroblastoma: a minimally invasive approach combined with radiation therapy. Otolaryngol Head Neck Surg 2007;136:104–7.
46. Koka VN, Julieron M, Bourhis J, et al. Aesthesioneuroblastoma. J Laryngol Otol 1998;112:628–33.
47. Rinaldo A, Ferlito A, Shaha AR, et al. Esthesioneuroblastoma and cervical lymph node metastases: clinical and therapeutic implications. Acta Otolaryngol 2002; 122:215–21.
48. Beitler JJ, Fass DE, Brenner HA, et al. Esthesioneuroblastoma: is there a role for elective neck treatment? Head Neck 1991;13:321–6.
49. Monroe AT, Hinerman RW, Amdur RJ, et al. Radiation therapy for esthesioneuroblastoma: rationale for elective neck irradiation. Head Neck 2003; 25:529–34.
50. Foote RL, Morita A, Ebersold MJ, et al. Esthesioneuroblastoma: the role of adjuvant radiation therapy. Int J Radiat Oncol Biol Phys 1993;27:835–42.
51. Nakao K, Watanabe K, Fujishiro Y, et al. Olfactory neuroblastoma: long-term clinical outcome at a single institute between 1979 and 2003. Acta Otolaryngol Suppl 2007;559:113–7.
52. O'Connor TA, McLean P, Juillard GJ, et al. Olfactory neuroblastoma. Cancer 1989;63:2426–8.
53. Austin JR, Cebrun H, Kershisnik MM, et al. Olfactory neuroblastoma and neuroendocrine carcinoma of the anterior skull base: treatment results at the m.d. Anderson cancer center. Skull Base Surg 1996;6:1–8.
54. Zappia JJ, Carroll W, Wolf GT, et al. Olfactory neuroblastoma: the results of modern treatment approaches at the University of Michigan. Head Neck 1993; 15:190–6.
55. Daly ME, Chen AM, Bucci MK, et al. Intensity-modulated radiation therapy for malignancies of the nasal cavity and paranasal sinuses. Int J Radiat Oncol Biol Phys 2007;67:151–7.
56. Nishimura H, Ogino T, Kawashima M, et al. Proton-beam therapy for olfactory neuroblastoma. Int J Radiat Oncol Biol Phys 2007;68:758–62.
57. Kim DW, Jo YH, Kim JH, et al. Neoadjuvant etoposide, ifosfamide, and cisplatin for the treatment of olfactory neuroblastoma. Cancer 2004;101:2257–60.
58. de Vos FY, Willemse PH, de Vries EG. Successful treatment of metastatic esthesioneuroblastoma. Neth J Med 2003;61:414–6.
59. Cerilli LA, Holst VA, Brandwein MS, et al. Sinonasal undifferentiated carcinoma: immunohistochemical profile and lack of EBV association. Am J Surg Pathol 2001;25: 156–153.
60. Ejaz A, Wenig BM. Sinonasal undifferentiated carcinoma: clinical and pathologic features and a discussion on classification, cellular differentiation, and differential diagnosis. Adv Anat Pathol 2005;12:134–43.
61. Smith SR, Som P, Fahmy A, et al. A clinicopathological study of sinonasal neuroendocrine carcinoma and sinonasal undifferentiated carcinoma. Laryngoscope 2000;110:1617.
62. Stelow EB, Bellizzi AM, Taneja K, et al. NUT rearrangement in undifferentiated carcinomas of the upper aerodigestive tract. Am J Surg Pathol 2008;32:828–34.
63. Gallo O, Graziani P, Fini-Storchi O. Undifferentiated carcinoma of the nose and paranasal sinuses. An immunohistochemical and clinical study. Ear Nose Throat J 1993;72:588–90.
64. Mendenhall WM, Mendenhall CM, Riggs CE Jr, et al. Sinonasal undifferentiated carcinoma. Am J Clin Oncol 2006;29:27–31.

65. Miyamoto RC, Gleich LL, Biddinger PW, et al. Esthesioneuroblastoma and sinonasal undifferentiated carcinoma: impact of histological grading and clinical staging on survival and prognosis. Laryngoscope 2000;110:1262–5.
66. Rischin D, Porceddu S, Peters L, et al. Promising results with chemoradiation in patients with sinonasal undifferentiated carcinoma. Head Neck 2004;26:435–41.
67. Greene F, Page D, Fleming I, et al, editors. American joint committee on cancer. nasal cavity and paranasal sinuses. (AJCC Cancer Staging Manual). New York: Springer-Verlag; 2002. p. 61–2.
68. Levine PA, Frierson HF Jr, Stewart FM, et al. Sinonasal undifferentiated carcinoma: a distinctive and highly aggressive neoplasm. Laryngoscope 1987;97:905–8.
69. Chen AM, Daly ME, El-Sayed I, et al. Patterns of failure after combined-modality approaches incorporating radiotherapy for sinonasal undifferentiated carcinoma of the head and neck. Int J Radiat Oncol Biol Phys 2008;70:338–43.
70. Musy PY, Reibel JF, Levine PA. Sinonasal undifferentiated carcinoma: the search for a better outcome. Laryngoscope 2002;112:1450–5.
71. Tanzler ED, Morris CG, Orlando CA, et al. Management of sinonasal undifferentiated carcinoma. Head Neck 2008;30:595–595.
72. Deutsch BD, Levine PA, Stewart FM, et al. Sinonasal undifferentiated carcinoma: a ray of hope. Otolaryngol Head Neck Surg 1993;108:697–700.
73. Kramer D, Durham JS, Sheehan F, et al. Sinonasal undifferentiated carcinoma: case series and systematic review of the literature. J Otolaryngol 2004;33:32–6.
74. Silva EG, Butler JJ, Mackay B, et al. Neuroblastomas and neuroendocrine carcinomas of the nasal cavity: a proposed new classification. Cancer 1982;50:2388–405.
75. Renner G. Small cell carcinoma of the head and neck: a review. Semin Oncol 2007;34:3–14.
76. Galanis E, Frytak S, Lloyd RV. Extrapulmonary small cell carcinoma. Cancer 1997;79:1729–36.
77. Barker JL Jr, Glisson BS, Garden AS, et al. Management of nonsinonasal neuroendocrine carcinomas of the head and neck. Cancer 2003;98:232–8.

Index

Note: Page numbers of article titles are in **boldface** type.

Hematol Oncol Clin N Am 22 (2008) 1317–1326
doi:10.1016/S0889-8588(08)00160-3
0889-8588/08/$ – see front matter © 2008 Elsevier Inc. All rights reserved.

hemonc.theclinics.com